CIGARETTES AND SOVIETS

A volume in the NIU Series in
Slavic, East European, and Eurasian Studies
Edited by Christine D. Worobec

For a list of books in the series, visit our website at cornellpress.cornell.edu.

CIGARETTES AND SOVIETS

Smoking in the USSR

Tricia Starks

NORTHERN ILLINOIS UNIVERSITY PRESS

AN IMPRINT OF CORNELL UNIVERSITY PRESS

ITHACA AND LONDON

First published 2022 by Cornell University Press

Library of Congress Cataloging-in-Publication Data
Names: Starks, Tricia, 1969– author.
Title: Cigarettes and Soviets : smoking in the USSR / Tricia Starks.
Description: Ithaca [New York] : Northern Illinois University Press, an imprint of
    Cornell University Press, 2022. | Series: NIU series in Slavic, East European, and
    Eurasian studies | Includes bibliographical references and index.
Identifiers: LCCN 2021056976 (print) | LCCN 2021056977 (ebook) |
    ISBN 9781501765483 (hardcover) | ISBN 9781501765759 (pdf) |
    ISBN 9781501765766 (epub)
Subjects: LCSH: Smoking—Soviet Union—History. | Soviets (People)—Tobacco
    use—History. | Cigarettes—Soviet Union—History. | Tobacco—Soviet Union—
    History. | Tobacco industry—Soviet Union—History. | Tobacco use—Soviet
    Union—History.
Classification: LCC GT3021.S69 S83 2022 (print) | LCC GT3021.S69 (ebook) |
    DDC 394.1/40947—dc23/eng/20211203
LC record available at https://lccn.loc.gov/2021056976
LC ebook record available at https://lccn.loc.gov/2021056977

The dank smell of the station in Negoreloye—the odor of wet sheepskin coats, of sawdust spread on the floors to absorb moisture, of disinfectant, of pink soap, of human sweat, and of the cheap Russian tobacco known as Makhorka—still remains for me the smell of the Soviet Union.

—Charles E. Bohlen, *Witness to History, 1929–1969*, 1934

Contents

Illustrations

Acknowledgments

When I first went over to the Soviet Union in 1990, people advised me to take condoms and cigarettes for trade. Both were considered worth more than the ruble, and neither was made in good quality or supply. I not only gifted cigarettes but inhaled them with abandon. Be it a *Marlboro* or a *Kosmos*, I did not need a ration ticket for cigarettes. Tobacco became my companion through the dismal twilight of a dying regime played out across the long, dark Leningrad winter. After I returned home, I found a *Pall Mall* to be light, and when I began to cough up blood, I quit. Snap. Only later did I realize how lucky I was to shed my habit so easily. My return left me with no addiction to tobacco but an obsession with the material conditions of life in Russia and the Soviet Union that continues to drive my research.

This research project germinated in personal experience, but it flowered with aid from a National Library of Medicine and National Institutes of Health Grant for Scholarly Works in Biomedicine and Health (Award Number G13LM011893), along with funds from the Kennan Institute for Advanced Russian Studies at the Woodrow Wilson Center, the University of Illinois's Slavic Research Lab, the Fulbright College of Arts and Sciences and the Department of History at the University of Arkansas, and support from Lynda Coon, Jim Gigantino, Todd Shields, Kathryn Sloan, and Calvin White. I appreciate the aid of these people and organizations, but the arguments and ideas herein are solely my own.

I owe thanks to many others. Natalia Lvovna Pushkareva, and her entire family of historians, always provided excellent advice and a warm kitchen. My friend Liza Gorchakova introduced me to the lovely Sanduny baths in Moscow and the always fascinating Leonid Sinel'nikov, who generously answered all my tobacco-related questions. The formidable women of the Russian State Library, especially of the Graphics Department, shared books and images and tea. And the staff of the State Archive of the Russian Federation and the State Archive of Movie, Photo, and Audio Documents were all helpful and patient. Closer to home, the University of California San Francisco's Center for Tobacco Control Research gave me training to access the 1998 Tobacco Master Settlement Agreement archive. The staff of the Interlibrary Loan office at the University of Arkansas searched for so many things and delivered so many more. I was lucky to meet Larry Zeman and Howard Garfinkel of Productive Arts, who shared images of cigarette pack collections. Nikolas Cornish of the Stavka photo archive searched through his extensive archives and reproduced amazing photographs. Vladimir Davidenko delved into the Zosa Szajkowski papers at the Bakhmeteff Archive at Columbia University Libraries to reproduce materials there, and Harold M. Leich informed me about, and helped me with, the fabulous Anatolii Zakharovich Rubinov Papers at the Library of Congress.

In writing the book, I have exploited even more people. At conferences organized by Fran Bernstein, Chris Burton, and Dan Healey; Grégory Dufaud and Susan Gross Solomon; Aleksandra Brokman and Claire Shaw; Cynthia Buckley and Paul McNamara; Christopher J. Gerry; Matthew P. Romaniello and Alison K. Smith; Julia Obertreis and Heidi Hein-Kircher; Claire Shaw and Anna Toropova; Dora Vargha, and the people of ASEEES, I was lucky to get the input of brilliant researchers and listen to papers that broadened my horizons. I am indebted to the work and advice of tobacco researchers Carol Benedict, Iurii Bokarev, William Clarence-Smith, Ellen Leen-Feldner, Julia Obertreis, Kenneth A. Perkins, Kathryn Stoner, and Mateusz Zatoński. Mentors and colleagues David L. Hoffmann, Paula Michaels, Kenneth A. Perkins, Judyth L. Twigg, and Elizabeth A. Wood provided letters and excellent advice. Faith Hillis, Stephen Jug, Aaron Retish, Brandon Schechter, and Alison K. Smith all gave valuable references and comment. Roger Haydon and Amy Farranto have both generously advised me in fashioning from an initial monster of a draft a reasonable manuscript, and a round of anonymous reviews produced by heroes during the height of the epidemic helped me further. Karen M. Laun and Carolyn Pouncy provided keen eyes and superior care for the manuscript. I was lucky to have their help.

Yet again, I relied on Lynda Coon and Matthew P. Romaniello. Lynda, even while pulling off a stint as the hardest working dean(s) at the University of Arkansas, still found the time to review and weigh every word. Readers can thank her for the 40 percent reduction in em-dashes and a 90 percent increase in punchy prose and luscious visual analysis. Matt suffered through multiple drafts and passed judgment on what was sad or confusing, allowed the adequatious and cromulent, and praised the amusing and interesting. His near encyclopedic knowledge of, well, everything is my crutch. Thanks again to you both.

I owe the most to the fam. The boys have patiently listened to Mom's rants about tobacco and put up with research trips poorly disguised as family vacations. Dick and Sharon Starks and Don and Pat Pierce helped through the hard times. More than anyone, I owe Mike Pierce. His ruthlessly effective editing and hard questions have made me a better scholar and writer, but his generosity to all and fearless passion for doing the right thing make me strive to be a better person. The world is a better place and my life is immeasurably happier because of him. Love you all.

Abbreviations

BAT	British American Tobacco
DGTF	Don State Tobacco Factory
GARF	Gosudarstvennyi arkhiv Rossiiskoi Federatsii
GiZRS	*Gigiena i zdorov'e rabochei sem'i*
GiZRiKS	*Gigiena i zdorov'e rabochei i krest'ianskoi sem'i*
Glavtabak	Glavnaia tabachanaia upravleniia tabachnoi promyshlennosti
mg	milligram
Minzdrav	Ministerstvo zdravookhraneniia
Narkomzdrav	Narodnyi kommissariat zdravookhraneniia
NASA	National Aeronautics and Space Administration
NEP	New Economic Policy
PMI	Philip Morris Incorporated
RGAKFD	Rossiiskii gosudarstvennyi arkhiv kino-fono-foto-dokumentov
RGASPI	Rossiiskii gosudarstvennyi arkhiv sotsial'no-politicheskoi istorii
RJR	R. J. Reynolds
Sovnarkom	Sovet narodnykh kommissarov
TsAODM	Tsentral'nyi arkhiv obshchestvennykh dvizhenii Moskvy
US	United States
USA	United States of America
USSR	Union of Soviet Socialist Republics
ZNB	*Za novyi byt*

Note on Transliterations and Translations

The book utilizes the Library of Congress transliteration system except for names recognized in standard western styles. All translations are my own, except where noted. To capture some of the snap and whimsy of slogans or pitches, there are occasional nods to western colloquialisms rather than strict word-for-word exercises.

CIGARETTES AND SOVIETS

THE REVOLUTIONARY SOVIET SMOKER

After the February Revolution of 1917, Vladimir Il'ich Lenin and nearly three dozen other displaced radicals began a trek across war-torn Europe. They sped back to Russia to agitate for even greater change, barreling through hostile territories in a special train car where real German guards monitored the chalk lines that denoted their space of fictive Russian soil. But more than suspicious glances and phantom borders divided the travelers. As the revolutionaries passed through the fields of one war, Lenin fired the first salvo in a battle that few had anticipated—an attack on tobacco.[1]

It was no secret that Lenin abhorred tobacco, but many of his colleagues embraced the habit. Surrounded by puffers, Lenin imposed no-smoking zones for their steam-powered isle of Russian territory—tobacco use would be allowed only in the bathrooms. For the thirty-some activists pressed together for days of travel, this sanitary authoritarianism nurtured the seeds of discontent. Soon enough the bathrooms became clogged with smokers, lines snaked down the corridors, and bickering erupted. Lenin stepped in, "with a sigh," issuing bathroom tickets for two types of clients—smokers and users. For every three conventional uses, he issued one smoking ticket, rationing tobacco time and smoothing over the difficulties he had created.

A queue persisted, but things got back to a more normal state of affairs as discontent turned to discussion of absent comrades—and what they would say to Lenin's tobacco tyranny. Karl Radek joked, "It's a pity that Comrade Bukharin isn't with us." Others agreed that Nikolai Bukharin could surely have enlightened the waiting group on the placement of tobacco on the varying "levels of human necessity," because he was an expert in the Marxian-value theories of the Austrian economist Eugen von Bohm-Bawerk. Lenin's thunderous return became the subject of many books, yet no one seems to have recorded if the revolutionaries finally settled the necessity of tobacco.[2]

After his return to Petrograd, through the fall of the Provisional Government, and following the success of the Bolshevik Revolution, Lenin's disgust for tobacco did not wane. The revolutionary Vladimir Bonch-Bruevich joked of Lenin, "He could not stand the smoke . . . Wherever he was—by himself in the office, at home, at a meeting, or a discussion, even as a guest—he energetically protested smoking . . . hanging signs everywhere saying, 'here it is forbidden to smoke,' 'please don't smoke' . . . [he] resented when smokers did not follow these requests and . . . told them that if they themselves could not stop . . . why must others put up with and breathe this disgusting, stupefying-to-consciousness poison."[3] At the meetings of the Soviet of People's Commissars (Sovet narodnykh kommissarov—hereafter Sovnarkom), Lenin exiled the smokers to the fireplace, forcing them to blow their smoke up the chimney and mocking them as "charred cockroaches."[4]

Although Lenin's smoking prohibitions tended toward securing his personal comfort, he found an ally for a broader fight against tobacco in Nikolai Aleksandrovich Semashko. Semashko was the leader of the newly created Commissariat for Public Health (Narodnyi kommissariat zdravookhraneniia, est. 1918, abbreviated Narkomzdrav, and after 1945 Ministerstvo zdravookhraneniia, Minzdrav). As the leader of the world's first national health administration pledged to universal, unified, prophylactic care, Semashko placed the Soviets at the forefront of twentieth-century socialized medicine and, importantly for this story, smoking cessation. Semashko waged a war against tobacco unprecedented for its intended scope and exceptional in range, making the Soviets the first country in the world, in 1920, to entertain a national health program to curtail tobacco production, sales, imports, exports, and use with the goal of eventually stamping out tobacco. Semashko did not achieve his full utopian ideal. Political and economic regulations languished, but the Soviets established the earliest national anti-tobacco campaigns and funded the first public cessation clinics.

Despite this early start, the animosity of the architect of the revolution, and the support of the leader of the first national health service in the world, tobacco remained integral to the Soviet experience and grew in use. By the 1960s–1970s, Soviet medical authorities estimated smoking rates of 45.0 to 56.9 percent among men and 26.3 to 49.1 percent among women.[5] Despite recent successes, the numbers caught in dependency and suffering are still high.[6] In 2020, 50.9 percent of Russian men and 14.3 percent of women used tobacco, most in cigarettes. For comparison, smoking rates in the United States (hereafter US) crested in 1965 at 52 percent of males and 34 percent of females and currently hover around 15 and 13 percent, respectively.[7] Considering that regular tobacco use kills half (or more) of its users with a smoking-related illness, it should not be surprising to learn of the nearly 329,000 tobacco-related deaths in Russia in 2020 or overall about 30 percent of male and 6 percent of female deaths.[8]

Tobacco may seem a small, even negligible thing—Leon Trotsky termed the butts an objectionable "trifle of life"—but as he noted, "Trifles, accumulating and combining, can constitute something great—or destroy something great."[9] *Cigarettes and Soviets* surveys the accumulation and combination of tobacco's effects on people, government, and culture across the Soviet era and the destruction it has left in its wake.[10] This analysis concentrates on the priorities of many different actors—from the government, tobacco producers, and public health administrators to workers, smokers, and the nonsmoking public—to unearth the culturally specific, politically contingent origins of Russia's current tobacco problem. The resulting stories engage debates on the history and rise of the global tobacco epidemic that challenge the centrality of capitalism to those narratives and reveal how changing technology influenced experiences and behaviors. At the same time, Soviet tobacco is more than just a global story. Smoking permeates Soviet identity creation, gender definition, physical experience, and cultural values. Tobacco's production, consumption, management, conception, and condemnation reaches into Soviet politics, economics, and society. Understanding how the state might both produce and resist tobacco showcases the influence of consumption and popular tastes on Soviet policy and undercuts visions of a unified state of coherent policies. Analysis of Soviet tobacco cessation and therapy highlights the difference of Soviet health care, its style, and its basic tenets. Gathering and interconnecting these stories of tobacco indicates smoking was more than just a trifle. Smoking outlasted Lenin and Semashko, endured and even triumphed under Stalin, survived the war, heated up through the Thaw, and persisted and intensified after the Bolshevik experiment collapsed. The revolutionary state withered away, but smoking, stubbornly, remained.

Lenin and Semashko's attention to tobacco reflected not a quixotic fight against an imaginary enemy but a reaction to its prevalence in revolutionary Russia. Despite an initial resistance in the 1600s, Russians had strongly taken to tobacco by the nineteenth century.[11] In 1898, the anti-tobacco author Dr. A. I. Il'inskii claimed that in Russia, a country infamous for its prodigious drinking, "the number of smokers is ten to twenty times greater than the number of people in alcoholic excess."[12] Although other types of tobacco use were available in Russia and then the Union of Soviet Socialist Republics (hereafter USSR), by far the most common mode of intake was the unique Russian cigarette—the *papirosa* (singular -a; plural -y). The hollow cardboard tube affixed to a tissue-paper-wrapped cartridge of leaf accounted for almost half of all processed tobacco in Russia by 1914; by 1922 the number was 80 percent.[13] For comparison, on the eve of World War I only 7 percent of tobacco in the US went into cigarettes.[14] Most Russian tobacco went to papirosy or loose tobacco for self-rolled smokes, and most Russian males smoked. Official consumption statistics, based on taxes, assumed 143 papirosy per person per year, but observers estimated much higher usage.[15] Industry analysts claimed that a pack a day (about twenty smokes) was standard for almost every Russian male.[16] The use of tobacco stretched across the empire, through its social fabric, and across its cultural divides, a democratic dependency that still allowed differentiation of status with brands, accessories, and styles of consumption. The more than one thousand Russian papirosy brands recorded by 1913 implied a market of diversity and size.[17] Even women smoked in large enough numbers to merit custom marketing, specialized brands, and exquisite Fabergé accessories.[18] It would be years, decades in some cases, for similarly mass use of cigarettes to develop in other markets.[19]

Not only did Russians consume tobacco in large numbers and in a unique form, most lower-class users, the vast majority, smoked a singular type of tobacco called *makhorka*. Makhorka (*Nicotiana rustica*) is a nicotine-laden, highly fragrant tobacco varietal smoked, loose and self-rolled, by about two-thirds of Russians at the time of World War I.[20] For the peasantry easily grown, worked, and smoked makhorka offered a cheap, untaxed, and untraced way to smoke. In the city, the use of aromatic, rough makhorka differentiated class, as makhorka was cheaper than the oriental/Turkish leaf (*Nicotiana tabacum*) preferred by well-heeled smokers. American-style bright leaf appeared rarely.

These two conditions exceptional to late imperial Russia—the large portion of tobacco smoked rather than snuffed, piped, or chewed and the availability of nicotine-heavy makhorka—made the Russian smoker revolutionary in another way. They created the possibility for more powerful tobacco dependency. Inhaled tobacco, as with cigarettes rather than pipes, quickly impacts the smoker. Dragged into the lungs, inhaled smoke delivers over 90 percent of the nicotine to the blood in less than thirty seconds, giving a quicker fix and increasing the possibility of dependency. Not only did Russians take to a more addictive means of tobacco use, but the tobacco smoked by the majority was incredibly strong. Makhorka contains nearly twice the nicotine of other tobaccos, and contemporary accounts all point to it being inhaled, despite the harsh experience this must have imparted.[21] These two factors are likely to have pulled Russian, and then Soviet smokers, into a quicker, more intense, dependency earlier than those in other tobacco markets.[22]

Whether the smokes were grown and worked at home, then self-rolled into "goat legs," or factory-rolled papirosy bought from a street seller, a tobacco haze enveloped revolutionary Russia, flavoring every aspect of life. Smoked tobacco, especially from makhorka, produced an almost palpable stench, and in the close confines of the city, the smell of smoke impacted bystanders and the diaphanous tendrils from papirosy showed visibly from afar. After use, smoking marked bodies with stale breath, yellowed teeth, stained fingers, musty hair, and burned and foul-smelling clothes. The smell from cheap makhorka or more dear oriental differentiated class and pretentions. Smoke anchored the "scentscapes" of Russian cities and homes delineating spaces of respectability, danger, work, and leisure with either odor or stench according to personal predilection.[23] The detritus of tobacco—musty spaces, ubiquitous butts, crumbs, and ash—blanketed streets and homes. When Russia experienced its liberal revolution in February 1917, followed by the Bolshevik Revolution in October of the same year, the politics changed, but every rally reeked of smoke. Spent papirosy and crushed packs littered the floors and tables of the numerous, endless meetings.[24] When the journalist John Reed described the postrevolutionary gathering of the soviet in Petrograd, not just Lenin and Trotsky took over the stage but so too did the rank miasma: "There was no heat in the hall but the stifling heat of unwashed human bodies. A foul blue cloud of cigarette smoke rose from the mass and hung in the thick air."[25] The smell of revolution was tobacco, its sensibility smoke.

This early start made smoking more noticeable and socially accepted and expected earlier, but the reasons and ways that the Soviets opposed tobacco also differed from those of the west. The Bolshevik seizure of power created opportunities for the maintenance of public health, even as heavy state interference in the production and sale of goods became policy. Connections to lung cancer or addiction were years in the future. Instead, Semashko's and Lenin's animosity to tobacco stemmed from the mass imposition of its smell and an opinion among some revolutionary-era doctors that nicotine was a poison that attacked the nervous system. In addition to viewing the danger of smoking differently, Soviet medical authorities held unique attitudes toward public health, had a singular set of professional conditions in medicine, embraced therapeutic techniques born of their native reflexology, and expressed concerns over a contextually specific, perceived decline in the population's health and virility.[26] In the decades that followed the revolution, the Soviets forged innovative cessation techniques dependent on social interventions and chemical therapies and penned inventive arguments regarding the social costs of smoking and the dangers of secondhand smoke.

Despite this push for cessation from some government actors, others supported tobacco production, use, and export. This was not quite the disconnect that it initially appears. On the one hand, not all were convinced tobacco was dangerous, and none considered it addictive like opium or alcohol. On the other hand, many thought smoking would cease on its own. Semashko tied smoking (and drinking) to capitalism and believed that revolution would defeat tobacco as social conditions eased and cultural levels rose. Representatives of industry and trade argued that for the moment, tobacco had to be produced and pursued heightened output to counter black marketing and public anger over low supply. The calculus, established early, maintained for years. Over the decades, state planners centered, celebrated, and even sacrificed for tobacco, and medical figures proved horribly wrong about smoking's eventual demise. By the end of the twentieth century the newly independent Russian state would be home to one of the highest smoking populations in the world, with horrific consequences for popular, especially male, health.

The events of October 1917 destabilized more than just political systems. Revolution rearranged the basic building blocks of society and expectations for male and female behavior. Tobacco use or abstention—freighted with social meaning, political ideas, and gendered concepts—became integral to the creation of a new Soviet self. Soviet family law evolved over the decades and campaigns at the factory and in the battlefield transformed the image of the ideal Soviet citizen. Just as expectations for masculine and feminine behavior fluctuated, so too did tobacco's meaning transform. If a woman smoked, what she smoked and how, where, and with whom was sticky with meaning. For males in the revolutionary era, tobacco could be a sign of un-Soviet attitudes in cartoons, a mark of distinction in advertising, an attribute of the hard-core Bolshevik in public, or a sign of resistance to the past even as health literature depicted it as a disgusting source of impotence.[27] In war, type of tobacco could signal military rank or authenticity as well as connections and status. By the 1960s smoking became so expected an aspect of male behavior that to attack it was seen as stripping away everything that made a Soviet man a man.

Not simply a cultural signifier, used and manipulated by people to communicate status or fashion, papirosy acted upon the body. Most basically, tobacco creates chemical dependency that can alter behavior and mood with both its presence and its absence. Further, smokers' gestures and habits for lighting, holding, inhaling, and extinguishing papirosy bring comfort in their familiarity and can convey vehemence or promise intimacy in their completion. Lack of tobacco can increase anxiety or spur anger. And smokers are not the only players in this drama. Papirosy are also social and political actors.[28] The sight of tobacco or an accessory could prompt desire to a habituate or trigger revulsion to a confirmed quitter without the smoker even being aware. For some an offered smoke invited comradery, for others the imposition of its smell denied a shared humanity.

Deficits of tobacco, and the discontent this caused, raised riots and forced policy shifts. At various times the papirosa has been a currency, measure of progress, diplomatic bridge, or shot at the enemy. Take makhorka. In the wake of the revolution the self-rolled makhorka smoke (and smell) could signal, depending on setting and smoker, a man of low class and poor education, a woman with radical interests, or a person of political authenticity and strength. During the wars it came to identify collective experience, national distinction, steely resolve, attainment of maturity, and comradery. Still later, makhorka turned into a sign of backwardness compared to filtered cigarettes of western style. In the post-Soviet era a nostalgia for a seemingly lost, vigorous, Soviet manhood softened the perceptions of makhorka's smell and taste to make it desirable again.

More than a master of meaning or prompt to behavior and understanding, the papirosa itself transforms. Production innovations, agricultural developments, scientific research, increased mechanization, and new standards of quality control changed the taste, burn, and experience of even established brands. The Soviet standard *Belomorkanal* papirosa produced in the 1930s was not the same as one from the 1960s, nor, to the communist connoisseur, were the *Iava* filter cigarettes made at satellite factories in the 1960s, '70s, and '80s comparable to those made at the main factory in Moscow. Changes in packaging, paper, filters, and leaf transformed burn, taste, smell, and effect. Competition from new styles either produced at home or imported from abroad transformed the familiar. Smoking a *Marlboro* just once changed the way a *Belomorkanal* tasted ever after. Soviet smokers luxuriated in their smokes and found ways to distinguish quality, purchase with discrimination, and display their knowledge and taste even when choices were few and supplies scarce. High quality and abundance were not necessary to the experience of communist connoisseurship. Smokers distinguished themselves from others in knowledge and valued and appreciated differences of taste and quality. Even in war or in exile, distinction could be found.[29]

Making the papirosa active in smoker behaviors, sensible in daily life, transformed by time, manipulated by ideology, and malleable in meaning challenges simplistic understandings of addictive behavior as largely biochemical and unchanging. It infuses cultural, social, and psychological factors into the history of dependency.[30] It also contributes to scholarship describing the full impact of material culture and sensory experience to understanding identity, the construction of the social, the meaning of modern, and the transformation of daily life.[31] In revolutionary Russia, the body was a constant for a world in flux. Physical experience and bodily health would remain even after the old world and its institutions, culture, art, and architecture were swept away or withered.[32] The body would be the foundation of the new Soviet state through the creation of a new Soviet man.[33] Even as this revolutionary person was discussed, many tried to fashion their behavior and speed the revolution by living it—moving from thoughts and words to experiences, sensations, and the material.[34] Tobacco, as it was actually brought into the body and transformative of its function, was intimately connected to that process of identity creation even as it functioned as a signifier to outsiders. Securing tobacco, displaying it, or offering it held psychological and physical significance for users.[35]

Cigarettes and Soviets reveals smokers' motivations and tobacco's meanings, but it also illuminates the priorities of top leadership and how these changed over time. Even as the Soviets opposed tobacco from 1917 to 1991, they also, for reasons running the gamut from countering popular discontent to exploiting mass addiction for revenue, produced it. This mirrored the similarly fraught relationship the tsarist, and then Bolshevik, government had with alcohol. One 1990s Russian analyst lambasted state production of tobacco, like alcohol, as reaping "the political loyalty of the masses with the help of psychoactive substances."[36] But the depiction of tobacco as the true opiate of the masses assumes a passive smoking population and a state in total control. The potency and popularity of papirosy prepared the Soviets to have a massive market for any tobacco they produced, and for the state to interfere in the biopsychosocial bond between smoker and tobacco held danger. Soviet actions to secure tobacco exposed the ways popular, consumer demand could overturn, manipulate, or even dictate state priorities. The volatile reactions of smokers to deficits and quality problems, and the uneasiness of authorities over tobacco worker anger and user demands show a more complex relationship than pusher and user. Despite the Soviet control of both the economy and the public health agenda, prohibition did not present an easy choice, and experience taught many that it would fail.

Responses of Soviet citizens to the scarcity of tobacco, or the poor quality of it, were often volatile, as mobs and rioters in the 1920s, 1930s, 1960s, and 1990s attest. The state worked to secure a steady tobacco supply and facilitate its equitable distribution with, at different times, nationalization, rationing, price controls, troop movements, and hard-currency investments. Consider the diplomatic dimensions of tobacco. Smoking and war were intertwined from the nineteenth century, and during military actions the Bolsheviks and their enemies deployed tobacco and rolling papers to destabilize the opposition. Placating smokers was an issue of national security. By World War II the Soviets were making extraordinary sacrifices to secure tobacco for their troops, and after their triumph, brands like *Pobeda* (Victory) allowed smokers to relive the Nazi defeat, on average, twenty to forty times a day. Later, Cold War success was measured in quality and availability of western-style filter cigarettes over the passé papirosy. Comparisons to the west were framed in terms of the strength of eastern tobaccos, the deficits of filter cigarettes, or poor-quality Soviet packaging. In the days leading to the 1991 collapse, tobacco riots joined pro-democracy rallies in destabilizing the system.

Bolshevik policy and politics dictated a different relationship to tobacco and assured that the growth of tobacco use in the USSR strayed from the standard narratives of market development elsewhere. Instead of vertical integration, extensive mechanization, aggressive marketing, and easy availability leading to increased tobacco use, the number of smokers in Russia, and then the USSR, grew without any of these factors.[37] No "vice-industrial complex" or voracious "limbic capitalism" powered by "accessibility, affordability, advertising, anonymity, and anomie" manufactured the addictive impulses of the Soviet population.[38] No entrepreneurs of pleasure preyed on the Soviet citizen, nor did industrial designers scheme to create the most seductive delivery and product feel for a modern "packaged pleasure."[39] Instead, communist ideological resistance to product fetishization tempered marketing and branding. Rudimentary agriculture limited leaf quality and quantity. Machinery shortages and obsolescence assured no mass supply, and the disinterest in increasing markets meant no manipulation of nicotine and design to increase dependency.

The Soviets' more lackadaisical attitude toward industrial design and product engineering challenges standard understandings of the onset and experience of dependency. The Soviets often sacrificed quality for quantity and laid taste on the altar as well, yet even so producers remained unable to satisfy the population's tobacco hunger.[40] Scarcity elevated product appeal even as conventional capitalist tricks for market expansion were thrown into the dustbin of history. The emphasis on heavy industry over consumer goods influenced supply in the best of times. The aftermath of war, revolution, civil war, and then war again on their own lands and often on the very fields that produced their leaf created shortages that at times were so severe that homegrown or ersatz tobacco became the norm. Producers struggled to simply meet demand, let alone increase it. But even without marketing, the number of smokers grew and the ever-agile papirosa took on new meanings. Tobacco availability turned into a marker of past good times or the sign of goals for future prosperity. The Soviet association of tobacco supply with periods of stability may have encouraged its prime place in production plans, while the allure of an often-scarce product likely reinforced individual dependency. In other markets the abundance of high-quality tobacco products has been depicted as the foundation of tobacco addiction, but the Soviet case indicates scarcity can inflame the desire for a smoke, too. The narratives of tobacco uptake are not universal or rooted in capitalism.

Culture, politics, and economics all distinguished the growth of smoking in the USSR, and they influenced the Soviet reaction to research from the 1950s connecting tobacco to cancer and other diseases. Whereas the British and Americans issued reports and promulgated new regulations in the 1960s, the Soviets would not. Despite their early start with cessation and tobacco resistance, a return to Semashko-style proposals to limit sales and production would not come from the Soviets until the late 1970s. This was partially because the Soviets had long maintained that smoking endangered health, and cancer was simply added to the list of dangers. But in the 1970s decreasing male life spans, a general deterioration in popular health, and increased international competition over living standards fueled grassroots animosity to smoking. Editorial actions at leading journals inspired a new, antismoking generation. Under the combined pressure of bad press and popular calls for action, the state and medical establishment renewed cessation work. In a departure from the experience of the west, production representatives voluntarily started warning labels and did not, seemingly, obstruct public health messaging. Unfortunately, popular anger from smokers, smuggled and black-market cigarettes, halfhearted support from Soviet doctors, and a general lack of enforcement hobbled cessation. With the opening of the market to full western advertising and production after 1991, relationships changed. Western tobacco manufacturers found an eager market where tobacco scarcity was rife, tobacco quality uneven, medical authorities distrusted, and advertising virtually nonexistent. The resulting availability of tobacco and aggressive hunt for new users was disastrous for short- and long-term health.

Cigarettes and Soviets presents the relationship among state, production, profit, health, culture, gender, biology, use, image, and users at different points from 1917 to the present. This is not an all-encompassing history of tobacco production throughout the seventy-odd years of Soviet power or of public health or the cultural strength of smoking. Nor does it engage all the ways that tobacco could be snorted, chewed, smoked, and ingested. Instead, it investigates the most widespread type of tobacco use in the Soviet period and emphasizes those points where Soviet smoking deviates from the global story, those features of the habit that were peculiar, those aspects of treatment that were unusual, and those times that were uniquely powerful for communist smokers. It is at once a study of Soviet tobacco deeply enmeshed in its social, political, and cultural context and an exploration of vagaries from the global tobacco experience.

The analysis starts in the foundational era for Soviet health policy and attitudes. The chapters "Attacked," "Resurrected," "Sold," and "Treated" each provide background to a different aspect of the early Soviet relationship to tobacco— from the perspective of the health system, producers, culture, and reluctant smokers. The chapters "Unfulfilled," "Mobilized," and "Recovered" show how the state embraced tobacco, sacrificed for it, and invested in its production from the 1930s to the postwar era as good tobacco increasingly served as a marker of the good life. Moving from the late Stalin years through to détente, "Partnered" explores the early incursion of western manufacturers into the Soviet market, while "Pressured" details the toll of increased use and outlines the resurrection in the 1970s and 1980s of anti-tobacco arguments first made in the 1920s. As detailed in the epilogue—"The Post-Soviet Smoker"—rules and players change after 1991. Privatization, aggressive marketing, mass availability of western blends, fresh approaches to health care and messaging, and new attitudes toward products, manufacturing, and consumption meant a different relationship to tobacco. Putin, a nonsmoker himself, has pushed campaigns to stamp out alcohol and tobacco use with seemingly impressive results. Fines and the closure of smoking rooms have reconstructed the space of smoking and the scentscapes of contemporary Russia. A century after Lenin established his no-smoking zones for his fellow revolutionaries on the sealed train, Russians are finally, seemingly, leaving tobacco behind.

ATTACKED

Commissar Semashko and Tobacco Prohibition

In 1959, after a lifetime as a leader in disease prevention, N. A. Semashko cast a jaded eye onto an early episode of his career. He recalled how, in 1920, Lenin prodded him: "Why not start a fight with that weed tobacco? I will support you." Goaded by Lenin, Semashko approached Sovnarkom with a two-pronged attack incorporating propaganda and economic sanctions. He recalled great success in smaller discussions but was surprised to be met "with bayonets" when things came to a vote. As the opposition piled on, Semashko looked to Lenin for his promised support and got a dipped head and a "sly" smile. Semashko wryly remarked that Lenin's challenge, and the policy debates that it unleashed, led to "one of the more comic episodes of my life."[1] But if the episode was "comic," it was a dark comedy. And for public health, it was a tragedy. Semashko's initiative was unique in its timing, scope, and reasoning. He audaciously attempted the first national antismoking campaign in the world—aimed at agriculture, production, and distribution and conceptualized before firm links had been made between smoking and cancer.

But Semashko's memoir gave only half the story. Defeated in Sovnarkom, Semashko began an expansive anti-tobacco campaign that he bundled with the general hygiene campaigns of Narkomzdrav. At the head of an agency devoted to prevention of illness and convinced of the social origins of disease, Semashko attacked smoking as a lifestyle illness akin to drinking and similarly responsive to changing social conditions. Communist ideology, which informed the public health agenda, made certain that this antismoking message would take on a red hue. The Bolshevik faith in propaganda coupled with the collectivist, materialist bent of Marxist ideology and the general reverence of the Soviets for the transformative power of science produced propaganda that highlighted societal dangers, collective responsibilities, and communal benefits. Although anti-tobacco pamphlets explored individual health consequences, it was the danger to the collective from secondhand smoke, smoking breaks, or antisocial smoker behavior that resonated with Soviet utopian rhetoric. In a continuation of prerevolutionary anxieties, cessation rhetoric focused on the poison of nicotine and its connection to nervous exhaustion. Fears over sensory exhaustion fed into a perceived epidemic of neurasthenia and concerns for virility and fertility. The policy context of the revolutionary response to tobacco was emphatically Soviet.

Semashko's Decree and Anti-tobacco Legislation

Russia entered World War I ill-prepared for a modern, industrial conflict. As war brought on shortages and the military stumbled, the tsarist government proved unable to deal with the battles against foreign enemies and internal disorders. The country roiled with first a liberal revolution in February 1917 and then, when that government proved unpopular and unstable, the imposition of Bolshevik power in October 1917.[2] Typhus, influenza, and cholera—fostered by war, destruction, and revolution and fanned by famine and dislocation—tore through the population, killing millions and threatening stability.[3] Narkomzdrav emerged in 1918 as an answer and fulfilled utopian, revolutionary promises to improve people's lives. Beyond stability and Marxist tenets, Bolshevik theorists believed that the bettering of worker health would bring with it the robust, vigorous bodies that would house minds primed for communism.[4] Semashko pursued policies driven by the philosophy of Soviet social hygiene—that is, that social conditions from material deprivation lay at the root of diseases like tuberculosis or syphilis and abuse of alcohol or tobacco.[5] Semashko, a longtime Marxist revolutionary, conveyed these ideas in speeches, essays, and pamphlets.[6]

Semashko's attack on tobacco started at a Small Sovnarkom meeting in late 1920. The Small Sovnarkom, a revolving group of three to four officials, met several times a week to speed decisions, generally for economic matters. With Lenin's signature, their decisions took on the authority of full Sovnarkom rulings. In cases of dispute, deliberation moved to the full Sovnarkom.[7] Tobacco came to the agenda through a report from People's Commissar for Trade and Industry Viktor Pavlovich Nogin. Nogin, who had been a professional revolutionary among Poltava tobacco workers, arrived at the December 14 meeting with a proposed decree concerning "the maintenance of tobacco production" through increased sowing and creating a general raw materials fund to supply factories.[8]

What began as a routine economic matter hit a roadblock in Semashko. After what was undoubtedly a lively debate not fully detailed in the minutes, a commission was created under Semashko for "the investigation of the question of the danger of tobacco and the possibility of gradual measures for diminishing and in the future destroying that culture." Semashko was charged with gathering representatives from the Commissariats of Agriculture, Trade, Food Supplies, and the Higher Soviet of National Economy and conveyed this charge to Narkomzdrav.[9]

Semashko's attempt for a revolutionary change with the flick of a pen was not without precedent. As Trotsky explained, Lenin wanted "to unfold the party's program in the language of power . . . The decrees were more propaganda than actual administrative measures. Lenin was in a hurry to tell the people what the new power was, what it was after, and how it intended to accomplish its aims." In 1922 Lenin commented: "There was a time when the passing of decrees was a form of propaganda. People used to laugh at us and say that the Bolsheviks do not realize that their decrees are not being carried out."[10] Even in a time of symbolic rulings, Semashko's plan must have seemed more audacious, because it did not quickly pass. Over the next two weeks, the commission met three times.[11] The head of the tobacco workers' union asked to be included, joining other representatives from Narkomzdrav.[12] The group got off to a rocky start. The absence of anyone from agriculture led to tabling discussion of cultivation. Semashko came out swinging, arguing for stopping tobacco exports because the Soviets should not "supply the international market with items that poisoned people." Trade and economic representatives resisted, and, in the end, the meeting minutes reported that these groups "stood in complete opposition to this opinion and strongly defended, in the present and in the future, the ability to export tobacco." The committee was unable to come to a vote.[13]

At the next meeting, on January 5, 1921, representatives from trade, economy, tobacco workers, and agriculture were now joined by a Narkomzdrav sanitary epidemiologist.[14] Economic representatives championed a fight against tobacco speculation, and this proposal was approved. Other tobacco questions stalled. The discussion regarding diminished sowing led to a debate "which took on a very volatile character." Semashko wished to forbid the distribution of seeds and plants for personal production, but the tobacco union and agriculture representatives pushed back. Semashko urged the restriction of tobacco cultivation to Crimea, the Caucasus, Riazan, Tambov, and by the Volga Germans. The meeting ended with a resolution to propose both ideas to the full committee.

Semashko must have felt optimistic, because he drafted a decree "for the diminution of tobacco smoking," including restricting where tobacco could be grown and forbidding the distribution of seeds and seedlings.[15] Export bans disappeared, but new proposals were introduced for limiting tobacco imports, stamping out speculation, restricting the military tobacco ration to smokers, ending ration cards for those under twenty-one or nonsmokers, limiting public smoking, and fostering "energetic agitation" against tobacco.[16] The file included a handwritten account of German youth smoking regulation, an indication of the influence of international examples.[17] Before the revolution, activists had lamented the absence of anti-tobacco movements in Russia like those in the US, Britain, and France, and Russian pamphlets and journals included foreign research.[18] Foreign anti-tobacco work continued to appear in Soviet publications.[19] Later Soviet reformers praised policies, especially bans on youth smoking, in Egypt, Japan, Portugal, Spain, Switzerland, and the US.[20]

Semashko presented his draft decree at the Small Sovnarkom meeting of February 3, 1921.[21] Industry and trade representatives did not hold back their disapproval, tabling points regarding limiting agriculture, production, and trade. Semashko was left with only the anti-tobacco agitation points. The protocol ended with the decree being transferred to the full Sovnarkom.[22] With no further entries, Semashko removed the decree from discussion at the large Sovnarkom meeting of July 1, 1921.[23] The battle for substantive economic anti-tobacco legislation at Sovnarkom was over, but debate over prohibition and efforts for smoke-free spaces continued. The anti-tobacco activist A. A. Press served on the Commission to Fight Smoking alongside the prominent psychologist and alcoholism specialist Professor Vladimir Bekhterev. The audience or authorizing agency for the report was unclear. The commission produced a proposal "On Measures for the Fight with the Extreme Distribution of Smoking." According to the report, Press termed it a critical time and railed against the irrational waste of labor and materials to produce tobacco. He optimistically thought the end could be achieved quickly, just as China had conquered opium and Russia had rooted out alcohol. The commission's conclusion that "the fight with it will not be that difficult as it seems many of these are weak-willed," was confident.[24]

Others called out government inaction and the fact that every meeting took place "under a fog of smoke."[25] In 1922 one anti-tobacco author wrote approvingly of Semashko's effort to eliminate smoking, moaned that propaganda and lectures were inadequate, and urged closing all tobacco factories, stopping military tobacco provision, eliminating smoking at hospitals, markets, and railroad facilities, and establishing smoking sections at work.[26] Other authors, guided by perceived failures of tsarist and Soviet alcohol prohibitions, distrusted bans as authoritarian and ineffective.[27] Nicholas II had prohibited alcohol in 1914.[28] Recognition of the pressures of bootlegging and the consumption of alcohol substitutes (cologne, lacquer, etc.), prompted the Provisional Government to relax the law. These same worries compelled the Soviets to liberalize liquor law gradually with the lifting of prohibition on wine in 1920 and then full-strength vodka in 1925.[29]

Mindful of prohibition's problems, other authors denounced coercive state tobacco measures.[30] The prolific health pamphleteer I. V. Sazhin, for example, proclaimed that the draconian policies of Tsar Aleksei Mikhailovich had done nothing under Russia's unique seventeenth-century tobacco ban.[31] Slitting nostrils did not dissuade people. He reasoned: "It is not the point that tobacco and spirits are sold, but it is that they are *wanted, searched for, paid for, and for not a little money. With that end we must begin.* Here, and in general for building a new life, we must begin with cultural revolution."[32] A 1926 pamphlet from a Dr. Nezlin similarly dismissed past prohibitions as ineffective in the face of popular demand and despaired: "Now because everything is in the hands of the state, it should be easy to destroy tobacco to its very core, close down the crops and close tobacco factories. But . . . simply to forbid smoking will not uproot it. In previous times even severe punishment did not uproot it. Even death sentences did not help in the past."[33] Nezlin pointed to how through the war and civil war smoking had not decreased. Although "makhorka could not be found for any amount of money . . . people did not quit smoking. At first, they smoked any trash, all sorts of nuts and leaves, and after they began to grow tobacco and . . . smoking did not diminish but rose and became all the more dangerous."[34] Another doctor held that the smoking of substitutes—"leaves, moss, and even manure"—showed that prohibition would not work.[35] Nezlin observed that without understanding the root of the compulsion to alcohol or tobacco, "to implant abstinence in the people is impossible." Instead, it was important to understand drinking and smoking because "no simple restriction will help while we do not recognize the roots and finally tear them up."[36] Policy followed the same course. A November 14, 1920, meeting of the War-Sanitary Commission contained a report regarding tobacco's negative effect on medical care. The commission decided that no further regulation was needed, as sanitary enlightenment work was already "organized and reasonable."[37]

Isolated groups explored prohibitions. In 1918 the Third All-Russia Congress of Soviet Workers in Petrograd, an event for some two hundred attendees, had a banner at the front of the hall reading, "Please Do Not Smoke."[38] A 1921 article regarding the prohibition of smoking at schools, kindergartens, and nurseries in Kazan implied this was out of the ordinary.[39] Soviet youth groups included anti-tobacco oaths in their pledges.[40] Articles in the popular press repeated these recommendations.[41] In 1924 *Izvestiia* reported a Moscow beauty salon forbade smoking, and another article detailed offices doing so.[42] The health cell, a subcommittee for the Moscow District Commission, forbade smoking, but it was not until 1926 that the Moscow Regional Health Authority did, with a fine of fifty kopecks per papirosa. This ruling followed a discussion of whether providing smoking rooms and breaks constituted an undue privilege.[43] Some workers tried to create designated smoking areas in dormitories.[44] In 1926 a special commission of pedagogues and parents considered banning smoking in schools. Fire safety generated some successful prohibitions. A 1924 story highlighted how smoking in theaters endangered patrons and had cost nearly three thousand rubles in just four months.[45] Smoking on boats was forbidden in 1926, including on loading docks and points of debarkation.[46] Fire safety also won out at building sites.[47]

Social Hygiene and Lifestyle Illnesses

Stymied in the Sovnarkom, as head of Narkomzdrav, Semashko retained a powerful platform. But Narkomzdrav had its own troubles caring for the health of a devastated population while plagued by shortages of medical personnel, dogged by insufficient funding, and weathering a dearth of supplies.[48] To make the most of scarce funds, Semashko focused on providing prophylactic care utilizing inexpensive, innovative propaganda and urging workers to "take hold of their health."[49] Posters were cheaper than practitioners, and observers commented on their variety, ingenuity, and omnipresence.[50] Visiting foreigners left convinced that Soviet health methods represented the future.[51] Pamphlets, posters, slogans, and lectures flooded the population with information on how to live, work, and rest. Museums, banners, and sandwich boards surrounded urban dwellers while trains, boats, and traveling displays toured the countryside. Workers' clubs staged lectures, films, slide shows, and agitation plays with new lifestyle messages. One author posited using tobacco products themselves for propaganda by decorating packs with tobacco dangers rather than brightly colored scenes and enticing names.[52] Between 1919 and 1922 the state published over thirteen million pieces of public health materials.[53] In 1923 there was a surge in interest on issues of daily life as part of Trotsky's campaign to improve party discipline and culture. In 1926 publications surged as part of the general campaign for a new Soviet lifestyle, and novel groups spread hygienic messages.[54] Authorities told parents to enroll their children in the Soviet nursery, kindergarten, or school, where health and hygiene were part of daily regimens alongside politics and party. At the end of the school day children were to join the Octobrists (up to age nine), Pioneers (age nine to fourteen), and Komsomol (age fourteen to twenty-eight) for tips on healthy leisure and to participate in campaigns to build the new, healthy, Soviet life.

Publications and programs spread messages about new balanced, rational, and progressive behaviors while uprooting backward, selfish, and irrational habits like smoking. In 1922 Bukharin spoke before the Komsomol on the need for better behaviors and against rough manners. He called out Komsomol members who mocked anti-alcohol and anti-tobacco campaigns because, while under capitalism smoking had been a means of resistance, now it could not be justified from a "physiological and educational standpoint."[55] In a May 1924 speech before the Komsomol, Grigory Zinoviev, an old Bolshevik and the head of the Petrograd party organization, connected the solidification of the revolution to the battle for an abstemious lifestyle: "If we create a sober generation . . . that can fight against bootleg liquor, alcohol, [and] smoking, then we will make a significant step in the consolidation of the gains of the revolution . . . We cannot pass a resolution against smoking and then secretly blow smoke up our sleeves. We cannot start a fight against alcohol, so that we can later joyfully drink to the occasion."[56]

A cornerstone of prophylactic propaganda lay in battling "lifestyle" illnesses, which transformed individual sickness into social and political danger.[57] Semashko's campaign against lifestyle illnesses coincided with his belief in social hygiene—that is, that eradication of illness was possible with the elimination of capitalism and perfection of the social system.[58] When disease persisted, theorists explained that although Soviet power had transformed Russia politically, the population had not yet caught up socially and culturally. To usher in a new age would require reeducation, and advice combined political, cultural, and social agendas with hygiene.[59] Some social hygienists, following the lead of Lenin and Semashko, expanded lifestyle disease like alcoholism and syphilis to include smoking. As one author determined, "it is visibly evident that tobacco appears on a level with alcohol, tuberculosis, and syphilis as one of the evils with which it is essential to energetically and unceasingly fight."[60]

The idea that smoking was a result of social conditions influenced cessation. As Dr. Nezlin explained, the workers and peasants did not live well under capitalism and tobacco became a way to distract them as "the worse he lived, the greater the need for escape." Nezlin cited the experience of the front, where soldiers "suffered more for lack of makhorka than for bread . . . The poor man drinks and smokes from sadness and despair. The rich man from greed and alarm for his wealth and thirst for pleasures." He finished, "The construction of a new, better life . . . is the most trustworthy way to fight with all drugs and included with that is tobacco."[61] Semashko similarly condemned alcohol and tobacco as holdovers of an oppressive, bourgeois system.[62] But smoking proved more deeply rooted than capital. By 1926 Sazhin concluded that smoking and drinking could not be attributed to harsh social conditions because times had changed and besides, women had it much harder than men and did not smoke.[63] One author proposed that tobacco was a greater, more widespread problem than vodka.[64] Another felt smoking had turned from an individual problem to a "social evil," noting that: "The spread of tobacco has been aided . . . by the complete ignorance of the population to the danger," so that "the lack of prohibitive measures and the uncultured population apparently aid tobacco poisoning, and the nonsmoking population, standing and breathing that same air, are also sullied by tobacco smoke."[65] One author recounted, with disgust, a train trip with a wagon full of invalid women and children, all suffering from coughs and fevers, who were further tortured by a smoker who would not be shamed into stopping.[66]

Smoke's social danger drifted across divisions of space and time, public and private, and work and leisure.[67] The story of a French doctor who blamed a father's smoking in the kitchen as the cause of the daughter's illnesses in the bedroom became a staple of Soviet pamphlets.[68] Leningrad's Dr. Bliumenau reminded men to consider the health of their wives and children before lighting up.[69] The anti-tobacco therapist A. S. Sholomovich condemned the tobacco that "poisons the air of peasant huts and worker homes, worker apartments in city institutions, mills, and factory premises, and what is worse than all, school buildings and crowded rooms where children live and sleep."[70] Lenin advised, "Believe me, your work will be more productive if you wander in the forest for an hour or two than if you sit in a stuffy room, mercilessly rub your forehead, and swallow papirosa after papirosa."[71] One author quantified the danger: 67 percent of the smoke of a papirosa befouled the surrounding air.[72] Overcrowding intensified problems, and heating oil shortages meant apartments were not aired. A. A. Press complained that when an average apartment of five rooms held fifteen people, and of these a third were smokers and at least one or two chain smokers of up to fifty papirosy a day, the atmosphere was suffocating. He continued that everywhere, "You are constantly surrounded by smokers . . . and you must breathe this spoiled air without a stop," and "forcibly and constantly" imbibe nicotine. He lamented he was "smoked out in all sides at meetings, sessions, and not infrequently in apartments." For smokers to continue their habit showed "lack of culture . . . rudeness . . . unforgivable disinterest."[73]

Authors considered tuberculosis a result of smoking, dismissing the prerevolutionary belief that smoking killed infections.[74] One author proposed that inhaling tobacco smoke filled the lungs with soot, making it harder for gasses to pass through, bringing in gasses of no benefit to the body, forcing them to do extra work, and making the lungs ripe environments for the tuberculosis bacillus.[75] Another author placed his warning in bold: "**He who smokes tobacco more easily falls ill with tuberculosis.**"[76] Nezlin observed: "Consumption, of course, has its cause not in tobacco but in infection. But smoking prepares a way for the infection and eases its penetration of the lungs."[77] Sickened smokers were transformed into disease vectors. A doctor called out overcrowding and the housing crisis as spreading tuberculosis and a reason to quit. He challenged children to press their parents: "To whom are you a friend? Tuberculosis or children? With whom do you march: with tuberculosis against children or with children against tuberculosis?"[78] Another doctor maintained that 95 percent of those with tuberculosis were smokers, plagued by smoking-induced mucus, which they then spit on the street to infect others, including youth who picked up the butts and got tuberculosis, or even syphilis.[79] A 1923 article claimed that the infection stayed on a butt for up to two weeks.[80]

Public smokers harmed others with their habit.[81] Sazhin mentioned Viennese researchers who proved nonsmoking restaurant workers suffered from nicotine poisoning and sailors developed heart problems from tobacco smoke on ships.[82] Another highlighted the rights of nonsmokers as opposed to the "large egoism of the inveterate smoker—who wishes that all, in condescension to his weakness, take into their very cores his filthy smoke, which he has just expelled from his nostrils?!"[83] He further accused smokers of "an immoral act . . . [and] a small evil, which gains great spread and may become a national disaster."[84] Press concentrated on the smoke that plagued the eyes of hairdressers or the danger to typographers, who already suffered from tuberculosis and nervous illness, forced to deal with smoke at work or in the dormitory. He advocated forbidding smoking in public spaces, imposing fines, and research on "a general plan for the fight with tobacco immorality."[85] As Sazhin concluded, "Smokers are social pests."[86]

In addition to endangering others, smokers wasted acres of land, piles of goods, and hours of labor to supply their tobacco.[87] Sholomovich claimed that papirosy squandered "hundreds of thousands" of acres of land and the labor of twenty-six thousand workers.[88] Another author bemoaned the land and machinery wasted that could produce food or useful goods.[89] Others laid out in tables and statistics the disproportionate illness of tobacco workers, who were 69.3 percent female.[90] In a 1921 *Pravda* piece, Semashko lamented that tobacco workers suffered from lung disease and society shouldered the cost.[91] Tuberculosis deaths among tobacco workers were 50 percent higher than in textiles or leather production. Dust, considered a major cause of tuberculosis, was declared the prime danger in tobacco work. Other authors detailed higher miscarriage rates, infant death, and general ill health among the largely female tobacco workforce.[92]

Anti-tobacco propagandists brought up smoking's negative effects on productivity—a precious resource of the workers' state.[93] Nezlin cited research claiming that a cigar cut the strength of a smoker by a quarter.[94] Another author maintained that tobacco weakened muscular strength.[95] Anti-tobacco authors advanced international studies that showed tobacco as detrimental to productivity, attention, and accuracy to counter the common belief that tobacco increased stamina and sharpened attention. One grumbled: "Great people become great, of course, not because they smoked **but in spite of the fact that they did**. No one has shown (and of course, cannot) that papirosy bring genius."[96] Another observed that one papirosa might help a person work late, but that over the years it would take its toll. Computing the difference in the pulse of smokers and nonsmokers, he estimated that smokers lessened their lives by eight years and two months.[97] Smoking breaks merited special ire.[98] A 1926 *Pravda* article estimated smokers wasted two hours of their workday in breaks, and in 1927 a similar work-loss discussion mentioned, "Smoking, conversations, reading newspaper, and going to the bathroom, etc., reduce the constructive use of work time."[99] Aleksei Gastev and the Scientific Organization of Labor groups that he inspired spurned irresponsible behaviors such as being late or smoking and emphasized beneficial leisure like physical culture. One of his groups urged members to "quit smoking within the next week."[100]

Even the economic arguments against smoking often emphasized the toll on collective advancement. One author detailed the costs of makhorka for a peasant (three kopecks per day) and papirosy for a worker (thirty kopecks per day) with a consequent cost of eighteen rubles a year for peasants and almost 120 rubles per year for workers. For a peasant, ten years paying for tobacco would "build a new house, buy a pair of horses and a thresher." Nezlin painted a picture of an idealized future where "trusts and cooperatives . . . will sell healthy things instead of papirosy—let's say vegetables and fruit, books and pictures. Then no sweeping prohibition will be needed." He continued: "Even from the first it is clear that smoking harms the pocket of not just the individual person. Tobacco carries devastation to all of the national economy."[101]

Visual propaganda emphasized collective danger. The early 1920s poster "Vodka, Hashish, and Tobacco" from the Political and War-Sanitary Command of the Turkestan Front provides an iconographically styled calculus of the dangers (Figure 1.1). The individual bears responsibility in each—a drinker, a toker, and, finally, a smoker (or part of one—the heart). In the realm of consequences, the user fades and society's withered outcomes are emphasized. At top the prosperous farm of the nondrinker contrasts with the dilapidated hut and broken equipment of the vomiting drunkard. For the hashish user, the anticipated burden to society is in the addict's incarceration in either the mad house or prison. The bottom panel instructs, "The Red Army man, with the money he monthly wastes on makhorka could buy the pictured items [soap, tooth powder, etc.] and collectively subscribe to a newspaper [*Krasnaia zvezda*]." Alcohol use/abstention is an individual threat or boon. The hashish smoker's choice to indulge is a burden on society. The smoker could either be a threat to themselves or become the new Soviet man or at least could have the accoutrements of good hygiene (brush, soap, and toothpaste), enlightenment (pen and notebook), and political literacy (*Krasnaia zvezda*). The lineup implies that drinking might be one man's tragedy, but tobacco held back society.

The poster "Quit Smoking" similarly targets a male, military audience and accentuates socio-economic over personal consequences (Figure 1.2). The

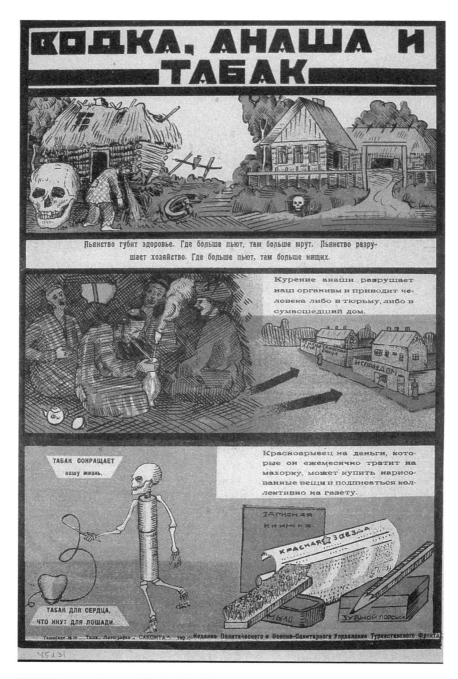

FIGURE 1.1. Poster. "Vodka, Hashish, and Tobacco," 1921–1925. Courtesy Russian State Library.

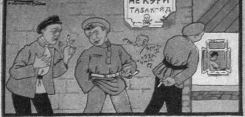
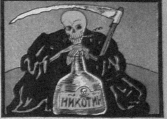
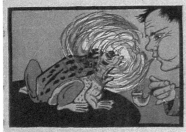
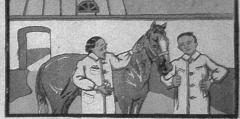
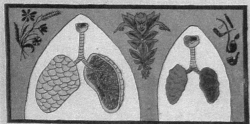
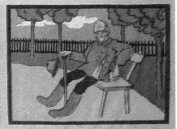
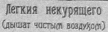

FIGURE 1.2. Poster. "Quit Smoking," 1921–1925. Courtesy Russian State Library.

smoker's introduction comes from social pressure as boys teach one another to smoke, the image hinting at older theories connecting smoking to criminality.[102] The Grim Reaper's embrace of his nicotine vial hints to the wages of indulgence. The death to frog and horse occupy the center panels, and the disembodied lungs, like the tethered heart, contrast to those of a nonsmoker. Only one panel features an individual smoker, and he is past his prime, twenty years a smoker, and sickened with the extremely severe, almost always fatal "central nervous system tuberculosis." Just as the lungs next to him are excised from the body, he is cut from society. Even though he now sits in a park, he cannot enjoy the fresh air in his wasted body. The bottom text underscores the social dangers of tobacco: "Comrades, if you wish to be healthy, quit smoking. It will save your life and money, which is vainly wasted on tobacco. You will free up for more healthful labors thousands of workers, who unproductively work in tobacco factories."

Soviet society returned to prerevolutionary antismoking arguments that emphasized the expense of fires caused by careless disposal of butts. Old tales held that Tsar Mikhail forbade smoking because of the danger of fires. In the 1920s authors fixated on rural fires caused by careless smoking.[103] Nezlin had an entire chapter on "The Red Cockerel," noting that "Smokers blow up mines and homes," offering as proof a vague story of surreptitious smoking that caused a mine explosion and a more concrete example from Moscow of a munitions explosion that killed ten in 1923.[104] The story of the conflagration at the Brussels exhibition of 1910, the result of one cigarette, also made the rounds.[105] Pieces in *Izvestiia* throughout the decade connected workplace fires and smoking.[106]

The cover for the 1926 I. M. Varushkin pamphlet *Why Tobacco Is Harmful* emphasizes tobacco's dangers to the countryside (Figure 1.3). In the image, vibrantly rendered in bright red and contrasting green, an old, hunched man with no shoes, balding, and sitting on a pile of straw exhales a swirl of green smoke. The sickly coloring, along with his gaunt features and exaggerated hands and feet make him a grotesque and pitiful figure, and his actions bring forward even more disgust. Passively, or even passive-aggressively, he continues to smoke as behind him the village goes up in flames. For this old man, tobacco's purported individual dangers seemingly have passed. The focus is not on prevention or even healing. The emphasis is on the social danger of his individual habit. He has become a double burden. Past the age of contributing to society, he is actively destroying it.

Even in discussion of the individual dangers of smoking, the social problem loomed. The prolific health writer L. M. Vasilevskii warned that smoking harmed the voice, one of the most important features of the activist.[107] Nezlin, after outlining the ways in which smoking dried the larynx and harmed the vocal cords, took his health arguments in a surprisingly political direction, proposing that

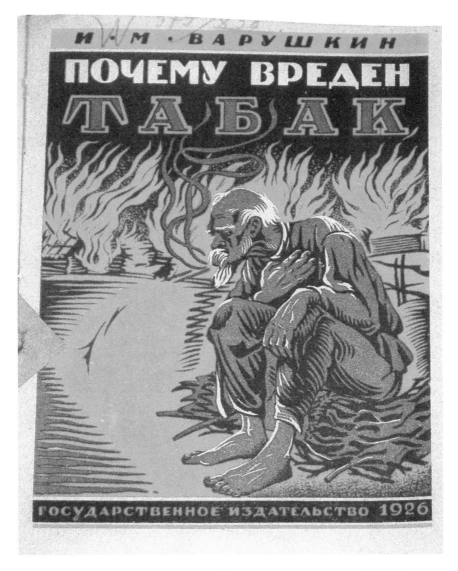

FIGURE 1.3.   Book cover. I. M. Varushkin, *Why Tobacco Is Harmful* (1926).
Courtesy Russian State Library.

"every person must protect his voice, as the voice is what distinguishes man from beasts. A healthy voice is what is needed for defense of your opinion at a meeting, or at a gathering, or in your case at court." The individual danger of a cracked, sore throat led to a social problem—diminished political participation.[108] For women, the irritation of tobacco on the throat lessened the feminine qualities of their voices, according to Sazhin, degrading their attractiveness and endangering their social duty as future mothers.[109]

A related, if seemingly minor, issue emerged in the campaign against papirosy butts and littering. In a diatribe on slovenly and uncultured throwback habits, Trotsky singled out the litter from smokers as a drag on revolutionary progress.[110] He was not alone in seeing a connection of culture and smoking. A 1920 *Krasnaia gazeta* article observed that the dining hall of Petrograd's Porkhov textile plant was a paragon of "discipline in word and deed . . . Here there is not a speck of ash or a papirosa butt. A sign reads 'No smoking'—and no one smokes."[111] A 1928 article pointed to the inhospitable conditions of a barracks with particular attention given to the rubbish and papirosy butts on the floor.[112] A 1929 *Krokodil* cartoon used butts to critique the lack of political consciousness within the Komsomol. The drawing portrays two youths in black boots and collared shirts—one spitting on the floor and the other smoking and surrounded by butts and cartons. These two slovenly youth interrogate a third well-dressed young man, asking him, "Why haven't you shown up for the culture campaign?" In typical fashion for *Krokodil*, the words and actions of authority figures are discordant.[113] Internal documents of the Komsomol showed similar critiques of hypocritical behavior campaigns.[114]

When smoking so endangered society, to quit became a political act. One pamphlet summed up cessation's revolutionary effects:

> Now, when the task of new building requires the physical and mental abilities of every member of society, all means of liquidating smoking will be waged as a benefit to not just the smokers themselves.
>
> The liquidation of smoking will release our children, our youth from a great burden hanging upon their physical and moral health. . .
>
> Individual and social manners, corrupted by the abnormal consciousness, will be refined.
>
> Thousands of the best acres of land will be freed for the growing of socially healthful products.
>
> Hundreds of factories will be able to be changed gradually into the production of essential social manufactures.
>
> A great deal of paper used now for tobacco products will become books and newspapers and serve the great need of enlightening the country.
>
> Thousands of workers will be freed for other socially helpful, and not dangerous to themselves, production.
>
> The smokers will save their time for helpful labor and rational leisure.[115]

The transfer of so much onto the action of smoking was at once empowering and burdensome. When individual actions could be so revolutionary, to remain passive bordered on treason. Transforming individual hygiene could revolutionize all of society, or as Nezlin put it: "Smoking is a trial for not just the individual. All the people and the state suffer because of the smoker."[116]

Individual Behavior and Secondhand Danger

Although by the 1920s some researchers had made the connection between tobacco and cancer, they linked only certain cancers—lips, tongue, and mouth—to irritation caused by tobacco.[117] "Safer" smoking entailed holders that kept the papirosa farther away to lessen irritation. A Narkomzdrav report listed many irritants that caused cancer, including "smoking, alcoholism, not extracting decayed teeth, ulcers, fistulas, chronic skin diseases, warts, leukoplakia of the tongue (white spots), animal parasites, chemical tumors, thermal and mechanical stimuli, unsanitary situation of home and soil, cancerous lesions, and cancerous tumors."[118] One author recommended avoiding excess in drink, food, or smoking to avoid cancer.[119]

Instead of cancer, Nezlin outlined the poisonous action of nicotine, starting with the use of tobacco as an insecticide by native Americans, providing a rundown of nineteenth-century anecdotes—oversmoking causing death, a list of the many animals that could be terminated with nicotine, and secondhand smoke's dangers.[120] An early 1920 army-medical pamphlet outlined the symptoms of nicotine poisoning, including, "headache, dizziness, nausea, palpitations, pulse irregularity (arrhythmia), salivation, general weakness, fainting, trembling, dilation of pupils, difficulty breathing, vomiting, diarrhea . . . unconsciousness, convulsions, death from paralysis of heart and breathing, and . . . poisoning."[121] Others concentrated on the amount of nicotine in different tobacco sorts, perhaps with a greater emphasis on animals or physical effects, but the focus stayed on nicotine.[122] One author maintained nicotine "hardens and dries out" the vessels—that is, causes sclerosis—and consequently stops blood from nourishing the extremities, and the "entire body starts to age." He observed, "smokers therefore age earlier, prematurely wear out, and without a doubt, shorten their lives."[123] Russian experimental biologists, biochemists, and others theorized that aging occurred when toxins built up in the body. If these toxins could be drained or lessened, they suggested that aging could be slowed.[124] One doctor cautioned worker youth that without proper relaxation, they "do not succeed in clearing all the poisons of the previous workday" and exhaustion set in.[125] Semashko denounced nicotine for leading to "exhaustion" when fresh air could "revive" the body.[126] In *Pravda* Semashko warned that youth wrung out by "alcoholism, smoking, early and incorrect sexual life" would not have the energy to contribute to a revolutionary new life.[127] Another author cautioned that while for most tobacco did not cause ill effects, with other "abnormalities of life of modern man" including abuse of alcohol, coffee, and tea, it "wears out the organism."[128] Another noted that only rest cured exhaustion and ideas that tobacco could were "delusion."[129]

Nicotine's effects on breathing, the heart, and digestion also merited attention.[130] Sazhin warned that smokers risked "heart attacks, interruptions in correct rhythm of the heart, sinking of the heart, a sense of anguish, fear, lack of air, and unbearable pain in the heart, radiating into the left arm and shoulder blade."[131] One 1919 author cited research on the heart disorders associated with smoking, which could result in pain radiating down the left arm and even into the fingers.[132] Nezlin recorded the onset of palpitations, weakness, irregular heartbeat, and *angina pectoris*.[133] Sazhin claimed that smoking wore out the heart, so that the heartbeat of a smoker at forty-three was the equivalent of a nonsmoker at fifty.[134]

These antismoking concerns tapped into a general anxiety about exhaustion, toxins, and nervous disease. Sazhin proposed that nicotine "above all and more strongly than anything, strikes the sympathetic nervous system," manifesting in weakened memory, unclear thoughts, and tremors.[135] The connections of tobacco to nervous problems came not just from Russian theorists.[136] One doctor referenced Richard von Krafft-Ebing when he argued: "Tobacco smoking often serves as the cause of nervous illness. It brings weakness of sight leading to blindness, nervous beating of the heart, neuralgia, and sexual weakness."[137] The Viennese psychiatrist Krafft-Ebing greatly influenced tsarist and Soviet hygienists in their contemplations of sexually transmitted diseases, homosexuality, and congenital diseases as well as nerve diseases, like neurasthenia and its connection to tobacco. They also relied on the psychiatry professor P. Kovalevskii, who observed that chronic nicotine poisoning might occasion "weakened attention to work, inadequate uptake, disquiet, fussiness, leaping from subject to subject, unclear ideas, and weakening of memory."[138]

Tobacco-induced nervous disorder could be observed in either heightened sensitivity or loss of sensitivity.[139] A 1920 pamphlet, aimed at the military, pointed out that smokers often experienced "tobacco blindness," loss of hearing or deafness, and even loss of speech, all of which indicated neurasthenic onset. The author proposed that chronic nicotine poisoning appeared as heightened sensitivity, so smokers should be seen as "sick 'obsessive' people."[140] A 1926 article in the journal *Meditsin* presented an anecdote in which a young woman smoked half a papirosa and lost visual perception. The author reported, "Many doctors notice in smokers also a lowering of the senses of touch, taste, and smell."[141] Others argued that smoking caused "amblyopia [reduction of sight in one eye] and the lowering of the senses of taste and olfaction."[142] A 1927 article proposed that color blindness came from smoking.[143] Tobacco's perceived ability to assuage another sense, hunger, had been a boon in time of famine but now showed smokers' declining sensory perceptions brought on by nervous disorder. Smokers suffered from loss of taste, dental decay, drying of the larynx, excess spittle, and stomach upset. They became "unable to desire nutritious, sweet, and tasty foods."[144] Unnourished, the body wearied and more easily "develops anemia, general weakness, thinness and as a result of these comes the dread disease—tuberculosis (consumption)." Yet if they followed the doctor's advice and quit, the smokers improved.[145]

The connection of the poison of nicotine, rise of smoking, and perceived epidemic of neurasthenia had broken onto the scene in the last decades before the revolution. Neurasthenia's flexible symptoms allowed for easy diagnosis of many patient complaints—from aches and pains to insomnia and gout. By 1880 over fifty symptoms could lead to a diagnosis of neurasthenia.[146] After 1917 anxieties about rapid industrialization, urbanization, and exhaustion alongside the stress, irritability, and weakness that plagued the party made neurasthenia an appealing culprit.[147] Several high-profile deaths and increased diagnoses of exhaustion spurred the Bolsheviks to perceive nervous diseases as devastating the party and see tobacco as a causal factor.[148] Physicians believed that most people had suffered a nervous disease, which might have precipitated hysteric or neurasthenic symptoms.[149] A popular theory connected neurasthenia to the buildup of toxins, which then caused auto-intoxication. This easily melded with the theory of smoking as slow poisoning.[150] The move from physical to office work; the use of alcohol, tea, and coffee; and the ready availability of lascivious entertainments joined in understandings of the causes of the neurasthenic epidemic.[151] In 1925 a book for the Sverdlovsk Department of Public Health connected mass neurasthenia among clerical workers to smoking.[152]

For the Soviets, from smoking to neurasthenia to madness was a slippery slope. One psychiatrist hypothesized a "strong tie between the contemporary development of neurasthenia and immoderate smoking," which he connected further to "psychasthenia [phobias, obsessions, and anxiety] and concluding with suicide."[153] Sazhin observed: "habitual smokers display an unstable unbalanced state of mind. Easy agitation, mood swings, irritability, confusion, in a word, all that which in medicine is called neurasthenia."[154] Another pamphlet reported the diagnosis of "nicotine psychosis," which had been used in Germany in the 1890s.[155] A doctor theorized that psychologically unhealthy people gravitated toward intoxicants as a means to shoulder "heavy burdens and sorrows," which provided "suitable soil" for nervous disorders because of their "psychopathological, hysterical, and psychologically ill constitutions."[156] Another doctor dismissed this question as unimportant: "Whether smoking is used for entertainment or to soothe the irritable brain, it is the same—a great evil."[157]

Anxieties over neurasthenia emerged during a period of hypermasculinization of culture, and tobacco was implicated in sapping the strength, vitality, and sexual potency of the Soviet male.[158] A 1927 article charged that "*papirosy* appear to simultaneously be the cause and outgrowth in the appearance of lack of masculinity."[159] Sazhin referenced the autopsies of animals that revealed gonads ravaged by nicotine.[160] Not just men were afflicted. Another pamphlet cited the experiments of a German doctor who placed nicotine under the skin of different animals, creating sterile females and changes in the gonads of males.[161] Other doctors cited studies of chickens and rabbits that showed decreased fertility with nicotine, using French and British research into the lower birth rates and higher infant mortality among female tobacco workers.[162] Another charged that women were more sensitive to nicotine than men because of "the cycles of women's sexual life."[163] One doctor diagnosed male sexual weakness from smoking and female infertility and miscarriage from handling tobacco or living with a smoker.[164] Like others he documented the nicotine that then traveled into breast milk, poisoning nursing infants and causing seizures, illness, and death. Sazhin cited a statistic gathered from Leningrad that of one hundred children born to tobacco factory women, fifty-five died in the first year of life.[165] Vasilevskii condemned women's smoking just as he did women's handling of tobacco, claiming that weak women were more susceptible and nicotine-laden breast milk killed infants; he warned that young women jeopardized their status as "future mothers" when they smoked.[166]

Medical experts before the revolution had worried that nervous disorders might pass from parents to children, and Soviet authorities cautioned of smoking's generational danger.[167] One warned that smoking by the parents produced epilepsy in children.[168] Another maintained that smoking parents inspired children and the tendency toward smoking might be passed on, because "a large role, actually, is played by heredity, and a tendency to poisoning with narcotic items is often passed on to the next generation . . . Smoking by parents prepares their children to take up the exact same habit."[169] Articles documented the large numbers of smoking orphans who moved from smoking to drugs, delinquency, and criminality.[170] A *Pravda* article on rehabilitation programs for street kids used the common trope that the first step on the road to criminality was stealing papirosy.[171] Authorities tried to get smoking out of schools because it was considered detrimental to physical and social development.[172] The child's body and character were not yet hardened and more susceptible to toxins. As Nezlin cautioned, "Nicotine slightly poisons their brains, and they become lazy to science."[173] Sazhin and others commented on how smoking children made for poor students.[174] Using American studies of smoking's influence on memory, behavior, and development, including research published in 1923 supposedly using seventy thousand schoolchildren, another argued that smoking youth were more prone to nervousness, weak will, and laziness, in addition to being less robust physically.[175] A study of worker youth in Leningrad determined that smoking increased sickness by 5.4 percent and that tuberculosis, in particular, was 58 percent higher among smoking worker youth than nonsmokers.[176] The author concluded: "The majority of older smokers, like the humpback whale, just send to the grave. But to the young, we must pay attention."[177]

Encouraged by Lenin, spurred by mass smoking, and supported by a new public health system, Semashko tried to take on tobacco. Although he failed in his biggest policy aim, stamping out tobacco production and trade, he did include cessation in his campaign to instill new behavioral norms and create a healthier society. It was an uphill battle complicated by the horrible effects of war, revolution, civil war, and economic collapse but aided by the resources of a new agency dedicated to prophylactic care, the elimination of social diseases, and the popularizing of healthful lifestyles. Narkomzdrav pushed cessation through a massive, inventive propaganda campaign exploiting innovative media and reverberating through a variety of novel Soviet institutions devoted to creating a new Soviet man, woman, and child.

The first national state-backed antismoking campaign spoke in the language of Bolshevism. Propaganda attacked smoking with a socialist, collectivist agenda by spreading the message that tobacco was a great social evil with political, economic, cultural, and generational harms. Tobacco's costs in terms of lost productivity and misdirected resources figured heavily in propaganda focused on the Soviet concern for the collective. Even in the personal effects of smoking, the emphasis was on poisonous nicotine as a trigger to neurasthenic decline, and although neurasthenia certainly had individual effects, it was seen as a society-wide danger, sapping the vigor of the revolutionary state as part of a larger set of social concerns over male vigor and female fertility. Social costs also loomed large. Although Semashko had pushed for an even broader attack, his propaganda campaign was unlike anything else in the world and revolutionary in its national scope, institutional support, and collectivist message.

RESURRECTED

Nationalized Factories and Revitalized Industry

In 1857 V. I. Asmolov opened a tobacco workshop in Rostov-on-Don with just three thousand rubles and seven workers. By 1880 he had the largest makhorka factory in the country, and in 1913 the three thousand Asmolov workers produced some twenty-six billion papirosy. Lenin cited Asmolov as an example, in his 1899 *Development of Capitalism in Russia*, of the phenomenal growth of Russian industry.[1] But by 1920 war, revolution, and civil war had devastated production. As the factory history recalled, "retreating, the white guard destroyed the factory . . . reserve material . . . [and] equipment. The building was ruined."[2] Trod under foot, unsown, or unharvested in the chaos, leaf harvests declined. All work took place by hand and workers had to walk to work, sometimes traversing several kilometers a day, because transport was overburdened. In 1920, the factory produced only 40 percent of its prewar levels.[3]

Beyond tobacco, the entire economy suffered. Faced with decreasing agricultural yields exacerbated by civil war and drought in 1920–1921, the virtual standstill in industry, and the mass depopulation of the cities, Lenin chose to change course, replacing the policies of War Communism with the New Economic Policy (NEP) in March 1921.[4] The policy developed from the recognition that the Soviets would not be aided by a worldwide revolution. Faced with the prospect of going it alone, Lenin decided to retreat, regroup, and rebuild with the aid of capitalist markets. NEP ended grain requisitioning, introducing a tax in kind, and allowed the revival of private trade yet kept the "commanding heights" under state control.[5]

Nestled in the commanding heights was tobacco. Even as NEP allowed a rein-troduction of small-scale capitalist development in the hopes of bringing indus-trial and agricultural production back up to prewar levels, the nationalization of factories and revitalization of agriculture sparked a recovery for tobacco.[6] At the now state-owned and newly renamed Don State Tobacco Factory (hereafter DGTF, né Asmolov) the policies meant a crackdown on labor deserters, inten-sification of output, and rising individual productivity. Reconstruction began in 1922 and proceeded slowly with the popular, if "modestly" packaged, *Nasha marka* (Our Brand) papirosy, along with *Shury-mury* (Sweet Nothings), *Ekh, otdai vse!* (Oh, Give It All Away!), *Grivenniki* (Ol' Ten Kopeck) and others. The factory returned to near prewar levels by 1926 and in 1927, with 4,572 workers, surpassed them.[7]

DGTF also served as a base for worker integration into the new state. The pre-revolutionary tobacco industry had been notorious for its harsh conditions and its vociferous, largely female, workforce. As DGTF rebuilt machinery, it recon-figured labor relations. Factory representatives went to Moscow to study, to hear Lenin, and to return to inspire their fellows. The factory Komsomol organized help for orphans, agitated for work discipline, engaged in antireligious activi-ties, and served as a conduit for new party members. Literacy and other eve-ning classes helped workers advance and a choir, string orchestra, drama circle, and workers' club with an eleven-thousand-volume library enriched off hours. Inspiration was important because tobacco's revival did not come as a result of massive capital investment or widespread mechanization but through the labor of a largely female workforce, little changed from before the revolution and little aided by improved machinery. Tobacco workers were some of the most radical groups before the revolution and continued to be vocal critics of policies after it. Stabilizing their jobs meant calming their anger. Health facilities, a night sanato-rium for lung patients, a general sanatorium and a house of leisure for vacations all provided benefits to counter disgruntled attitudes and hazardous conditions.[8]

Investment in the tobacco industry did not just secure employment for thou-sands of volatile female workers. Producing tobacco satisfied a "durable" demand and secured needed revenue. Government moves to stabilize tobacco catered to a large, and at times angry, market of smokers, many of whom were in the military or government and settled in urban centers of power. Tobacco excise taxes, a holdover of the tsarist government, contributed to the bottom line. Espe-cially from 1914 to 1925, when alcohol prohibition held the "drunken budget" in check, tobacco taxes provided an important alternative revenue stream. As a 1928 anti-tobacco pamphlet concluded, "We cannot at present forbid [tobacco] production, as it is important to the national economy. Only with the further strengthening of our socialist economy can we move . . . to that period when production will be only one of those things needed for the support of people. Then the tobacco business will fall as will the use of tobacco."[9] The argument, even from industry, remained that once society was fixed, then tobacco use would automatically decline. It was not simply a choice of economic health over public health. Many in public health similarly believed that economic stability would decrease tobacco use. It was, however, a capitulation on an all-out assault on tobacco. Just as Lenin had chosen NEP over continued revolution, so did revitalizing industry, and placating workers and users, win over a revolutionary path in cessation.

Tobacco Production and Revolutionary Change

Tobacco came to Russia during the seventeenth century under Tsar Alexei Mikhailovich. He promptly banned it, meting out notoriously brutal punishments—slitting of nostrils and beating with the knout.[10] Peter the Great overturned the ban in pursuit of profit, and by the nineteenth century Russia had established its own tobacco agricultural traditions and a growing group of small workshops that turned leaf into snuff, cigars, loose tobacco, and papirosy.[11] From 1861 to 1900 newer, larger firms consolidated control, and the production of papirosy increased by almost thirty times, from 0.3 billion to 8.6 billion items, and the proportion of tobacco as papirosy more than doubled.[12] Output rose without raising product costs largely because of the increased use of lower-paid female and child labor rather than mechanization. From 1890 to 1914, in just twenty-four years, papirosy production increased by over seven and a half times as the average production per factory rose by 350 percent and the number of workers per factory rose by almost 40 percent.[13]

Foreigners hailed Russia as Europe's largest producer of tobacco.[14] From 1890 to 1904 exports of papirosy—to the southern border (Persia), the east (Mongolia and China), and the west (Germany and Finland especially)—increased by 1,100 percent.[15] St. Petersburg housed most tobacco production in the empire (81.5 percent), and Moscow stood in second place (17.3 percent).[16] Materials for the factories of Moscow and St. Petersburg—the paper, the cardboard, and the flavorings—came from across the empire, but the areas associated with quality leaf production were the Caucasus, Crimea, and along the Don. Makhorka production rose most precipitously in the years before 1914 dominating local consumption and an increasing portion of factory-prepared tobacco.[17]

The war and civil war decimated tobacco growing areas. The author Isaac Babel bitterly condemned the Mensheviks for nearly destroying the incomparable tobacco crops of Abkhaziia, but everywhere leaf production was down.[18] A 1918 piece in *Pravda* warned that without "heroic measures" all factories would stop production within four months.[19] The state nationalized tobacco raw materials, but this did not stop factory closures.[20] The industry analyst S. Narkir'er detailed the dire situation in a set of charts in 1921 (Table 1).

By 1921 the "catastrophic" decline in harvests in Southeast Russia made tobacco "a valuable source for trade with the countryside, where demand for tobacco is strong."[21] A report in *Rabotnitsa* attributed the problem to the fact that "the hottest events of [the civil war] occurred in the raw material growing areas—Crimea, Kuban, and Sukhumi."[22] The 1921 makhorka harvest was at 20.8 percent of the 1914 yield, and output in other tobaccos was at 42.4 percent of 1914 (Table 2).

As Narkir'er concluded, "The decline of seeding was such that if compared to the prewar levels, then by the end of 1921 we may say that there was almost no tobacco farming."[23] The *Rabotnitsa* report claimed the resurrection of production "rests entirely on the restoration of the raw material base."[24]

Despite shortages, production continued because factories had stores of leaf, which had been curing for sometimes two or three years. A bumper crop in 1917 for Kuban, Crimea, and the Caucasus aided in the buildup.[25] Additionally, because exports collapsed with the war, more leaf stayed in the country. In 1918 *Izvestiia* reported that the industry was working with materials from 1916, 1917, and even 1915 and was kept going only by the careful planning of the workers

TABLE 1. Percentage declines in tobacco products, 1913–1919

PRODUCT	1913	1914	1915	1916	1917	1918	1919
Tobacco	100.0	87.3	79.5	94.4	82.6	61.3	41.1
Makhorka	100.0	110.6	124.3	115.9	99.4	74.6	37.2
Cartridges	100.0	106.6	101.2	105.0	99.0	40.3	31.0

Source: S. Narkir'er, *Proizvodstvo tabachnykh fabrik RSFSR v 1919 godu (v tsifrakh): Po materialam Statisticheskogo otdela Glavnogo pravleniia gosudarstvennoi tabachnoi promyshlennosti* (Moscow: Vysshii sovet narodnogo khoziaistva, 1921).

TABLE 2. Tobacco and makhorka production, 1914–1921

	1914	1917	1918	1919	1920	1921
Loose tobacco and/or papirosy equivalent in billions	21.94	20.02	14.37	8.26	9.30	12.80
Makhorka in 1,000 kg (tonne)	57,560	54,973	25,650	16,953	11,981	7,059

Source: S. Narkir'er, "Tabachnaia promyshlennost' i snabzhenie naseleniia tabachnymi izdeliami v gody revoliutsii," *Vestnik tabachnoi promyshlennosti*, no. 1 (1922): 19–30.

themselves.[26] Stored tobacco made all the difference, as "these resources saved the tobacco industry from collapse."[27] Even when materials could be found, personnel shortages, particularly of specialists, led to problems.[28] Other issues troubled the industry. The Balkan Star Factory of Iaroslavl struggled with distribution because of the overburdened rail system and the loss of skilled workers to the front. A *Pravda* article of November 1918 mourned the closure of several Moscow factories, including those of Gabai and Dukat, because they had no heating or electricity.[29] At times, higher state organs manipulated distribution to help certain factories maintain production. A report from April 1918 in *Pravda* mentioned Soviet requisitioning of one hundred wagons of raw materials to aid the production of factory shops.[30] Shortages of wood for cases and rolling papers caused some factories to move to production of simple crumbled tobacco for smoking in pipes or with papers.[31] By the 1920s papirosy exceeded 80 percent of worked tobacco in Russia, but large amounts of production had moved to loose tobacco.[32] A 1921 set of draft provisions for factories made clear that without a quick restart of agriculture by "next fall the makhorka factories will truly start limiting work as a result of raw material shortages and the makhorka users of the northern districts, where it is almost impossible to grow it, will begin to smoke any kind of surrogates."[33] Against a general reduction in all industry to just 15.9 percent of prewar levels by 1920, the decline of tobacco production to just 46.1 percent appeared comparatively healthy.[34] Industry downtimes meant difficulties for workers as lack of materials closed factories. Narkir'er reported that in 1919 the number of workdays per tobacco factory had decreased to just 259, and at makhorka factories it was still worse.[35] As late as 1924, the Balkan Star Factory maintained five months of downtime because it lacked raw materials to sustain continued production.[36]

Despite troubles, the market remained strong.[37] A 1918 *Pravda* article estimated that 600,000 Muscovites smoked, and of these 360,000 chose prepared papirosy in a population between 1.3 and 1.7 million.[38] The industry analyst S. Egiz proposed: "In the absence of statistics, simple universal observation boils down to the opinion that the Soviet Russian population smokes more than the prerevolutionary . . . tobacco endures, and demand continues—and growth too."[39] In this "enduring" demand, Egiz indicated makhorka's preeminence.[40] Urban markets found more ready-made papirosy in either loose or pack forms, but rural inhabitants grew their own makhorka that they dried, chopped, and smoked self-rolled or in pipes without ever reporting it for statistics.[41] This resembled the market system of prerevolutionary Russia, where untaxed use remained invisible and resembled the situation in contemporary China, where urban and rural smokers consumed differently because of access to factory-produced cigarettes and the money to buy them.[42]

From 1910 to 1920 official makhorka production grew by 48 percent as the smoking population increased by two or three times.[43] Narkir'er attributed this to a variety of factors:

> The demand for tobacco in the war years was very big. On one side was the stopping of vodka sales and the need to fill the void with some other narcotic. On the other there was a mass of users—the army. A whole line of circumstances connected to war such as the nervous intensity of warriors, the large amount of free time during the endless sitting in one place, sitting in a trench, waiting, etc., endlessly widened the circle of smokers in the army. People who before had never smoked began to smoke. Tobacco became for them an indispensable item, and when it was not available there were sharp complaints. As a result, the commissariat included tobacco in the items of their procurement and supply of the army.[44]

The war years provided many lessons on how maintaining tobacco helped preserve order. British and French soldiers rioted over tobacco shortages.[45] In Russia, shortages created volatile circumstances. In Viatka in 1914, six thousand local peasant conscripts rioted against the draft, demanded vodka, and grumbled over rising tobacco and grain prices.[46] In the 1917 zemstvo elections in Viatka, Peasant Union groups purportedly tried to buy votes with tobacco.[47] In the aftermath of the civil war, Polish forces printed propaganda rolling papers under a cover that suggested Red Army soldiers read the slogans as they smoked.[48] The papers inside offered different anti-Bolshevik, antisemitic, or antiwar invective (Figure 2.1). If soldiers had no tobacco to roll into these propaganda papers, the medium and message likely had even greater ability to foster discontent.

Military men, early adopters of smoking in Russia, readily turned to tobacco when denied alcohol, but the war disrupted supplies.[49] According to Narkir'er, if it was assumed that about a quarter of the population smoked, then each smoker consumed about eight *funt* a year in 1913 (about three and half kilograms). By 1918 this amount was six, and by 1921 it had been reduced to two. He did not blame falling demand.[50] Narkirer's math assumed even distribution, but the mass of tobacco went to the military; in 1920 this sum was nearly 30 percent of worked tobacco and 80 percent of makhorka. The remainder of each type was distributed to preferred workers in transport and government officials.[51] To meet popular demand, cultivation of makhorka on private plots rose, and one author concluded that this fully made up for industrial deficits.[52]

Rationing policies and skyrocketing prices told a different story.[53] According to a 1918 report, the monthly ration for smokers was 275 papirosy (about half

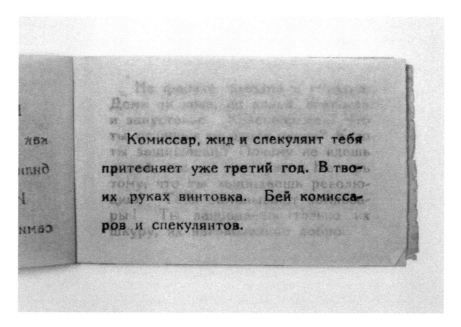

FIGURE 2.1.   Photo. Anti-Soviet cigarette papers book, interior, "The commissar, Jew, and speculator have oppressed you already three years. You have a rifle in your hand. Kill the commissars and speculators." Zosa Szajkowski Collection, Box 1, Folder "Fliers and Open Letters," Bakhmeteff Archive of Russian and East European Culture, Rare Book and Manuscript Library, Columbia University Libraries.

a pack a day) and 3 boxes of matches.[54] In 1919 *Pravda* outlined the decree of the Sovnarkom for tobacco rations—250 smokes for workers and white-collar employees and 100 for other citizens. In makhorka it was a quarter *funt* for agricultural workers and one and a quarter *funt* for soldiers. According to the article these amounts were based on "real" supplies and not "fantasies." Seventy percent of the supply went to workers.[55] Articles kept track of where to find tobacco throughout 1920.[56] Even when found, tobacco might be too expensive. Makhorka jumped fifteenfold in price between 1914 and 1920, from 50 to 750 rubles per *funt*. Makhorka costs rose more precipitously than the prices for beef, chicken, milk, butter, and kerosene.[57] As late as 1924 the government continued artificial prices, trying to bring the market in line.[58]

Smokers dipped into a shadow market of illegal or unlicensed sales.[59] In 1918 *Izvestiia* reported a speculator who had taken thirty thousand papirosy from the Gabai Factory and tried to sell them for profit.[60] "Bagging," usually associated with grain but also common with tobacco, arose in response. Baggers traveled to an area (or factory), purchased tobacco, hauled it to the city, and sold it. Makhorka baggers working out of the regions of Tambov, Riazan, and the Volga Germans. They transported 150-pound sacks of makhorka to sell in smaller quantities. State authorities tried to clamp down, claiming that bagging evaded official channels and clogged transport, but for tobacco producers baggers proved a more reliable buyer, and in some regions baggers were primary distributors.[61]

Strong demand and uneven production meant stress on sales. In 1918 retail outlets for tobacco were brought under municipal control, as were other retail stores. This change was partially in response to the rise in speculation and non-traditional sales.[62] Goods were on the shelves, but since few had discretionary income, it was usually the cheapest goods that were in shortest supply and subject to massive inflation. More expensive goods were found in abundance, and state and party officials received tobacco allocations, which the nonsmoker could trade or sell for other goods.[63] Some industrious sellers took to the streets as profiteers, unloading old papirosy that had been made before the revolution or homegrown, home-cured makhorka. Invalids from the war who had saved their tobacco rations could turn a profit.[64] According to observers, the lines of people waiting for tobacco, usually filled with soldiers, had a happy mood as most were expecting they could resell the tobacco later.[65] Tobacco made it onto the exchange market in other ways. During the civil war, employers offered payment in kind, especially in the textile, footwear, and tobacco industries. Reselling was illegal, but workers paid in galoshes had no other options.[66] Tobacco workers and those on vouchers faced similar choices. A cartoon and short satirical piece in *Krokodil* in 1924 showed a nursing mother at the cooperative with her state-supplied vouchers, finding nothing but candy and papirosy. The mother quipped that her baby was a "nonsmoker." *Krokodil* recommended that the authorities provide money rather than vouchers to avoid making people take goods that they would then only have to pass on.[67]

During the revolution, war, and civil war, markets collapsed as unemployment increased, the currency proved unstable, and shortages left no goods. Many fled the cities searching for food and work.[68] Overall, from 1913 to 1924 gross national income fell by 60 percent.[69] Tobacco factories made do or stretched what they had, and it would seem that many smokers grew their own. For those who had only recently left the peasantry or returned to the village, learning to work their own smoking tobacco would have been attractive and conceivable. An article in *Kooperativnoe delo* from 1922 described in detail how to make homegrown silver makhorka "smokable" from harvest to drying with simple instructions: heap the leaves under straw until they heated up from fermentation, and when two-thirds had turned golden dry, ferment again and its ready for use.[70]

State Intervention and Tobacco Taxes

To manage the troubled tobacco industry, the Bolsheviks nationalized all 136 tobacco factories on January 31, 1919, then consolidated them. Prerevolutionary owners became "exploiters" subject to removal or incarceration.[71] Members of the Dunaev family, who owned Balkan Star, ended up in the secret police camps; others fled; and the remainder took up work at a hotel in Tsargrad, which later became a House of Soviets.[72] Factories in the worst shape were closed. Whereas in 1905 there had been 144 factories, by 1914 this number diminished to 94, in 1919 to 30, by 1924 to 28 and by 1928 to 26.[73] The number of factories declined by 29 percent, with makhorka factories falling by 64 percent.[74] Some middle-size factories and workshops made it into the hands of private actors as the state experimented with renting factories.[75] The rest were consolidated into large "trusts" structured by region (Petrograd, Moscow, Ukraine, Crimea, Rostov-on-Don) and encompassing 85.5 percent of production by 1921.[76]

When the factories were organized into trusts, machinery went too. Unions and committees formed at factories to assess damages.[77] Of two thousand papirosy machines, eighteen hundred remained in the trusts, and many were seriously rundown.[78] *Izvestiia* reported in 1921 that at Dukat only 70 of 128 machines worked.[79] A worker at the Iava Factory in 1925 reported that there were still no conveyers or forklifts and everything had to be hauled with manpower.[80] Fewer factories meant fewer technicians could service more machines—an important consideration, since a massive brain drain of around two million emigrations between 1917 and 1921 had wiped out technical experts.[81] Of the sixteen thousand workers in the tobacco industry, thirteen thousand were under state trust control. The remaining three thousand were split evenly between midsized factories and small workshops. Together these factories, workers, and machines produced about half the amount of tobacco products of 1913.[82]

About the time that Semashko pulled the decree from Sovnarkom, production began to revive. A worker from Kharkov recalled that the introduction of a diesel machine in late December 1920 "saved" the factory. The mechanization of the most dangerous tasks in 1924 and the introduction of nine cartridge machines in 1925 allowed for growth of production and improvement in workers' lifestyles.[83] According to a 1923 expose in *Rabotnitsa*, it was often tobacco factories with poorer ventilation or other worker safety concerns that were phased out in favor of more hygienic facilities.[84] Despite the obstacles, starting in 1926 and ramping up in 1927 and into the 1930s, industry innovated. Iava experimented with new styles of papirosy, such as batting in the mouthpiece to "trap" nicotine.[85] A report in *Pravda* boasted of machines that produced 120,000 papirosy per day and were like those seen "only in England and America."[86] In 1927 *Pravda* announced a new research institute, which would work with tobacco chemistry and agronomy; the Krasnodar tobacco fermentation factory was the first in the world.[87]

Tobacco remained sought after, and inflated prices continued.[88] According to one 1926 observer, the only thing stopping increased use was output. He emphasized that "production will find solid and secure internal consumer demand."[89] To meet the problem of black-market sales and speculation, the state established new price regulations for "essential" consumer goods including salt, sugar, kerosene, and tobacco.[90] Surveys indicated growing supplies of tobacco were met by growing hunger. Higher consumption meant greater potential tax revenue and was a lesson for the Soviets from the tsars. The excise tax on tobacco began in 1838 as an assessment at the point of manufacture for the right to prepare and sell tobacco.[91] Personal use remained untaxed by the tsarist regime, and a weak inspectorate allowed for much tobacco to sneak out.[92] Still, from 1839 to 1899 the taxed amount rose by fifty times.[93] In 1889 excise taxes from tobacco generated twenty million rubles, and by 1906 they were nearly sixty million (59,903,000 rubles).[94] Tobacco taxes generated 92.8 million rubles in 1914, 114.2 million in 1915, and 169.6 million in 1916.[95] Tobacco excise taxes profited the tsars, if not as much as the alcohol tax. In 1895 vodka produced 230 million rubles for the state and in 1904, 576 million.[96] Prohibition dropped this to only 30.7 million rubles in 1915.[97] Bereft of the substantial alcohol excise tax, the tsar looked toward tobacco, especially low-grade but high-use makhorka, to fill the gap. Tapping tobacco taxes to prop up the state did not change immediately in 1917.[98] As *Izvestiia* put it in 1918, "The tobacco industry is not just a part of the state economic organization but also a direct source of income for the state treasury."[99] For the Soviets, tobacco served as a monopoly.[100]

Semashko opposed alcohol just as he had tobacco, but because prohibition temporarily removed the problem from his shoulders, it was not until 1922 that he came forward forcibly on the issue. In a 1922 commentary for *Izvestiia* Semashko argued that fiscal issues could not trump those of popular health, and as with the 1920 tobacco fight, he lost.[101] With prohibition overturned, alcohol proved especially profitable so that by 1927–1928, almost half of the state-collected excise taxes came from sales of spirits. This amounted to 12 percent of all state revenues.[102] Tobacco's tax revenue rose steadily through the 1920s (Table 3).[103]

Soviet analysts saw "passionate smokers" as reliable buyers who would "deprive themselves of the most essential items of use in order to smoke," but they noted that when confronted with rising prices, smokers would not reduce their smoking. Instead they would "transfer to cheaper sorts," showing that they were flexible on quality.[104] Many turned to homegrown or other alternatives. Faced with

TABLE 3.   Soviet excise receipts in million rubles, 1922–1928

PRODUCT	1922–23	1923–24	1924–25	1925–26	1926–27	1927–28
Wine/beer/alcohol	18.7	65.0	178.6	364.2	585.0	697.0
Sugar	22.4	51.6	117.8	177.5	244.7	245.0
Tea and coffee	4.8	13.9	22.0	22.7	31.5	29.5
Matches	5.0	9.4	15.3	21.1	21.0	25.0
Tobacco products	18.4	37.4	82.0	123.9	153.6	166.7
Cigarette tubes/papers	0.6	1.4	1.4	1.3	1.5	0.8
Perfume/toiletries	–	–	–	–	–	8.0
Salt	14.3	15.4	15.9	17.6	10.0	3.0
Petroleum products	10.8	17.8	24.1	33.6	35.7	41.0
Candles	0.5	0.8	1.5	1.8	2.6	2.6
Textiles	7.3	26.5	46.1	72.2	100.2	109.0
Rubber footwear	0.2	1.6	3.1	5.6	16.1	23.0
TOTAL	103.0	240.8	507.8	841.5	1201.9	1350.6

Source: Gregory Y. Sokolnikov, *Soviet Policy in Public Finance, 1917–1928* (Stanford, CA: Stanford University Press, 1931), 189.

TABLE 4.   Exports in million kilograms, 1922–1929

YEAR	EXPORTS IN MILLION KG	YEAR	EXPORTS IN MILLION KG	YEAR	EXPORTS IN MILLION KG	YEAR	EXPORTS IN MILLION KG
1922	3.4	1924	2.2	1925/26	0.5	1927/28	4.3
1923	2.0	1924/25	1.1	1926/27	3.3	1928/29*	6.3

*for only 1–3 quarters
Source: Evsei Kogan, "Sovetskii eksport listovogo tabaka," in *Sbornik materialov po tabachnoi promyshlennosti,* ed. A. A. Rozhnov (Moscow: Gosudarstvennoe tekhnicheskoe izdatel'stvo, 1930), 303.

shortages, domestic smokers had tried Virginia-style tobacco to fill the gap, but once supply recovered, they returned to oriental tobaccos over "the peculiar taste of Virginia."[105]

The Soviets looked to generate revenue from tobacco exports. One 1923 article lamented that the state was so focused on growth that it allowed former owners to do as they would and skimmed off the best tobacco to be exported abroad.[106] Another author obsessed about not exploiting exports well enough.[107] By the late 1920s things had stabilized and exports rose (Table 4). This increase came despite supply problems.

Demanding taxes did not mean being able to collect. As with alcohol, tobacco floated through the black market. According to data from 1924, illegal tobacco stood at the same level as excise-taxed tobacco.[108] Stories of counterfeit tobacco, black-market sales, or illicit trade continued even after supply rebounded.[109] Baggers, speculators, and black marketeers joined in with the many other tobacco sellers of the city. As one contemporary described it, tobacco products were everywhere and consumed by everyone: "There were hundreds and thousands of them, these street sellers of papirosy—nimble roguish boys, legless invalids, old men in general's overcoats, and sad women. And there were a hundred tobacco stores—from the elegant tobacco trusts to squalid little shops."[110] A foreign observer, Alexander Wicksteed, noticed the prevalence of tobacco sellers in Moscow in 1923 and mused: "Considering the enormous number of these cigarette sellers it is very difficult to believe that there is a decent living in it; you cannot walk fifty yards along any of the main streets without passing one."[111]

Street sellers typically fell into the vulnerable groups trampled in the NEP-era economy: women who were unemployed by either efficiency campaigns or the return of men to the workforce, and street kids who were orphaned or abandoned in the aftermath of war and revolution. These groups lived on the uneasy boundary of selling on the streets or selling themselves, as the scenario of the popular 1920s silent film *The Cigarette Girl of Mosselprom* intimated. Crowds of women could be found peddling in busier areas of the city. Both the poet Vladimir Maiakovskii and the constructivist artist Aleksander Rodchenko memorialized the female street sellers. A photograph by Rodchenko of a woman sitting next to her case of tobacco products hints at the ubiquity of street sellers and their precarity; within a minute the street seller could close up her case, collapse the stand, and move on to another spot (Figure 2.2).

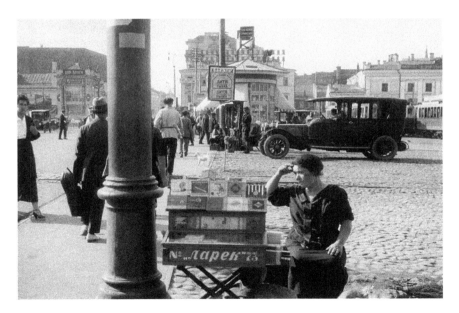

FIGURE 2.2.   Photo. Aleksandr Rodchenko, "Street Seller, 1920s," Courtesy Russian State Library.

Other shortages troubled smokers, including the deficit in quality rolling papers.[112] Smokers took to using any materials at hand, including propaganda leaflets, pamphlets, and posters.[113] Wicksteed observed: "when I first knew Russia it was the usual custom to use newspaper. I have often been told that the great popularity of the Bolshevik propaganda in the Kerensky ranks was chiefly due to this habit of making cigarettes out of any and every kind of paper that they could lay their hands on."[114] A functionary of the Central Committee's agitation-propaganda section bemoaned the tendency to sacrifice newspapers to a smoke.[115] Supposedly concerned that the peasants would burn up his October Decree on Land, Lenin sent out old calendars at the same time, hoping that the villagers would smoke those before the official government document, and in a *Pravda* article of 1921 Lenin complained of newspapers "wasted as rolling paper."[116] Cartoons in *Krokodil* lampooned propaganda going up in smoke as late as 1924. One cartoon—"Good Uses for Books"—sketches people using pages for toilet paper, starting a fire, wrapping a fish, or rolling smokes.[117] Another cartoon offers "Four Views of the Alliance with the Countryside" where an urban official romances a peasant maid, a peasant drinks vodka from the city, and another rolls up newspapers for smokes. Only the fourth panel offers the officially sanctioned friendship—an urbanite carrying books to a smiling, enthusiastic peasant.[118] The destruction of newspapers for tobacco rolling continued as *Krokodil* mocked another paper as only able to "shine" when lit up to wrap tobacco.[119] Another 1924 *Krokodil* piece told of a factory worker who was a "lit' smoker" because he smoked down the entire factory literary library before opening one of the books.[120]

As the 1920s progressed, state shops and cooperatives got a better handle on the market reflecting the gradual strengthening of industry. By 1925/26 the raw material base had nearly rebounded. Moscow and Rostov-on-Don firms began to appear in Leningrad, and by 1925 the old Laferm Factory, now named for Uritskii, was approaching prewar production levels.[121] Makhorka achieved prerevolutionary production levels in 1926, and tobacco products reached this milestone in 1928.[122] It was a national revival (Table 5). Larger percentages of tobacco now went into papirosy, a change from 46.3 percent in 1913 to 94.4 percent by 1927/28, and the public increasingly chose papirosy.[123]

Scarcity defined the Soviet tobacco experience as much as product differentiation and surplus characterized the British and American markets. Supply of loose tobacco and factory-made papirosy was up. Smokes increased, but the tobacco inside—probably makhorka enhanced by the taste of the smoldering newspaper, book page, propaganda poster, or leaflet—was probably difficult to inhale, though people still did. The different paper qualities—from brittle-thin, cellulose office papers to wood-pulp-enhanced book pages or thick, ink-heavy

TABLE 5. Tobacco production figures, 1913–1927/28

YEAR	SMOKING TOBACCO IN TONS (1 TON = 1,000KG)	PAPIROSY IN MILLION PIECES	ALL TOBACCO AND PAPIROSY	MAKHOHRKA IN TONS
1913	10,475	22,055	47,634	78,676
1914	10,803	25,725	52,106	84,654
1915	9,300	31,112	53,821	73,304
1916	12,744	29,346	60,465	82,330
1917	8,885	22,009	43,704	81,564
1918	6,917	12,703	29,593	28,468
1919	4,798	10,249	21,965	18,722
1920	7,525	4,850	23,225	21,384
1922/23	888	10,791	12,959	19,546
1923/24	530	12,994	14,226	30,599
1924/25	411	26,285	27,290	46,506
1925/26	782	37,284	39,161	81,458
1926/27	1,149	40,737	43,543	82,486
1927/28	1,186	48,990	51,885	83,815

Source: Bokarev, "Tobacco Production in Russia," 151–53; L. B. Kafengauz, *Evoliutsiia promyshlennogo proizvodstva Rossii (posledniaia tret' XIX v.–30-e gody XX v.)* (Moscow: Epifaniia, 1994), 156, 198, 240.

propaganda posters and leaflets—would have changed the burn, flavor, smell, and inhalation. Other quality issues resulted from uneven manufacture, storage, or transport. In 1919 government authorities investigated "moldy papirosy."[124] A 1924 *Krokodil* article reported that the leaf sent to the Eletz Factory included substantial quantities of dirt. *Krokodil* stepped in and contacted the syndicate for an explanation.[125] In 1926 an *Izvestiia* reporter complained: "the quality of contemporary papirosy and makhorka is markedly worse than before the war . . . Before anything you sense the smell . . . The burning in the mouth will irritate the mucous linings."[126] An error in packaging, where the low-quality smokes of one factory appeared in boxes for their higher-priced brand led to an investigation by Trotsky.[127] Other press reports decried the miscommunications from factories that resulted in a "Papirosy Graveyard" in Ukraine or the loss of six thousand papirosy a day from poor transport practices.[128]

Revolutionized Factories and Communist Lives

Although the story of the cigarette industry in the US centered on "Buck" Duke and his vertical integration, marketing innovation, corporate power, and factory mechanization, the industry's growth in Russia and the Soviet Union followed a different path. Prewar trusts and postrevolutionary state control streamlined procurement and production. Output expanded while workforce numbers did not increase or even declined, bringing down the cost per unit and allowing for the use of Soviet-made, rather than imported, parts for machines, which brought down costs. The standardization of the width and length of papirosy supposedly saved three million rubles.[129] Mechanization was limited or late in coming. At DGTF many packing and packaging machines from before the revolution made it through the 1920s, but by 1928 they could no longer be repaired and patched, so that they were "put out to pasture."[130] At the Balkan Star Factory, a successful smokestack reconstruction salvaged production.[131] Only in 1927 would the Iava Factory get the first mechanical carton machine, with specialists coming from Leningrad and Baku to help train workers.[132]

Because of prerevolutionary labor markets and postrevolutionary efficiency pressures and machine deficits, the industry remained largely low-paid handwork with an overwhelmingly female workforce.[133] Before 1917 employers believed that females would be more pliant, but women in the tobacco industry proved remarkably volatile, striking regularly from the 1870s onward and becoming a target for revolutionary organizers from all sides, although few would affiliate with the Bolsheviks.[134]

The postrevolutionary labor force, like the machinery, held a striking resemblance to the prerevolutionary group, although as the number of factories decreased, so did the number of workers (Table 6).

On average, from 1890 to 1905 tobacco factories employed thirty-six thousand workers, 70 percent of whom were women and children.[135] By 1914, 31 percent of the general labor force was female. The textile trades employed the largest number of female workers, yet the percentage of female workers in textiles was much smaller than in tobacco.[136] In 1921, 70 percent of the tobacco workforce remained female, but the percentage of youth did drop to below 1 percent.[137] The exploitation of women and children within the tobacco factory system had been notorious in the prerevolutionary period and inspired literary treatments, labor diatribes, and moral appeals. This strong presence of women in tobacco organizing continued after the revolution. In 1919 the Union of Tobacco, Cartridge, and

TABLE 6.   Workers employed in tobacco industry, 1885–1927

YEAR	NUMBER OF WORKERS	YEAR	NUMBER OF WORKERS
1885	31,000	1912	32,820
1899	38,590	1920	38,192
1904	35,108	1927	26,443

Source: "Chislennost' i sostav rabochei sily, zaniatoi v tabachnom proizvodstve," in *Tabachnaia promyshlennost'*, ed. S. A. Gol'dshtein (Moscow: RIO TsK VSRPVP, 1929), 6:69–70.

Makhorka Workers included 250 people, of whom 227 were women, most of them underage.[138]

Working conditions and wages were poor.[139] Emma Goldman, visiting the Laferm Factory in Petrograd, commented on the horrible conditions. "The air in the workrooms was stifling, nauseating," she reported. "There were some pregnant women at work and girls no older than fourteen. They looked haggard, their chests sunken, black rings under their eyes. Some of them coughed and the hectic flush of consumption showed on their faces." Goldman expressed her disgust with the conditions, the piece work, the lack of rest areas, and the disgrace of this all being after the supposed triumph of the worker state. She confronted her guide, Lisa: "'But if even such small improvements had not resulted from the Revolution,' I argued, 'what purpose has it served?' 'The workers have achieved control,' Lisa replied; 'they are now in power and they have more important things to attend to than rest rooms—they have the Revolution to defend.'" From the evidence of tobacco workers, Goldman remained unimpressed with the triumph of the Bolsheviks, "The thought oppressed me that what she called the 'defence [sic] of the Revolution' was really only the defence [sic] of her party in power."[140]

In 1918 the Main Tobacco Committee in Moscow inspected all factories in Moscow and Petrograd for their hygienic standing. The committee reported on the vulnerability of the largely female and underage workforce and the general "pale and yellowed . . . prematurely aged" nature of almost all.[141] Critics reported that the nicotine that workers touched and the tobacco dust released in manufacture led to lung, heart, nerve, digestion, and circulation problems and ailments like thrombosis, anemia, and tuberculosis.[142] At the first scientific conference for the Moscow Health Department Narkosection a Dr. Rozenbaum revealed the serious health effects of tobacco production for women—specifically on the breathing organs and the nervous system, later implicating tobacco work in tuberculosis, blood and breathing problems, digestion issues, and sexual irregularities.[143] Other authors singled out the dangers of tobacco dust even as anti-tuberculosis activists mounted a vigorous campaign against dust in all aspects of urban life.[144] Research on tuberculosis among tobacco workers indicated their increased susceptibility.[145] Together, anti-tobacco forces, pro-workplace safety movements, and infectious disease campaigns made clear the need for better ventilation.

In protest over conditions and governance, tobacco women turned to agitation and upheaval during the meeting of the tenth party congress in March 1921. The women of Laferm joined the soldiers of Kronstadt and other disgruntled citizens and revolted against the Soviet government and for freedoms of speech, the press, and association.[146] Tobacco had been a haven of anti-Bolshevik groups after October, and the women continued to be a source of disquiet.[147] A memo to Lenin and Stalin reported the spread of materials of anarchists at Laferm even as the state attempted to frighten the rioters back into obedience.[148] Despite a major crackdown, strikes and agitation continued.[149] The events of Kronstadt overlapped to some extent with Semashko's attempts at a tobacco ban but did not precipitate his initial defeat. The revolt and tenth party congress met just after Semashko was shut out of reform in the Small Sovnarkom and before the final pulling of the decree from discussion at the full Sovnarkom meeting. The revolt was put down, but popular discontent helped usher in NEP.

Although for most women NEP meant mass unemployment (50–70 percent of all unemployed were female), the tobacco industry had a different story.[150] If in 1921, 70 percent of tobacco workers were female, by 1927 the gender composition of the tobacco workforce had changed only slightly with 64 percent adult females, 33 percent adult males, and 3 percent youth of either sex.[151] The presence of most workers (95 percent) in state-run factories is likely to have kept underage labor more regulated.[152] Before the revolution grueling, labor-intensive tobacco handwork paid at piecework wages had been poorly remunerated. In the 1880s men earned eighteen to twenty rubles a month, women eight to ten, and children three to four. Families often worked together to make enough to live.[153] Better pay distinguished the postrevolutionary era, as did attention to some of the more deleterious aspects of production. The average monthly pay by 1927 was sixty-seven rubles and sex disparity less dramatic, with men making more at seventy-seven rubles and an adult female sixty rubles. Children of either sex earned almost half of that—twenty-seven rubles.[154] In 1928 in tobacco women earned 85 percent of a male wage at one of the most equal footings of any industry.[155] For tobacco women the emancipatory policies of the revolutionary state were not undercut by unemployment and lack of wages.[156] Instead, their factories developed and their opportunities expanded. As one worker enthusiastically recalled, "An interesting life arrived. Every day brought something new. They began to build new stations. The factory expanded. They brought new machines. They mechanized all handwork, labor for workers [female] stopped being difficult, or even unbearable for pregnant women. We understood that we labored not to feed a bunch of fat bourgeoisie but for our own sakes."[157]

Undoubtedly some of the praise was hyperbolic, but because of the closure of many older, dilapidated factories and the consolidation of machinery, the conditions of the shop floor had improved. Technological innovations made for better-ventilated, healthier workspaces.[158] A 1924 *Pravda* article described the Rosa Luxembourg Factory in Rostov-on-Don as "a woman's kingdom," not just by workforce but by the look of the shop floor, where "machines are decorated with red kerchiefs." The more than two thousand workers of the factory enjoyed "laughter and happy conversations" even as the sorting department with its new "gigantic ventilation tubes" revolutionized processes. The author enthused over innovated, lightened, and streamlined everything. American-style conveyer belts moved materials, box making was mechanized, and packing machines were employed. Worker productivity went up by 114 percent, and the workday was curtailed to seven hours. The article declared, "The workers love their factory. They have professional pride, and this explains why not only does labor productivity increase but also the quality is higher."[159] In the 1929 Soviet film *Man with a Movie Camera*, among the many women's workspaces featured was a tobacco factory where dexterous women folded boxes for papirosy and then deftly packed them by hand.

An article from *Rabotnitsa* detailed the work of one tobacco factory where women made up five hundred of the seven hundred person workforce. The author proposed that the recently installed ventilator and shields protected workers from many hazards and increased productivity.[160] The Iava Factory changed policies, keeping child workers out of preparation stations and installing ventilation systems.[161] A worker at DGTF recalled efforts to remove dust from the shop floor, commenting on how "amazing" the transformation had been: "On the shop floor you could breathe easily, and even among those unused to it, walking along the street, a person did not have the need to sneeze."[162] Although a decade later workers hailed the ventilation, a commentary at the time observed that they reduced only about half the dust, "because of problems on education on dust, tobacco working methods, and workers themselves."[163] The author claimed handwork "greatly increases the problem" and that workers needed to take the issue seriously.[164] In this way, the author blamed workers for any lingering job safety problems.

Other initiatives expanded or extended existing programs. The female workforce of tobacco had enjoyed benefits before the revolution including onsite medical and pharmacy services, nurseries, and clubs.[165] The Soviets began a number of programs to encourage social participation and cultural uplift. The Iava Factory history claimed that the factory founded the first kindergarten in Moscow in 1918 with thirty children. For older youth the first Komsomol cell began at the factory in the same year. It also had a medical treatment center, and a factory school started in 1922.[166] A Ukrainian tobacco factory claimed: "Social work among us is in good shape. We do not have one commission, not one organization, where women do not work in good number." The organizer noted, however, "The only poorly thing among us is the participation of women in club work."[167]

The gendered nature of the tobacco factory floor comes out in two photos from the period (Figures 2.3 and 2.4). In an image from the Dukat Factory,

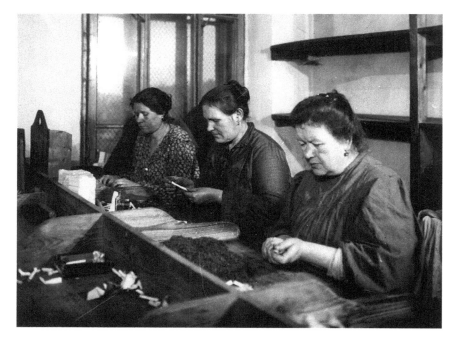

FIGURE 2.3. Photo. First tobacco factory, previously Dukat, hand rolling of papirosy, before 1930. Rossiiskii gosudarstvennyi arkhiv kino-fono-foto-dokumentov (hereafter RGAKFD), no. 1878, dated 1920–1930.

female papirosy rollers line up at their bench, shoulder to shoulder, laboring by hand, twisting the paper cartridges to stuff with tobacco before curling on the cardboard mouthpiece. Piles of tobacco sit in front of the women along-side stacks of papers. The women, intent on their labor, look well dressed and prosperous with earrings, hair accessories, and well-kept clothes. The second photo, shot in the same period but at the Uritskii Tobacco Factory, presents a triumphant brigade of eight kerchiefed female workers around a papirosa machine. Whereas on many shop floors men got the premium spots as machine operators, in this women's kingdom women ruled, wielding machine tools as scepters.

When Semashko pursued his ban in 1920, the government faced a decision of either reinvigorating a declining tobacco industry or investing energy and author-ity in a campaign against tobacco aimed at an exhausted population. The tobacco industry stood at its lowest point, plagued by production problems brought on by shortages of paper, fuel, and leaf and hampered by aging machinery, derelict buildings, and a workforce in revolt. The market had broken down to unofficial back channels, payment in kind, and virtually no exports.

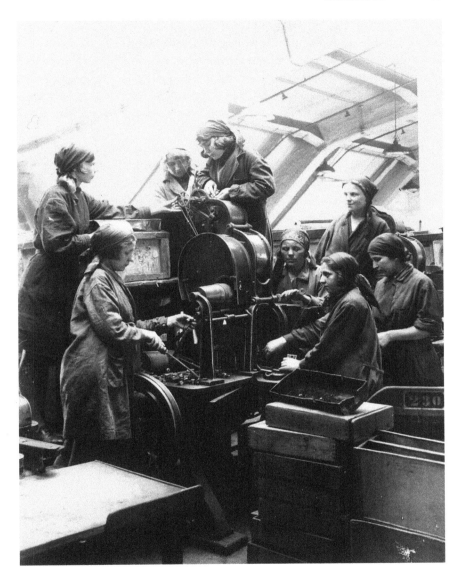

FIGURE 2.4. Photo. Women at production: A brigade of women organizing brigade work at the first tobacco factory in the name of Uritskii, RGAKFD, no. 235630, n.d.

Faced with the decision to kill or nurture tobacco, the Soviets took these factories, nationalized them, and invested in recovery. Factories were rebuilt, machinery consolidated, shortages managed, and needs met. To forestall an often-volatile female tobacco workforce, production was smoothed, workplaces cleaned, and benefits expanded. Tobacco workers enjoyed higher wages, greater social amenities, cleaner and safer workspaces, and more cultural opportunities. Securing tobacco production also satisfied the vast number of smokers even as it helped the general economy and enriched the state. As one author argued, "the development of tobacco production . . . depends exclusively on technical and raw-material ability and not in any way from the size of the internal market, which will swallow by the very least measure twice the current amount of production."[168]

By the end of NEP, Semashko's attempt to shut down tobacco culture, his campaign to discourage increased tobacco use, and his hopes for stopping the export of Soviet tobacco to the rest of the world had been definitively defeated. Semashko lost out first on tobacco, then alcohol. The choice of increased production over prohibition held deep implications for the fortunes of the population in the long term. While Semashko and others believed that smoking would disappear once the economy recovered and social problems were addressed, it did not. Instead, tobacco was snapped up as soon as it was produced and the market hungered for even more.

SOLD

Revolutionary Advertising and Communist Consumption

The early 1920s poster for Makhorka no. 8 from the Volga German commune peddled more than tobacco (Figure 3.1). Two peasants, a soldier, and a worker—each enjoying a smoke in papirosy or pipe—nod approvingly to one another over the taste and quality of their chosen brand. Framed by factories, these icons of political propaganda try to sell the public not on an idea or a policy but on a product, as the makers of revolution now emerge as the smokers of it. The borrowing of political imagery is not a one-way street. Flashing through the background and lingering in the glances, hints fly that Makhorka no. 8 carried political, social, and communal effects alongside the jolt of nicotine.

Stereotypically garbed as peasant on the far left, Volga German in yellow hat, Red Army soldier in greatcoat, and blacksmith in heavy leather apron, the smokers surround an enlarged package of tobacco, emblazoned with a red star, one of the earliest symbols of the Soviet state.[1] The soldier is not a comrade of the trenches of World War I but in the garb of revolution.[2] This tableau stands in front of yet another large red star and behind the comically large pack, which takes on the appearance of the draped head table at a political meeting. The players, the symbols, and the setting all intimate that Makhorka no. 8 would appeal to a smoker with a revolutionary worldview and could be consumed politically.

Despite the seeming equality of the foursome in the center of the poster, the Red Army man commands the scene. Standing full face to the viewer, he places his finger authoritatively on the table as if engaged in a fiery speech. The two peasants confer with one another, pointing to their tobacco, and the blacksmith faces away from the viewer. The Red Army man dominates the space, and his

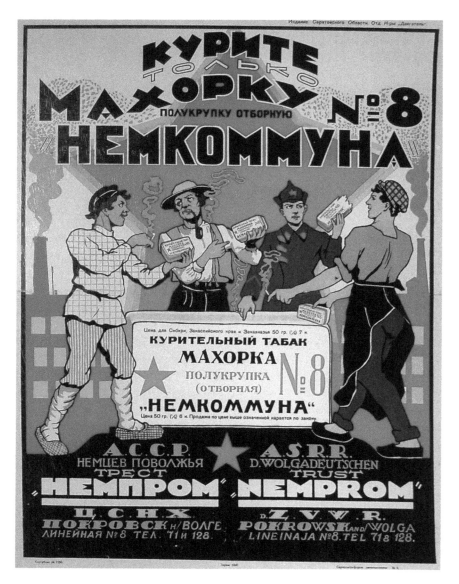

FIGURE 3.1.   Poster. "Smoke Only Makhorka no. 8," 1921–1925. Courtesy Russian State Library.

pack is the only one open, suggesting he guides the tobacco taste of his fellows. Leading the way, he encourages his brethren to take up Makhorka no. 8 alongside the struggle for worldwide revolution. Social interaction and the connoisseur's exchange of considered knowledge regarding taste and method for enjoying a product are wed to the political authority of the Red Army soldier.

The look of pleasant surprise from the peasant to the Volga German and the German's gesture to the pack indicate the rural man is being educated to the brand rather than enjoying a long-standing familiarity. The blacksmith turns with similar inquiry to the soldier, pointing down to the large pack as if in confirmation. The political action of participating in a meeting becomes entangled with the social act of smoking. The radical promise of the revolution, the exchange of in-depth understanding of taste, and the solidarity of shared tobacco create a new type of Soviet distinction different from bourgeois consumption—a communist connoisseur.

More meaning swirls in the smokers' exhalations and the factory's belching pipes. The act of consuming tobacco produced in the correct manner and advertised in a revolutionary way allows smoking to move from a leisure activity and unite with production in the workers' state. Star and factory shine in the same vibrant color scheme: a brilliant crimson envelops both, punctuated by the vital yellows of the factory outlines and the dazzling gold framing the Soviet star. Together, star and factory conjure a brave, new, Soviet dawn in which politically educated consumption intimately connects to proper production.[3] The communist connoisseur smoked brands produced in revolutionary ways by communal manufacturers. By consuming, smokers enacted and imbibed political consciousness. Tobacco connoisseurship before 1917 involved its own specialized knowledge with attention to leaf, blend, saucing, taste, and smell, accompanying appreciation for the agricultural origins of a product, the workplace politics of a factory, and the symbolism of the brand name. A proper Soviet citizen could attend to many of these same issues from a politically enlightened perspective. When confronted with the choices of NEP, a true communist connoisseur could select a brand from a state factory with a native-grown tobacco, advertised in a revolutionary name or in proper political frameworks that bespoke their party affiliations and political sophistication.

The connection of smoking to the political and social was nothing new. Nineteenth-century Russian advertisements linked tobacco to political imagery, though in that case it was the frontiers of the tsarist empire and their Cossack guardians, not the leftist frontiers of political ideology and their Bolshevik defenders. The 1919 violent program of de-Cossackization and the Bolshevik disavowal of empire assured the death of these old associations, but advertisements incorporated new figures and images imparting to consumption meanings that fit the radical scene.[4] Showing smokers as part of a community remained consistent with tsarist imagery, but in the 1920s messages of belonging had immense power. Confronted with the chaotic social and cultural landscape of revolution and the NEP era and given the frightening consequences that followed from choices of what, how, where, and with whom to associate, being able to just light up and belong would have been comforting.

Not all NEP-era posters for tobacco worked through visions of revolution. Other smokers joined the men of Makhorka no. 8 in posters showing Soviet citizens what to smoke and how, and not all were revolutionary. Images of elegant and exotic consumption, manly smoking, or leisurely puffing made it through the jumbled landscape and joined the flesh and blood inducements to smoke that surrounded people in the city, at work, on the shop floor, in the theater, at the museum, at the club, and in the dormitory. At meetings and speeches, many communists smoked, becoming examples to attendees. Movies showed heroes and villains, men and women, foreign and domestic, smoking. But the positioning of tobacco as a form of political, even communist, consumption stood out as new. Tobacco, a luxury good rather than a staple, should have suffered doubly as being not just consumption but petty entertainment built on the temptation of baser appetites that an active public health campaign depicted as an individual danger and social evil. But images of soldier, worker, and peasant smoking on posters, in films, and in life made smoking into a political act that promised physical comfort, psychological reassurance, and belonging in social and political situations. Papirosy served up the revolution in a wrapper.

Marxist Advertising and NEP Contradictions

In the world's first Marxist state, condemning advertising and product fetishization for creating artificial value disconnected from utility would seem an easy thing. Although the Bolsheviks immediately nationalized and limited advertising, in 1922 at the eleventh party congress, Lenin pressed for the sale of advertising space in *Pravda* to fund the paper's publication. Under NEP strictures, newspapers struggled to be cost-efficient while juggling high prices in paper, ink, and printing.[5] In the wake of the decree, several advertising firms entered the scene, and trusts and other government groups organized their own advertisements. Chief among these in Moscow was Mossel'prom, which in addition to beer and candy factories dealt in tobacco. In Petrograd a primary advertiser was the tobacco trust, which produced many popular prerevolutionary brands.[6]

By the mid-1920s more than fifty advertising firms had set up shop in Moscow alone. Some of these were independent, but many functioned within newspaper or governmental agencies, such as at Mossel'prom, the mail and telegraph, and city soviets and transport. At one point, advertising made up over 20 percent of the city's revenue.[7] The reliance of government agencies on advertising money led to pressure on manufacturers for "charitable advertising" aimed not at motivating and educating consumers but simply helping fund a group. Abuses of the system led to an investigation in 1926 that revealed gross corruption and mismanagement, and after that, disgust and distrust led to closures and diminished newspaper advertising.[8]

The debates over whether advertising should be allowed in official publications reflected a long-standing hostility to consumerism among the Russian revolutionary intelligentsia, who promoted asceticism and productive labor rather than frivolous leisure and empty pleasures. This antipathy to bourgeois acquisitiveness was brought into sharp relief in the complicated 1920s environment of NEP, when revolutionary principles jostled against market forces and figures. In literature, film, and advertisements NEP's excesses became personified in the overdressed, overindulged, and overstuffed figure of the NEP-man. His costume was that of the bourgeois and aristocrat, a tuxedo and top hat; his companions were symbolic of carnal consumption, the cigar and the prostitute. The NEP-woman displayed her wanton behavior as a sign of female sexuality unleashed. Her markers—red lipstick, fashionable clothes, and papirosy—betrayed her interest in the frivolous and sensual and showed her as an object for sale and an acquisitive consumer.[9]

The continuation of limited capitalism under NEP left the revolution incomplete and gave an opening for the new life to be contaminated by the old. In this environment of confusion, behaviors took on added danger. Individual, revolutionary, progressive habits could move all of society forward toward the communist utopia, whereas regressive, individualistic, selfish behaviors threatened to pull everyone back into the exploitative past. The institution of NEP, meant to ease material and social conditions, unnerved many who struggled to negotiate in their daily lives the contagions of capitalist consumption, bourgeois enrichment, and frivolous diversions that now infected the revolutionary world.[10] Transgressors endangered collective progress and risked personal punishment. The state took these proclaimed enemies of the people, these exploiters and saboteurs, and deprived them of rights, denied them privileges, or subjected them to incarceration and death.

The signs of improper behavior were not always clearly discernible. In reality, the NEP-men did not continuously wear tuxedos, and activists did not always agree on the way forward. Yet not knowing how to behave in a revolutionary manner could have deadly consequences. A profusion of advice literature on how to be a good communist in a semicapitalist world directed the Soviet public through the treacherous political, social, and cultural landscape. Guidance on health and leisure, sport and labor, and education and political activities appeared in newspapers and pamphlets, decrees and posters, and movies and speeches. These in turn were distributed by unions and factory clubs, youth groups and schools, or museums and city governments. No part of daily life avoided notice. Activists questioned whether a good communist should dance the tango, if an activist could wear makeup or a workers' club serve beer. Discussions probed intimate questions of sexual responsibility, the division of domestic duties, and child care. With so many different people and entities involved, the message to the public did not maintain a singular focus. The advice on behavior changed from entity to entity and, as economic conditions calmed and international issues intruded, from year to year.[11]

In addition to communist officials, literary figures, artists, and travelers fashioned their own revolutionary lives, and advertisers generated alternative visions of modern Soviet lifestyles that included consumption of certain products. Newspaper advertisements were the cheapest and ubiquitous, but their copy tended toward prosaic comment of where to buy what, although slogans and graphics could be eye-catching and suggestive.[12] A 1923 advertisement for the Crimean Tobacco Trust from *Izvestiia* acknowledged the universal nature of tobacco, declaring it "for every taste and every pocket," while pointing to the economic logic of their brands, where "there are more expensive, but none better!" The visual was simple but strong, showcasing eight packs. The implication of varied yet affordable products allowed viewers to consider themselves discerning users who might cater to their taste without indulging in impractical, expensive luxuries. The advertisement implied that principled, educated consumption could be the mark of a disciplined, conscious, Soviet consumer, not a capitalist glutton.[13] Able to employ larger, detailed color formats, posters hinted even more about proper behavior and how a communist might also be a smoker. Compositions showed goods being consumed and suggested appropriate settings. Advertisers provided comforting, educational messages of how to fit in and implied the many dangers of not doing the right thing, buying the right goods, or living the right way. For newly Soviet citizens, many rising quickly into the class of consumers with little prior acquaintance with goods, either because of location or because of want, advertisements were transformed from sellers' tools into manuals for viewers on how to behave in alien, confusing situations.[14]

Advertisers within official state entities bridged the line between political agitation and exhortation, combining the philosophies of high art with the aesthetics of mass publication. Politically motivated constructivist artists embraced poster advertising to reach the public, arguing that the artist was an engineer of beauty, inspired by the industrial, and bent on serving the working class. The constructivist artist Rodchenko teamed up with the Futurist poet Maiakovskii to design advertisements utilizing new techniques like photomontage and catchy slogans to burst into the popular consciousness.[15] Maiakovskii worked to transform inanimate objects into motivators of revolution, showing the potential of things to change lives and creating new relationships between humans and objects. He melded Soviet ideals with western advertising techniques to create agitational advertising, and in the summer of 1923, he and Rodchenko began the private firm Agit-Reklam to follow this course.[16]

The constructivists attempted to develop consumer habits that could generate cultural, social, and political changes—a type of productive consumption—and saw great potential in advertising with proletarian themes as a means of uplift. If artists could make everyday objects revolutionary, their advertisements could educate the public on how to negotiate the new life and drive the revolution.[17] Perhaps nothing was so quotidian as the papirosa. The 1923 advertisement for *Ira* papirosy from Mossel'prom typified constructivism's arresting graphics and bright colors, combined with witty couplets. The rhyming slogan—"The only thing of the old world here/is the papirosy *Ira*"—in strong block letters implies the capitalist world had been destroyed, but certain products could be resurrected— especially when found "nowhere like at Mossel'prom!" Even though Maiakovskii penned this and other memorable slogans and was an ardent smoker himself, he wrote anti-tobacco couplets such as the long-lived, "Quit your smokin'/Papirosy are poison!"[18]

The two capitals provided much of the artistic talent for poster advertising, and Moscow artists produced the work for brands made outside the center like the tobacco firm Urtak. The brothers Semion and Stepan Aladzhalov drew many of the fresh-looking advertisements for DGTF. In Petrograd Aleksandr Zelenskii revolutionized the look of the tobacco industry advertisements for established brands like *Trezvon, Peri,* and *Safo.* His images, with their distinctive smoke rings and clean designs, transformed consumer goods into works of art. M. Bulanov, attached to the Leningrad city advertising agency, designed for Mossel'prom and others, adding humor, exaggeration, and dynamic compositions. He also introduced advertisements sized specifically for inside trams, a modern acknowledgment of the relationship of space, viewer, and message.[19]

Most any surface could host a poster—a fence, a window, a building wall, the interior (or exterior) of a tram or wagon. Banners and billboards supplemented posters and hung in offices, hotels, and city squares and sometimes as decoration in apartments.[20] Electric billboards assaulted the pedestrians of Moscow, proclaiming the benefits of featured products. Political art, hygiene posters, and announcements for concerts and events joined these appeals. Posters and slogans for galoshes and powders in colors and lights surrounded urbanites, calling to everyone—NEP-man and communist—to look, to try, and to buy. Undoubtedly this visual cacophony did not reach full volume in the countryside and perhaps became a background hum to the accustomed urbanite, but its omnipresence allowed for citizens to hear everywhere, perhaps just on the edge of consciousness, commentary on what to do, where, and how to do it from state sources, economic concerns, and the occasional NEP-enabled private business.[21]

The pack of tobacco offered an additional, convenient space for messaging. Artists adorned the wrappings of loose tobacco and packs of papirosy so that a small piece of artwork accompanied the buyer home or served to impress others as smokers lit up at work, on the street, or in the club. Urban vendors of papirosy offered dozens of such boxes, packs, and port cigars. The tray became a miniature art museum showcasing pieces of portable, affordable, collectible, and usable art (Figures 2.2) Perusing the images would have provided a few minutes distraction for even nonsmokers waiting to cross the street or grab a ride. The British traveler Wicksteed observed the multiple ways in which tobacco packs functioned, commenting, "The real purpose of the different brands is, I think, to provide an outlet for the Russian inventiveness in designing new covers nearly all of which are gay and many really artistic, and to minister to the love of change of the Russian public."[22]

Packs were many things at once—protective cases, marketing, art, and collectible—but they also sparked sensory reveries of tobacco indulgence. The senses are intimately bound to consumption. Capitalist industrial designers exploited the senses to excite the buyer's desire—the sight of the graphic, the sound of the cellophane, the touch of the smooth paper, the smell of the fresh tobacco.[23] Soviet designs similarly enticed consumers with playful labels, bright colors, different blends, and innovative packaging, though constrained by material and production limitations. For capitalist or communist smokers, there was also a biological trigger—nicotine and its withdrawal. Packs could remind smokers of their habit and induce desire through their physical intrusion on the body and its movements. Packs held in the pocket, visible to others, or discarded in the gutter became more than inanimate objects—packs were transformed into actors in smokers' lives and cues for continued use.[24] The sight of a pack elicited a visceral and aesthetic response by triggering a biological compulsion in tobacco habituates and sparking aesthetic appreciation.[25] Packs further served as signifiers to users and others of political, social, and cultural affiliations. Prerevolutionary brand choice and pack display signaled attention to taste, style, gender display, and social etiquette. Proper Soviet citizens could, when confronted with the choices of NEP, select a brand that displayed their hopes for class advancement, desire for social acceptance, and/or pretentions of political affiliations.[26] By lighting up, the smoker became involved in not just an act of consumption but a new style of political consumption—a communist connoisseurship.

Advertising's positive portrayals of smoking provided a compelling counter to Semashko's propaganda, and the growing number of smokers showed which side was winning. A 1925 article estimated that 15 percent of the population smoked a little over a pack a day.[27] And the Bolshevik's core constituents smoked even more.

According to a Moscow Department of Health survey of 1926, 61 percent of Moscow Komsomol members smoked. A 1927 study claimed that among urban workers 68 percent of men and 45 percent of women smoked.[28] Other areas showed lower rates and greater gender disparity. A 1926 survey of consumption in Ukraine found around half of male and 4 percent of female white-collar workers smoked an average of 6,320 papirosy a year, or about a pack a day (Table 7).

Among workers, the researcher found even higher amounts of smoking for men, though among women the percentages remained lower (Table 8). Overall

TABLE 7.   Smoking among Ukrainian white-collar workers, 1926

PROVINCE	PERCENTAGE OF SMOKING WHITE-COLLAR WORKERS		
	MEN	WOMEN	AVERAGE
Kharkov	51.9	2.8	23.5
Kiev	47.9	6.5	23.1
Donbass	50.9	4.9	23.2
Ekaterinoslav	42.8	2.3	20.3
AVG for province	**49.2**	**4.3**	**22.9**

Source: D. Sokolovskii, "K voprosu o emkosti vsesoiuznogo i ukrainskogo tabachnykh rynkov v sviazi s piatilet-nim planom razvertyvaniia promyshlennosti," in *Tabachnaia promyshlennost' i tabakovodstvo*, ed. Ia. M. Gol'bert (Moscow: Mospoligraf, 1926), 7.

TABLE 8.   Smoking among Ukrainian workers, 1926

PROVINCE	PERCENT OF SMOKING WORKERS		
	MEN	WOMEN	AVERAGE
Kharkov	63.5	1.4	31.2
Kiev	62.5	5.6	31.2
Donbass	66.3	1.0	31.7
Odessa	63.0	1.5	31.2
AVG for province	**63.1**	**1.9**	**31.2**

Source: D. Sokolovskii, "K voprosu o emkosti vsesoiuznogo i ukrainskogo tabachnykh rynkov v sviazi s piatilet-nim planom razvertyvaniia promyshlennosti," in *Tabachnaia promyshlennost' i tabakovodstvo*, ed. Ia. M. Gol'bert (Moscow: Mospoligraf, 1926), 7.

TABLE 9.   Smoking among worker youth, 1926–1929

	MEN	WOMEN
Worker youth (data of this study)	50.2	11.6
Students, Leningrad Med. Inst. (1928)	56.0	22.7
Students, War-Medical Academy (1928)	62.6	-
Railway workers (1926)	75.9	-

Source: B. B. Kogan and M. S. Lebedinskii, *Byt rabochei molodezhi* (Moscow: Moszdravotdel, 1929), 71.

TABLE 10. Tobacco consumption among youth, 1926–1929

PAPIROSY PER DAY	MEN—277 ANSWERS		WOMEN—13 ANSWERS	
	#	%	#	%
1–9	41	14.6	7	54
10–19	118	42.7	5	38.3
20 or more	118	42.7	1	7.7

Source: B. B. Kogan and M. S. Lebedinskii, *Byt rabochei molodezhi* (Moscow: Moszdravotdel, 1929), 72–73.

smoking rates for women were lower, and fewer female workers smoked than female white-collar workers.[29] This may have reflected their reduced buying power as much as preference.

A survey of worker youth reported in 1929 found over 50 percent of males and almost 10 percent of women smoked. In some fields, such as railway workers, as many as three-quarters smoked (Table 9). Of these, the average male smoked around a pack a day. Women smoked far fewer papirosy on average (Table 10). The author of the study placed the blame for smoking's onset with the beginning of paid work, which gave workers means and opportunity to smoke.[30] Advertising and pack design incentivized it.

Gendered Smoking and Sensual Appetites

Not only revolutionaries made posters and consumed tobacco; NEP allowed others to preach consumption, luxury, and even decadence. In posters for the papirosy of the State Tobacco Factory of Vladivostok (1925), the firm A. S. Maikapar of Moscow (1924), and *Karmen* papirosy from DGTF (1925), elegant individuals took center stage (Figures 3.2, 3.3, and 3.4). NEP made for strange partnerships as state trust advertisers tried to woo the NEP-man and NEP-woman to their brands or tempt others who might aspire to a life that while officially derided took on all the trappings of elegance. They were featured in isolation yet in a public space, actively enjoying the product yet displaying no markers of engagement with the politics of the state or production. Each figure smoked at leisure—in evening clothes, at the theater, or on the beach. None are presented against the backdrop of the city, the revolutionary, or the militant.

For Vladivostok papirosy (1925), an individual appeal highlights the personal, sensual experience of a stylish, attractive user (Figure 3.2).[31] The glow of his match brings life to his tobacco companion, illuminates his face, and animates the scene. No other compatriots—soldier, blacksmith, or peasant—are implied by the setting, unlike in the communal, revolutionary experience of Makhorka

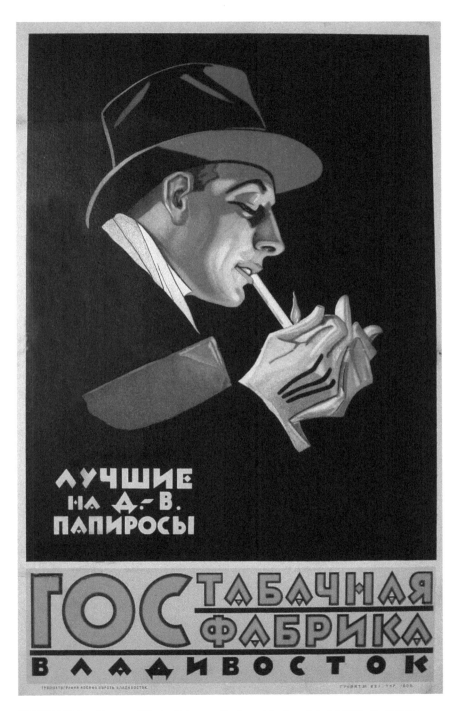

FIGURE 3.2. Poster. "State Tobacco Factory, Vladivostok," 1925. Courtesy Russian State Library.

no. 8 (Figure 3.1). His gloved, cupped hands impart an impression gentle and tender, suitable for an individualistic, private moment of pleasure. Like the pre-revolutionary connoisseur, the Vladivostok male savors "the best papirosy of the far east" displaying an understanding of the other accessories of the good life: fancy evening dress, top hat, gloves, fresh shave, and groomed brow. In propaganda, the NEP-man was rapacious, corpulent, and often disgusting, but this advertiser's alternative is a sophisticated, urbane consumer. This NEP-man seems ready to be emulated, not excoriated, and becomes an endorsement not just of tobacco but to the life of stylishness, grace, and luxury.

The joint-stock company of A. S. Maikapar fashioned an image of a genteel female smoker. She enjoys her papirosa in chic apparel, countering the salacious depictions of NEP-women (Figure 3.3).[32] A white fur coat drapes off her shoulders revealing a mauve dress with a daring décolleté highlighted by a large red flower. Whereas the male of Vladivostok enjoys his tobacco outside and in isolation, the woman of Maikapar smokes in the public theater but in a private box. Privacy, individuality, and exclusivity flavor these bourgeois appeals, an interesting choice given the crowded 1920s city and particularly the situation of many bourgeois in apartments subdivided in revolutionary redistributions.[33] As with the male smoker, this isolation did not imply a lack of companionship as tobacco took up the position of soul mate. Our smoker's attention is taken up by the open pack of papirosy. For well-to-do smokers, the posters highlighted the personal experience of consumption, and the sensual delight of smoking. These appeals echoed tsarist imagery of connoisseurship more than Soviet imagery. This may have been a result of their status as being outside the center (Vladivostok), appealing to international markets (Riga and Berlin) or artifacts of uncertain economic times (NEP).

The 1925 poster for *Karmen* papirosy from DGTF displayed the NEP-woman as an active consumer of tobacco, although not a productive person (Figure 3.4).[34] The commentary at the top of the pack that it is "papirosy of the higher sort" and the retention of the prerevolutionary name of the factory in the copy below and on the box, brought the bourgeois past of differentiated product values and ownership of the means of production actively into the advertisement. Named for the titular heroine of the 1875 Georges Bizet opera, the smoke itself suggests a dangerous and hedonistic, irrational womanhood, fully connected to the carnal. In the opera the character Carmen worked in a cigarette factory, seduced several men, discarded them, and ultimately was killed by a jealous lover. The promiscuous, active Carmen contrasts with the languorous and chic woman on the chaise, who protects her delicate skin from the sun with a massive parasol. In a sign of her stylish ways, her parasol coordinates to her outfit, which matches the small pouf on which her high-heeled shoes rest. Her pose insinuates the odalisque, and

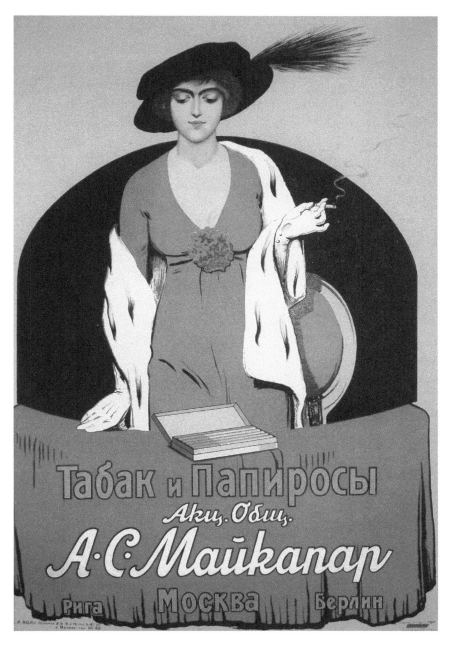

FIGURE 3.3. Poster. "Joint Stock Company A. S. Maikapar," 1924. Courtesy Russian State Library.

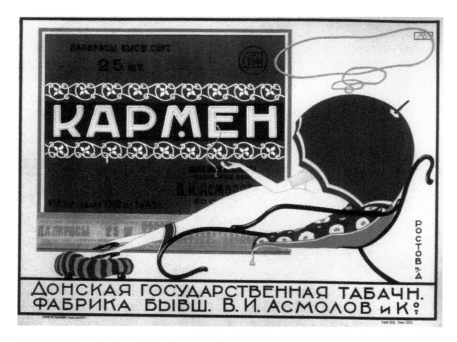

FIGURE 3.4.   Poster. "Advertisement for *Karmen*," 1925. Artist Aleksei Zaniatov. Courtesy Russian State Library.

she evokes a papirosa herself, a smoldering, white column lounging on its side. The visual link of the two comes in the smoke of her papirosa, entwined with the scrolling text.

Even more blatant in its appeal to tobacco as a pleasurable, even erotic, indulgence for women was the 1924 poster for *Safo* papirosy from the Leningrad State Tobacco Trust (Figure 3.5).[35] By A. Zelenskii, the poster showed his preference for the clear, graphic styles of the European modern tradition.[36] More so even than *Karmen*, the brand title *Safo* calls to mind the sensual delights of the ancient Greek poet from the island of Lesbos. The naming of the papirosa implies the substitution of tobacco for other pleasures, and the visual of the poster cements that link with a radiant blonde woman, eyes closed in reverie, inhaling her papirosa. The draped clothing, blushed cheeks, and her mussed, though stylishly cropped, hair convey a postcoital languor. The implication that tobacco sexually satisfies women in turn connects to the idea that smoking women were sexually available. Yet like other nonrevolutionary smokers, she is featured alone in frame, the source of her blushing cheeks and tousled hair can only be her satisfying *Safo*.

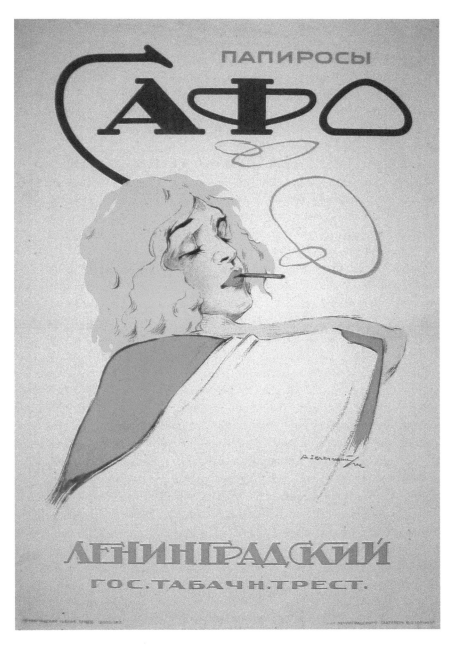

FIGURE 3.5. Poster. "Advertisement for *Safo*," 1924. Artist Aleksandr Zelenskii. Courtesy Russian State Library.

The female smoker had achieved her equality with men in advertising well before the revolution. Imperial Russian advertisers depicted active female smokers instead of using women simply to entice male buyers.[37] Women's brands, travelers' accounts, and angry commentary from antismoking advocates indicated that a sizable number of women smoked and generally enjoyed public acceptance for their habit, in ways parallel to women's smoking habits in China, where imagery of women's smoking indicated a bourgeois or decadent character.[38] In the 1920s the world's women began to light up and catch up, as international marketers changed tactics and blends. In the US, Britain, and other areas of Europe, women began smoking in larger numbers and became more visible.[39] Smoking in the tsarist period had been associated with political activism and public roles, and Soviet reforms broke women free of the family and pushed women into even greater connection to public and political life.[40] After the revolution, at least in the cities, Soviet women smoked in good numbers but became less visible in imagery. A rising emphasis on a New Soviet Man—who exemplified the values trumpeted by the state in terms of progress, development, science, and military strength—left little place for the female smoker, unless she adopted male looks and behavior. For some politically minded women, smoking did become part of the look of the serious activist.[41] Yet the smoking Soviet woman remained controversial. An extended commentary by Commissar of Health N. A. Semashko argued a smoking woman was "manly" with caustic mannerisms.[42]

Portrayals of smoking in film by women and men in the west have been blamed for glamorizing the habit and spreading it.[43] Soviet films and literature did have female smokers, but infrequently, and smoking continued to be a more polyvalent sign of female stress, depression, profession, protest, independence, or even counterculture leanings.[44] In *Kino-Eye* (1924), a "documentary" of street life in Soviet Russia, smoking is everywhere, at all times, and by men and women. A male baker smokes while working, a woman with a male companion and baby smokes in a crowd as they watch a magician, and a paramedic pulls the cigarette from his mouth to hastily depart for an emergency. The film *Oktiabr'* (1927), by Sergei Eisenstein depicts decadent tobacco use by members of the Women's Battalion of Death, who smoke, drink, and carouse in their negligees in the Winter Palace. The later film *Tsirk* (1936) featured the type of elegant female smoking more prevalent in western cinema when the beautiful protagonist played by Liubov' Orlova contemplatively draws on her cigarette in its long holder. Soviet advertisements, however, maintained a division between actively smoking NEP-women and abstemious communist women. The relative absence of positive models for female smoking outside of bourgeois, capitalist, or sensual female figures indicated a continued connection of women's smoking with indecent behaviors, unbridled sensuality, and uncultured consumption. Advertisers characterized women's smoking as entirely embodied and allied with nonproductive leisure, opulent fashion, and sexual promiscuity. This association fit within the larger communist discourse suggesting women were less revolutionary and generally backward.[45] Positive portrayals of users skewed male. Despite the Soviet campaign for women's equality with guarantees of equal pay, easy divorce, legal abortion, and a host of labor protections, the woman smoker remained separate.[46] It was not just smoking. According to a statistical study of posters from the 1920s, positive portrayals of general consumption are gendered, with 61 percent including only men, 21 percent male and female, and only 14 percent women alone (3 percent with children). More often women were represented as peasants rather than workers.[47]

The compromised position of the female smoker emerged from links of tobacco with licentious activity from its introduction in the seventeenth century until well into the twentieth. The presumed negative effects on morality occupied many anti-tobacco activists, but those who enjoyed tobacco made cheeky fun of the obsession with the "devil's weed" as the poster "And I Smoke!" for Ukraine's tobacco trust made clear (Figure 3.6). In the playfully bright graphic a suave devil puffs away on a papirosa with seemingly no care, only pleasure, perhaps because he already embraced the possible outcomes. This smoking Satan has a twinkle in his eye and a more debonair than demonic appearance. The disregard for the traditional religious case against tobacco coincided well with the new state's antagonism toward the Russian Orthodox Church as did Old Nick's red-hooded costume. That this antireligious stance came at the expense of a prohealth agenda seemingly was fine.

Certain advertisements challenged the cessation arguments trumpeted by Semashko and his state health service. A counter to arguments about the cost of smoking framed the appeal of the brand *Klad* (Treasure) from the early 1920s (Figure 3.7). *Klad* trumpets in bracing couplets and in pulsating, constructivist-style attributed to Rodchenko the many benefits of smoking their tobacco and earning premiums.[48] The peasant tractor driver and worker in peaked cap, smoke comically oversized papirosy. Capitalist marketing innovators introduced premiums, coupons, and other giveaways well before they had become part of the *Klad* pitch, but the economic arguments against tobacco that emphasized its cost lent this approach a political effect as well.[49] Examples of the prizes perch atop the packs, as with the country home and bicycle, or burst forth instead of papirosy, like the bull or stallion. The horse, the classic victim of nicotine poisoning from so many medical tracts, seems an especially pointed choice for a tobacco premium. Despite the acquisitiveness of the message, communist red saturates the entirety. Proceeds from the lottery, sponsored by Mossel'prom and the Commission for the Improvement of the Life of Children, went to orphans and homeless

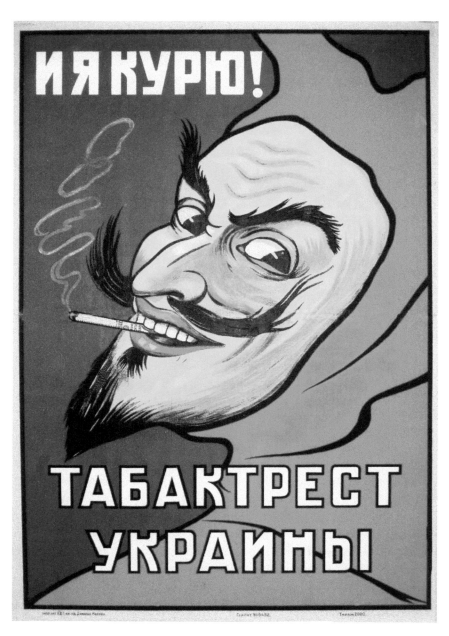

FIGURE 3.6. Poster. "And I Smoke!," 1921–1925. Courtesy Russian State Library.

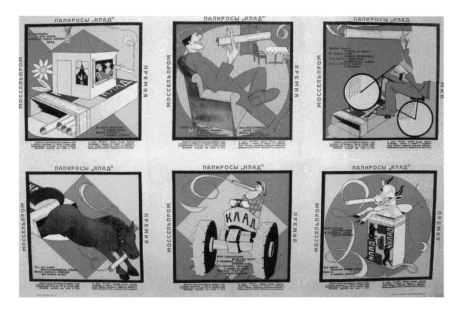

FIGURE 3.7. Poster. "Advertisement for *Klad*," 1921–1925. Courtesy Russian State Library.

children.[50] *Klad* transformed smoking into a form of consumption that could produce things for individuals and society's helpless.

Mikhail Bulanov's 1927 poster for the *Pachka* (Ammo) brand papirosy of Mossel'prom exuberantly refuted commentaries on neurasthenia and male weakness by depicting smoking as an exhibition of male bravado, military might, and even revolutionary consciousness (Figure 3.8). The drawing of a male worker, jubilantly astride his over-proportioned papirosa, blasting out from the cannonlike pack, humorously defuses decades of fevered commentaries on tobacco harming male virility.[51] Further testimony to his vitality hid in the brand name— *Pachka*. The term could refer to a pack of papirosy itself or an ammunition clip. In the same martial vein, the tobacco-filled segment at the end of a papirosa took its name from the militaristic-sounding *patron* (cartridge). The bellicose terminology had long been part of papirosy culture, reflecting the apocryphal stories of the origins of the smoke on the battlefield and tobacco's status as comfort for the fighting man. Years of war and revolution had only further solidified these links. Additionally, the advertisement thwarts the notion that consumption was a politically suspect activity. In a red blouse and leather boots the protagonist seems to be an urban dweller, but he is not the urbane smoker of the Vladivostok

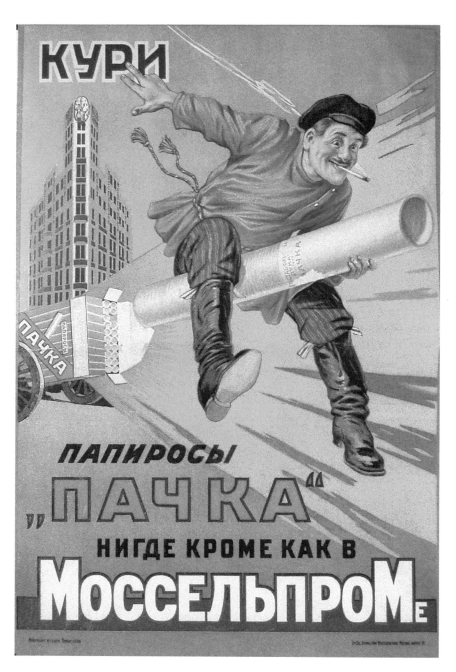

FIGURE 3.8. Poster. "Advertisement for *Pachka*," 1927. Artist Mikhail Bulanov. Courtesy Russian State Library.

advertisement. Instead, he engages in consumption that might fit into the politically connected ideas of cultured use. His *Pachka* dynamically shoots forth from the façade of the Mossel'prom store and the poster sports the slogan—"nowhere like at Mossel'prom." Located along Arbat near the center of Moscow, the building served as a landmark of city life and an indication of where one could obtain goods that were not politically suspect. The red blouse of the worker, red labeling of the brand, presence of Mossel'prom, and implied setting of the Soviet capital all brought forward the ways in which this worker had chosen to consume in a politically conscious manner.

Productive Consumption and Communist Connoisseurs

Appeals that connected smoking to revolutionary and modern industrial, communal, and political ideas were much more common than those using bourgeois imagery. The poster for Vladivostok State Tobacco Factory makhorka made for a startling counter to its tuxedoed NEP-man. Here tobacco links with production rather than leisure (Figure 3.9). A worker, clad all in red, smokes a self-rolled "goat-leg" of makhorka while leaning on an oversized pack of the same.[52] The pack, produced twice, would be easily identified in street sellers' cases. Billed as "strong," this makhorka likely appealed to the more recent immigrant to the city. The setting evokes the transitional status of the smoker by placing him at the liminal zone between two worlds, the edge of a large field with a factory-studded city behind. The political and industrial productivity of his smoking can be read through his proximity to factories and his red attire.

At times, language, not visuals, took up the heavy work of revolutionary suggestion, such as tobacco products named after patriotic events, persons, or concepts—*Oktiabrina* (October), *Trudovye* (Labor), and the Leningrad Tobacco Trust's *Sten'ka Razin*, named for the seventeenth-century peasant rebel.[53] Before 1917, famous statesmen and generals had their brands too, but the explosion of Soviet propaganda made certain that the figures, names, and symbols would be changed to appeal to a different type of patriotism. Such naming cloaked the negative connotations of consumption with comforting revolutionary attire.[54]

Smychka (Worker-Peasant Alliance), with its visually arresting dual-sided pack, served an educational, agitational, and advertising purpose (Figure 3.10). The pack physically represents the alliance of worker and peasant on its competing faces. On either side, a red background frames a laboring male actively involved in socialist construction. A peasant male, with clean-shaven "modern"

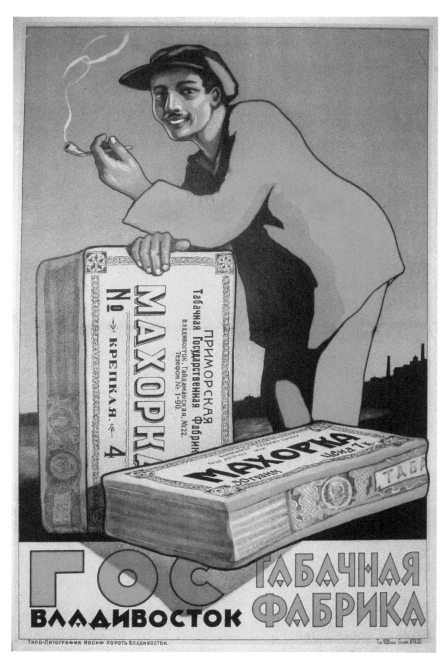

FIGURE 3.9. Poster. "State Tobacco Factory of Vladivostok Makhorka," 1926. Courtesy Russian State Library.

face but iconic cotton shirt and sowing basket, prepares to scatter seed onto a presumably freshly turned field. On the obverse, the stereotypical "every worker"—the blacksmith—readies his sledgehammer to assist in construction (or destruction?). For the buyer, the pack shows the link between worker and peasant in concrete terms—both labored together in a red-infused world. They are pictured in the act of doing rather than completing. The future of their labors is off-screen. The future of the consumer is shielded within the pack—twenty-five second-sort papirosy from the Leningrad-based Uritskii Factory, waiting to be ignited and inhaled while the revolutionary code of the visuals could be further contemplated. The message of *smychka*, unlike a piece of propaganda on the factory floor or on a city wall, came along with the buyers as a symbol of their politics and an education for the uninformed. Each pack implied an act of revolutionary sympathy with purchase and prompted continued consumption.[55]

Not everyone appreciated attempts to make tobacco revolutionary. A 1924 piece in *Krokodil* joked that the new papirosa from Leningrad Tobacco named *Oktiabrina,* with a beautiful woman on the pack, would soon be followed by one of a smoking boy named for the popular slogan—"Children are the future."[56] But just as there were those who resisted the marketing of tobacco, so did many oppose the marketing of health. Workers did not trust the abstemious communist, and some youth flaunted poor behavior and smoking as evidence of affiliation with the masses.[57] At the meeting of the fifth Komsomol congress, Bukharin disparaged the tendency of youth to overplay smoking as rebellious and scorn all norms—smoking four papirosy at a meeting, spitting on the floor, and being as rough as possible.[58]

Advertisers did not invent the association of tobacco with the revolution. Tobacco's addictive qualities helped it maintain users, but the social pressure of tobacco's near omnipresence among soldiers and the working class cemented its status as a habit of the people. Tobacco had fueled the Red Army and clouded the meetings of soviets.[59] Lenin himself realized, despite his personal animosity to the habit, the need for "food, tobacco, and other necessities" for the Red Army in its fight against Denikin.[60] The French visitor Henri Beraud depicted tobacco as a necessity of the revolutionary state: "The real misery of Sovietism is not in the street but in housing. Those acrid cigarettes in boxes of alien design, what a lot of them I have burnt as I sat on broken-springed sofas! In Moscow you smoke as much as you possibly can so as not to be conscious of the room. The samovar bubbles noiselessly. You try and fill yourself up with tea and tobacco."[61] The scent of cheap makhorka marked the spaces of the people allowing intellectuals to distinguish the true revolutionary groups.[62] Contemporaries recalled the smoke that hung over every meeting of the soviet in Smolny and the piles of butts that littered the floors and desks. Scent and litter marked the revolutionary

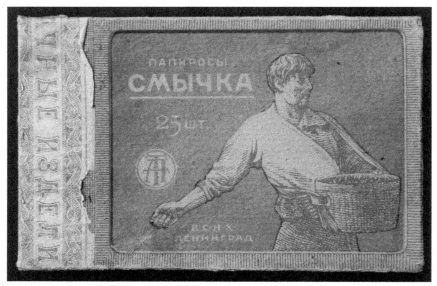

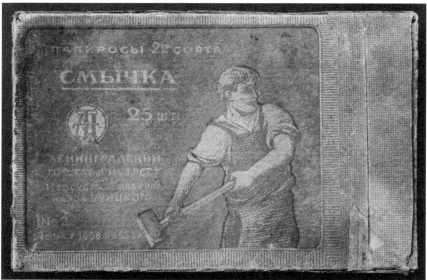

FIGURE 3.10. Photo. Two-sided pack of *Smychka*. Undated. Courtesy of Productive Arts. Russian/Soviet-era posters, books, publications, graphics—1920s–1950s. www.productivearts.com

space and in turn communicated the message that revolutionary activity smelled of smoke and looked chaotic. As N. N. Sukhanov remarked in his memoir, in Smolny "everything was dirty and untidy and smelt of cheap tobacco, boots and damp greatcoats."[63]

The connections were clear. Tobacco was named for communist events. Communists smoked tobacco. Smoking tobacco made one more communist. The poster for *Sovetskie* (Soviet) took this overtly political naming and deployed propaganda symbols, and even the prerevolutionary brand *Senatorskii* (Senators), as a political foil (Figure 3.11). The poster appeared early, somewhere between 1917 and 1920, an extraordinary time for advertising papirosy, since production was nearly at a standstill and paper scarce. Trying to build a market when papirosy were rationed seems an odd choice. In the poster a stereotypical figure personifies each of the brands. A diminutive, shriveled, old man represents *Senatorskie*. Balding and misshapen, he holds an oversized pack in one hand and a fuming papirosa in the other. *Sovetskie* brand's robust representative hoists this malformed man of the past aloft with one strong arm while cradling an even larger pack of his own papirosy in the other. The poster—with its dominant blonde and blue-eyed figure, smoking comfortably, stronger, younger, and with a larger pack of bigger papirosy—and the slogan make clear the political position and virile promise that came with the new order: "We don't smoke *Senators*—give us *Soviets!*" It also implied a different effect on health than Semashko's propaganda threatened.

The advertisement for the low-grade, loose makhorka *Moriak i chaika* (Sailor and Seagull) brought this makhorka into the new world by featuring in the background a fully outfitted battleship, plowing through rough, technicolor seas (Figure 3.12). Given the association of the best tobacco regions with areas of Crimea and the Black Sea coast, a sailor was an evocative choice, but the vibrant coloring and jubilant pose imply a smoke more joyous than combative. The poster also employs a long-standing association of tobacco with the military, and particularly with sailors, who believed it a preventative of scurvy.

The poster for Saratov Makhorka no. 8 moves the political message forward by deploying the revolutionary triumvirate, with the soldier at top towering over the two seated co-revolutionaries of lower status (Figure 3.13). The active positioning, plus the firearm and official uniform, make him the most powerful of the pyramid. The worker on the right wears the smock of perhaps a printer or blacksmith, indicating his membership in urban, politically conscious groups. He chomps on a papirosa suitably called *Proletarian*. The figure on the left enjoys self-rolled, low-grade makhorka from the packs advertised at top and bottom. His facial hair and bound leggings denote a peasant. His red shirt conveys his political consciousness. Again, tobacco brings together the men who made the

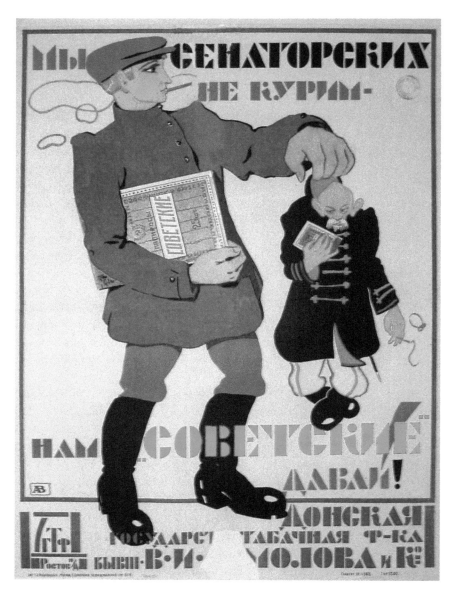

FIGURE 3.11. Poster. "We Won't Smoke *Senators!*," 1917–1920. Courtesy Russian State Library.

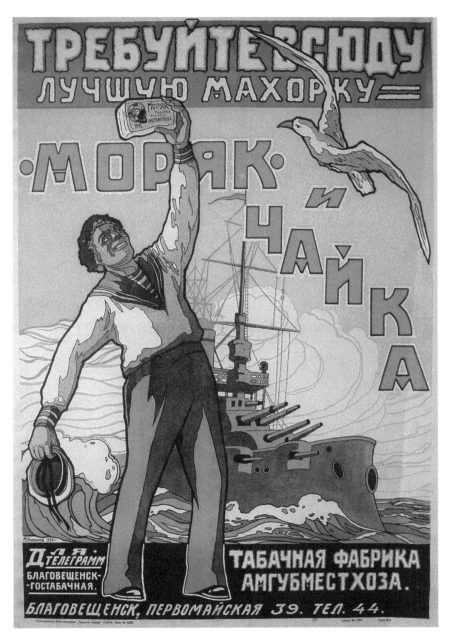

FIGURE 3.12. Poster. "Advertisement for *Moriak i chaika*," 1926–1929. Courtesy Russian State Library.

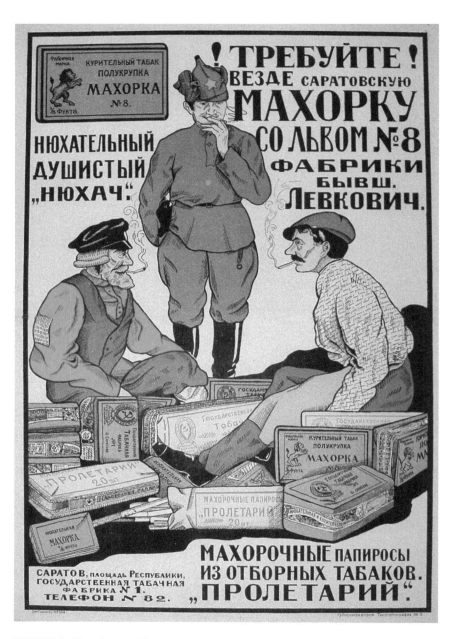

FIGURE 3.13. Poster. "Ask for It Everywhere—Saratov Makhorka," 1921–1925. Courtesy Russian State Library.

revolution, who now relax from the hard business of politics and production as they contemplate the taste of their politically suitable smokes.

Even as tobacco brought users together, the type consumed became a marker of revolutionary progress. In the crusade to make workers and peasants Soviet, even smoking patterns gained dialectics of progress and consciousness. This echoed earlier European concepts that the march of civilization could be seen in the assumption of more refined, discriminating tastes.[64] Communist consumption trumped the modest and utilitarian and showcased methods of production that lionized labor.[65] In 1926 D. Sokolovskii connected the smoker's progression through tobacco types as a cultural and political evolution. He claimed that peasants would "move undoubtedly with the rise of culture from using makhorka to yellow tobacco."[66] Economic planners attempted to force tobacco consciousness. Prices for lower and higher sorts of tobacco were manipulated to mold behaviors and attempt to change tastes.[67] In 1925 the Rosa Luxemburg Factory of Rostov-on-Don tried to discourage makhorka smokers by raising the price on it even as they decreased prices on higher grades. Reporting on the matter, *Krokodil* sarcastically depicted the factory administrators as ill-advised though well-intentioned.[68] Although the campaign against makhorka nominally engaged health issues, as with many hygiene campaigns, political and social concerns hid in the shadows. Author Mikhail Bulgakov brought life to the social progression of the smoker through products in his short story "The Rotten Intelligentsia." As the character moves through the NEP-man trajectory from university-educated doctor to working for an artel and profiting from the tainted capitalist economy, the protagonist goes from smoking roll-your-own makhorka to *Ira* papirosy, which he carries around in a metal syringe case. Here, instead of consciousness, progression in tobacco quality signified the character's creeping political rot.[69]

Alternatively presented as for health or culture, a more useful means of understanding the campaign against makhorka was control. In the campaigns against both home brew and makhorka there was a concern for tax revenues. While attacks were picking up on makhorka, the government battled peasants brewing their own alcohol—although there the quest for control was presented primarily as concern over grain loss. By encouraging the growing number of smokers to consume higher-quality tobacco that was more easily counted and taxed, the state could weather financial crises with a consumer item of near constant demand.[70] According to one anti-tobacco author, peasants smoked makhorka at a rate of what would have been eighteen rubles a year if they bought it from state dealers. They tended to grow their own.[71] Their self-sufficiency situated them outside state revenue streams.

Be it cultured smoker or peasant puffer, placing smokers within a community had been a tactic for some time. Prerevolutionary advertisements urged smokers

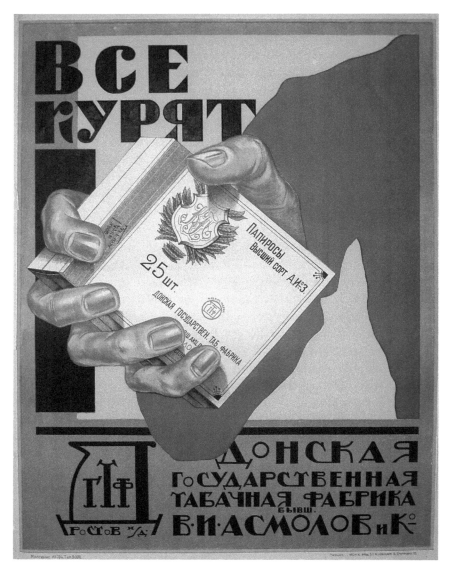

FIGURE 3.14. Poster. "Everyone Smokes," 1923. Artist Aleksei Zaniatov (attributed). Courtesy Russian State Library.

to become part of the in crowd, the urban group, or the fashionable set by smoking the correct brand. Gender, clothing, and setting signaled cliques to which one might aspire, and slogans cemented the deal. The artist Aleksei Zaniatov produced such a communal call in his 1923 poster for DGTF (Figure 3.14). The graphic arrests the viewers' attention with a massive hand thrusting out with a large pack of papirosy and a simple call—"Everyone smokes."[72] The slogan implies the popularity of the habit and the brand. The exclusion of any identifying markers for the user, and pusher, make smoking anonymous and transferrable. The way the elbow breaks the frame indicates a connection to the faceless, anonymous man across space. Every smoker could envision themselves as part of this group. No identifiable spokesperson guides the audience because the product, and the community around it, were bigger than one individual.

A vision of people working together to produce a larger outcome infused propagandistic treatments in the period, and a 1928 Crimean tobacco products poster borrowed this appeal (Figure 3.15).[73] Using the symbolism of dawn as the stand-in for the utopian, socialist future, the poster shows many small, faceless, nameless figures working together for a greater cause. Instead of laboring to raise a socialist dream world, the mass instead admires the outpouring from the future of "the best papirosy" including brands like *Klub* (Club), *Motor* (Motor), *Yalta* (Yalta), and more. The communist future, it seems, would include lots of tobacco. Even markers of class and gender are scrubbed from the silhouettes, with only their shared adulation for the products appearing and communicated to the viewer.

Tiny consumers similarly populate the poster of the Sukhumi State Tobacco Factory (Figure 3.16). Cartoonish workers, clerks, peasants, and even a NEP-woman in short skirt and visible stockings run toward the cascade of tobacco packs tumbling from the machine. Two stereotypically drawn Turkish figures haul the device, to some unknown purpose, as they smoke and look with delight at the darting figures. Here the makers and source of tobacco are merged because presumably the tobacco comes from the areas of the Black Sea. The poster set out a vision where the product dwarfs the buyer in importance. The figures drawn in two dimensions and illustrated in black and white pale in comparison to the detailed, vibrant drawings of the tobacco packs and leering Turks, underscoring, along with the size of the massive machine, the hierarchy of production over people.

The late 1920s poster for the *Nobless* (Noblesse) brand of Crimea cut out the consumer entirely in preference for a red-infused chain of technology, transport, and trains (Figure 3.17). For a throwback name like *Nobless*, perhaps it was best to ignore the implied buyer. Instead, the glories of the new Soviet system received red highlighting from the top right, including the stock train, the telephone operator, the factory with plumes of smoke, the truck, the docks, the seller, the handcart pusher, and the pink buildings, perhaps warehouses, at top left. Packs of tobacco circle the poster, but smokers are barely evident. There is seemingly only one smoker: the man hauling a box of *Nobless* at bottom right has a papirosa clenched in his mouth. No plumes of tobacco smoke loft about.

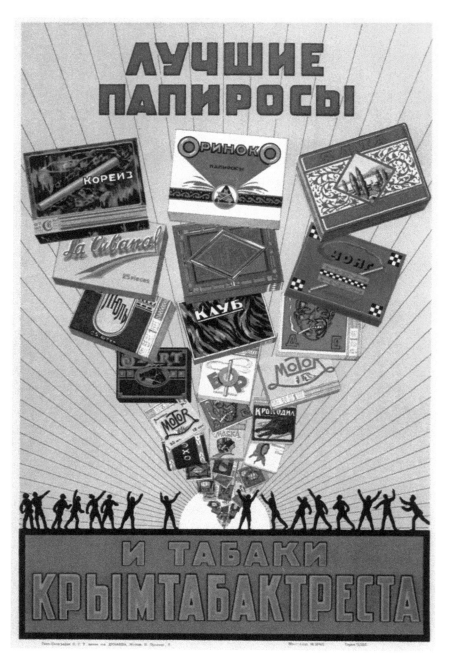

FIGURE 3.15. Poster. "The Best Papirosy," 1928. Courtesy Russian State Library.

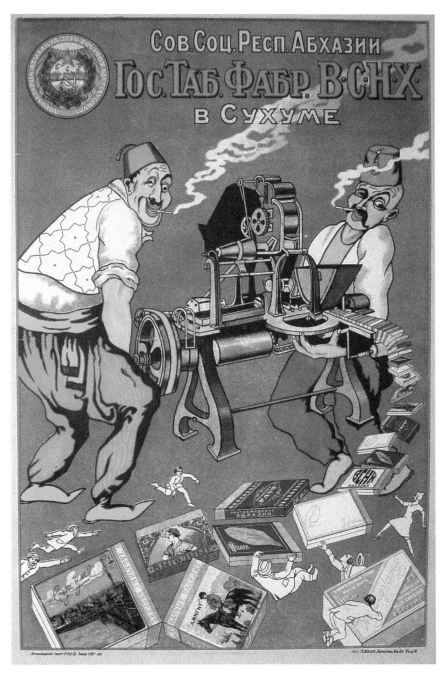

FIGURE 3.16. Poster. "State Tobacco Factory VSNKh," 1921–1925. Courtesy Russian State Library.

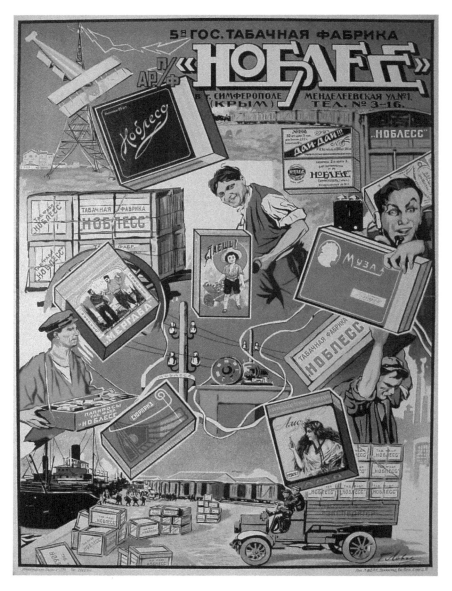

FIGURE 3.17.   Poster. "Advertisement for *Nobless*," 1926–1929. Courtesy Russian State Library.

The only things in the air are the crackle of a signal from a radio tower, the wire of the telephone and telegraph, and the yellow biplane. The entire production cycle receives detailed treatment, but consumption of the product is tangential. The message of productive consumption has come to the point of nearly cutting out consumption entirely.

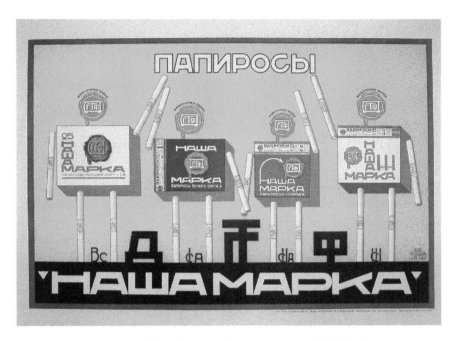

FIGURE 3.18.   Poster. "Advertisement for *Nasha marka*," 1926. Courtesy Russian State Library.

The 1926 poster for DGTF's *Nasha marka* (Our Brand) took the negation of the user in favor of production to its conclusion by replacing the buyer with the product (Figure 3.18). In the poster, which combines the tropes of revolutionary propaganda and styles of constructivist art, four boxes of papirosy personify revolutionary figures reduced to constituent shapes fashioned from papirosy tubes and rectangular packs. The two central packs indicate, spatially and physically, a stereotypical alliance of male and female, with one pack larger than the other and forward while the other appears more diminutive and set to the back. In their construction, these papirosy people echo science-fiction visions of robotic futures and machine men. The tobacco automatons join hands and raise arms. The packs on either side similarly raise arms in celebration or perhaps shared victory. Behind them, the factory acronym becomes a stylized version of the factory's buildings and pipes. The smoker transmutes into the product within a politicized composition with a politically motivated artistic form bent on bringing art and rationalization into production and consumption.[74]

Revolutionary art and tobacco unite in avant-garde visuals and buildings. The 1929 *Urtak* poster from Uzbekistan caricatures the smoker as product with his teeth the factory name, the smokestacks his monocle, and the jumble of packs

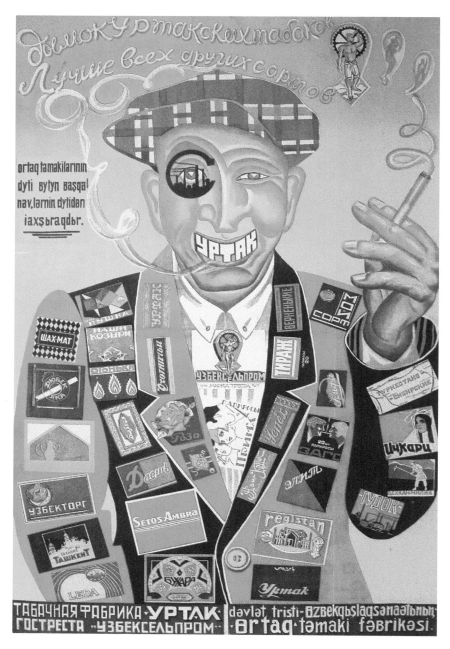

FIGURE 3.19. Poster. "Advertisement for *Urtak*," 1929. Artist Mariia Aleksandrovna Nesterova-Berzina. Courtesy Russian State Library.

combining to form him; he is a creation of the packaging—a kind of papirosa Frankenstein's monster (Figure 3.19). Even the smoke is performing multiple functions, becoming on top right the brand seal (as echoed in his tie) and at top left a slogan for the brand, "The smoke from *Urtak* tobacco is better than all other types." The same slogan appears in the Azerbaijani language in type at left. The female designer of the *Urtak* poster, M. A. Nesterova-Berzina, broke barriers with her life and art. Other avant-garde figures dabbled in tobacco. The iconoclastic architect K. S. Mel'nikov performed one of his first commissions with the Makhorka Pavilion at the 1923 All-Russian Agricultural Exhibition. The building— all angles and beams and ambition—turned heads and won him general acclaim and visibility for the makhorka syndicate. The year after, Mel'nikov won the right to design the sarcophagus for Lenin.[75]

A 1925 poster for DGTF encapsulates the fractured nature of 1920s tobacco visuals and advertisements—educating the consumer even as it attempts to woo (Figure 3.20). A procession of figures slide past an altar framed by a ludicrously sized pack from DGTF. The papirosy—*Nasha marka*—underscore the democratic availability of the product, and the pantheon of different people infers an equality of use, but the poster implies that not all consumers are created equal. Males stand at the highest and lowest levels of the ladder—gender does not clarify placement here. Nor did using the product. The two women are not smoking, even as the males are. The relationship of each figure to production, not consumption, guarantees their spot, showing the persistence of production as the underlying gauge of product worth.[76]

The various characters of the NEP era—male, female, worker, peasant—all march by the tobacco altar in a clear hierarchy. From left to right, they proceed from level of highest to lowest consciousness.[77] Males occupy the top rungs of the social ladder, each one clenching a papirosa in his teeth, cementing their status as the most enlightened form of citizen and dedicated smokers. The first two—the familiar Red Army soldier in uniform and boots, and the worker, in smock and wielding a hammer—are not surprising. An urbanite replaces the triumvirate's expected peasant. His glasses, briefcase, and hat betray him as a desk worker. This may have reflected the tensions with peasants regarding supply of tobacco and other agricultural products or perhaps recognition that city bureaucrats were more likely to consume prepared tobacco. Contemporaries recognized smoking as especially widespread, "among all workers of mental labors, so that they may appear, as it were, more professional."[78]

In the center, looking down at the pack, stands one of the two females. Clothing and placement indicate the status and social role for each. The woman at center, in fashionable bobbed hair and a smart hat, looks like a modern woman, and the red bow of communist sympathy and the folder of papers under her arm

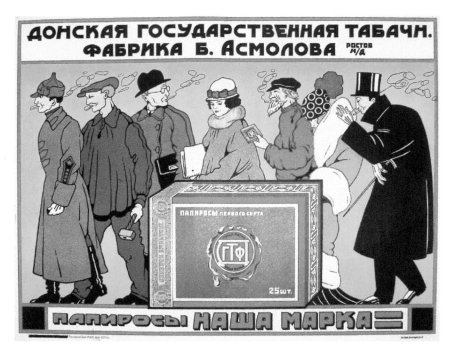

FIGURE 3.20.   Poster. "Advertisement for *Nasha marka*," 1925. Artist Aleksei Zaniatov. Courtesy Russian State Library.

indicate that she works, unlike the frivolous, parasitic, NEP-woman to her right. The composition separates her slightly from the clerk in front of her and the peasant behind her, signposting that she is not a member of the revolutionary leaders, but she is more conscious and not as denigrated as the three behind her. Her lack of physical proximity to the males, unlike the NEP-woman, suggests her personal distance from them and less sexually available nature. While she does not have a papirosa, she looks down at the pack with curiosity, and the peasant behind her offers up his. Perhaps she will soon be smoking or does not partake in public.[79]

The final three figures are not yet saved by smoking. In a parody of church rites, proximity to the altar of tobacco is an indication of communist redemption, and these three have not fully passed the portal of the pack into full consciousness. The bureaucrat's backward glance, directed at either the peasant or the NEP-man, intimates he may not yet have thrown off his backward ways. The peasant male, in red blouse and with a white beard, smokes but has not yet made it to the level of the working female. His liminal status coincides with other depictions in which both had yet to be fully divorced from the past. Still, there are signs they could be redeemed. His red blouse indicates at least his potential, but he is the only aged figure, a nod to the place of the peasantry in the past and not the future. The last two figures, both in the evening wear that associates them with nonproductive leisure, are further tainted by the indications of impropriety. The proximity of the NEP-woman to the peasant in front of her and the touch of the NEP-man's gloved hand on her fur collar indicate her physicality and sexuality. Her slight separation from the NEP-man and the near overlapping of her body with the peasant male hints that she might be redeemed. Even though he smokes, the bourgeois man is far separated from the others, perhaps a sign of how far he has to go to become a true communist connoisseur.

The Soviet smoker did not get the same inducements for tobacco as advertisers used in other global contexts because of the unique economic and social conditions of the 1920s. As the regime balanced between small-scale capitalism and revolutionary change, tobacco messaging fluctuated. Before the revolution, manly, militaristic images and appeals to a bourgeois connoisseurship held sway; after the fall of capitalism, such messaging remained in small part, but much of the market began to "speak Bolshevik" and triumph tobacco consumption that conformed to the prevailing ideology.[80] Perhaps this reflected the uneasy place of consumption within the NEP era. The NEP-men, bent on enriching themselves through capitalist means of getting and spending, were seen as necessary for the economic recovery of the state. They were building the industrial foundations for the eventual jump to socialism. Yet ideologically driven revolutionaries cringed from contact with these contaminated elements of a past exploitative system.[81] NEP-era tobacco advertisements strayed from international tobacco imagery, where smoking was often depicted in leisure settings or as a lubricant to social contacts. Instead, productive images wed to consumption allowed smoking to rise above base appetites and frivolous pursuits. The political aspects of Soviet smoking posters set them apart.

Despite the Bolshevik flavor, other elements of tobacco imagery are remarkably like prerevolutionary visions and those of western markets. Smoking was militarized. It was depicted as a habit that created inclusive communities. Tobacco choice could indicate shared values and aspirations. The image and packaging of tobacco was not important just as an inducement to smoke. Product choice, packaging, and display could make a communal identity that was legible to even a passing stranger with a glimpse of a pack. Tobacco use and choice remained an important part of creating a legible self in the anonymous city. Only now the self was red.

TREATED

Individual Will and Collective Therapy

According to the mental health specialist Dr. Aleksandr Sergeevich Sholomovich, smokers in Moscow had heard and understood the propaganda and wanted to quit. In 1928 he explained: "Each one of them feels the great danger of nicotine for their health. It tortures them. They are prepared to discard their disgusting habit, but they are unable to do so without the help of a doctor."[1] The Moscow Regional Health Department, often at the forefront of new public health initiatives, stepped in by expanding its specialized dispensaries devoted to treatment of abuse of alcohol and other intoxicants to aid smokers.[2] The dispensary model combined doctor consultations, nurse home visitations, and educational instruction, providing care for those with social diseases (e.g., tuberculosis, syphilis, alcoholism, etc.) while allowing patients to continue work.[3] The decision to fight tobacco in this system made sense considering the perceived similarities. One author stated that tobacco represented "the same persistent bad habit and disease" as "the abuse of alcohol, morphine, cocaine, and other narcotics."[4] This early provision of cessation therapy set Soviet smoking policy apart from the rest of the globe.

Sholomovich did not understate demand. So many smokers wanted to quit that they overwhelmed the system, and authorities had to replace individual therapy with mass sessions involving fifty to eighty people to one doctor. According to Sholomovich, this gave "serious and valuable results" and allowed the dispensary "to more widely satisfy the broad desire for this method."[5] Whereas in 1924 thirty to forty people a month signed up, after a district campaign applications climbed to a thousand per month.[6] With the treatment centers overwhelmed, therapy was limited to only those smokers with tuberculosis. Yet again patients outstripped facilities.[7] In 1927 three thousand smokers availed themselves of revolutionary, state-funded, anti-tobacco therapy at one of the two dispensaries that undertook such work.[8] In 1928 eight thousand smokers flooded the system, and enrollments were cut off.[9]

Despite the popularity of dispensary methods, success varied. A 1924 experiment at one of the dispensaries tracked one hundred smoking tuberculosis patients who were provided individual hypnotherapy from an experienced practitioner over the course of two to three months with nurse follow-up. Sholomovich determined, "hypnotherapy had no type of serious effect on smokers ... The large expenditure of time and energy by the doctor and patient emerged as ineffective, with only a 5–7 percent success rate, and that over time." Psychotherapy had a slightly better success rate of 6–10 percent.[10] A 1926 *Izvestiia* story reported: "Thousands of smokers came to the dispensary with the request for help ... Only 10 percent of patients have been able to heal from smoking, much lower than among alcoholics."[11] Sholomovich observed: "Despite the mass failures, many smokers seek out treatment, and we have many individuals engage in almost futile smoking therapy."[12] Even today, cessation is difficult, with only 5 percent of smokers able to quit on any one attempt.[13] Yet in 1928 Sholomovich reported that when accompanied by health lectures, explanations of the conditioned reflex, and workplace smoking prohibitions, the Soviet dispensary method enjoyed a success rate of 40–50 percent.[14]

The faith in communal influences for explaining why people started smoking, why they continued, and how they should quit fit with the Soviet emphasis on the collective. Antismoking authors theorized that societal pressures tempted youth to start smoking and kept them smoking. To counter this, they employed pressure from family members, social acquaintances, and therapy groups. Therapies also swayed to the science of the times, so that hypnosis and reflexology had their adherents, as did a neurasthenia-inspired focus on strengthening the will with physical culture and hygienic regimens. Contemporary understandings of tobacco as not addictive further influenced Soviet therapies and their dismissal of biological reasons for continued smoking. Although the dispensaries were popular, competing advice on how to quit or to smoke "safely" revealed the still contentious understanding of exactly how dangerous smoking was and what made people continue. Negative reviews from some dispensary patients further undermined the institution's cessation efforts.

Like the earlier attempt at anti-tobacco legislation, Soviet cessation clinics had a mixed legacy. Forward-thinking and unique in their early appearance, exciting in their identification of the problem, innovative in their combination of social and psychological methods, they still failed to live up to their promises. These efforts, however, left a tantalizing vision of the possibility of early public health intervention against tobacco had it continued. It was not to be. The changeover in leadership at Narkomzdrav, coupled with diminishing anti-tobacco propaganda and increased production of tobacco, signaled a major change in government attitudes toward supporting and encouraging cessation.

Neurasthenic Decline and Childhood Uptake

Soviet medical authorities did not recognize tobacco as addictive, or even unequivocally harmful. Addiction—continuation of use despite knowledge of harm—was a complicated issue in a period when tobacco was not universally understood as harmful and when withdrawal symptoms from nicotine were unrecognized. Most anti-tobacco authors contended that tobacco dependency was a problem of mind/will, not brain/body, and therefore an issue of nerves and psychological weakness, not biological dependency with recognized withdrawal symptoms (like cocaine or alcohol).[15] The story of Lenin's youthful flirtation with tobacco, penned by the popular satirist Mikhail Zoshchenko, revealed the general attitude toward tobacco uptake, dependency, and quitting among the Soviet public and medical community. According to the tale, Lenin began smoking as a schoolboy to fit in with the young men around him. Confronted by his mother over the cost of tobacco and the strain on her meager pension, he put down the pack, never to smoke again. Zoshchenko enthused that "weak-willed people" turned to tinctures that changed the taste of smoke or suggestions from doctors to strengthen their resolve, but "Lenin had an enormous will. Without any doctors, he decided to quit smoking. And he quit for real. And never again smoked. He was a strong person with an iron will. And all people need to be just like him."[16]

The prolific health author D. N. Lukashevich gave similarly terse advice on how to quit. In his 1925 *"The Harmless Habit" (Tobacco Smoking)*, he elevated tobacco to the point of a national threat. To answer the question of why Soviets smoked, Lukashevich turned to an 1890 essay from the Russian author and moralist Lev Nikolaevich Tolstoy. Lukashevich gleaned from Tolstoy's "Why Do Men Stupefy Themselves?" a conclusion that tobacco, like alcohol, functioned to relieve feelings of disquiet, whether of moral failing or monotony, and appealed to all levels of society. Instead of relying on research in the fields of psychology, physiology, reflexology, or even statistical data, Lukashevich jumped from Tolstoy's depiction of smoking as a moral failure to dismiss smokers' tales of compulsion as minor. He argued: "it is just a habit, and not a physiological need . . . the difficulties of stopping smoking are overblown. When a person's health is suffering and he says that smoking is burdening him with too serious a cost, he always finds in himself the strength to quit."[17] His therapeutic recommendations were basic—fresh air, physical culture, and vigorous rubbing with a wet towel.[18] He proposed that no replacement therapy or slow easing was required: "An authentically conscious, authentically masculine and decisive person does not participate in such self-delusion."[19]

Just as the papirosa butt signified a cultural decline greater than the object itself, so too did continued smoking betray a greater difficulty—the decline of will, crisis of masculinity, and onset of neurasthenia. As Sholomovich pointed out, "the vast majority of smokers are unhappy with their habit and feel its danger, and all are ready to stop tobacco. [But] without the willpower to stop, they become unhappy, irritable, bilious neurasthenics."[20] The emphasis on the willpower of the smoker as a root cause allowed for smoking to be a manifestation of social issues and required the least resource-intensive treatments—exercise, self-control, and sport.[21] Authors maintained this was easier with smoking than with alcohol and within anyone's strength.[22]

One pamphlet compared tobacco to alcohol's physical and social effects and warned "early smokers also are early drinkers," cautioning that "tobacco and spirits are good friends." The author attributed this kinship to physical changes, since "a smoker does not like sweets and often loses taste and appetite. In exchange he receives a strong desire for spirits. Smokers almost always drink. . . [and] bring to their health a double danger."[23] Even the public emphasized the two together. A letter to the newspaper *Izvestiia* proposed that the fight against public drunkenness should be joined by a battle against public smoking.[24] Authors argued both endangered order, health, and political progress.[25] Ia. I. Lifshits warned pioneers they must fight tobacco and alcohol as they "soften consciousness," imparting feelings of "ease and joy" while "degrading work ability and health." Ultimately, "smoking and drinking free a pioneer from the self-control of political consciousness and discipline."[26] Reasons for smoking were usually backed up with anecdotes or ideology, not statistics. One author guessed that smokers continued not for any chemical compulsion but because of various character failings or the convenience of tobacco: "tobacco drowns their remorse at poor life choices . . . they smoke so as to forget some type of sorrow or suffering that they carry in their soul. Or they smoke simply from boredom or festively, without the free time to fulfill a more healthful pastime, thanks to the fact that tobacco items take up so little space that they may be taken in one's pocket (alcohol is more difficult to carry always with oneself)."[27] A 1926 manual echoed a similar reasoning. Tobacco carried away "depressing thoughts and worries."[28]

The difficulty was teasing out what sickness was a result of smoking and what of society. According to one author, although sickness could come from many factors, the fact that smokers were often sickly implicated tobacco.[29] Others situated the problem in society, especially the social effects of capitalism. Just as alcoholism rose from "circumstances of labor, low pay, disgusting housing and poor food, lack of means for maintaining family and raising children," so did it cause smoking. He argued that the "predatory capitalism of the city and its smoke and soot, with its furious movement, with its immeasurably high demand on the strength and endurance of a person" brought on exhaustion, nervous fatigue, and the deterioration of the organism. To whip up declining strength, a person became addicted to tobacco smoke or guzzling "miraculous" vodka.[30] According to the prolific health author Sazhin, like the religion utilized by capitalists to hinder worker consciousness, so too did alcohol and tobacco serve to keep workers insensate, sluggish, and complacent. Sazhin conceded that the habitual smoker might discover "satisfaction, and also some kind of use," in smoking, but science "finds that this is incorrect. There is no type of use [to smoking,] and the dangers are very many."[31] Authors maintained that older smokers deluded themselves into continuing their habit through irrational commentaries on "usefulness." Nezlin snapped, "Only people who are not accustomed to deep thought consider that they smoke for the taste and satisfaction."[32] For B. S. Sigal, a prolific author of health pamphlets, tobacco was irrational from all perspectives. It was a food product without nutritional value. It risked industrial accidents and hampered productivity. It served as a means for damaging the health of workers and consumers. It fouled the air and ruined social gatherings. Sigal concluded that there was no utility to tobacco, and the only reason people continued to smoke was because it "stupefies."[33]

Although many dismissed anything besides irrational preference, others proposed some compulsion to continued smoking. Violin called smokers "sick, 'obsessive' people" who needed help "weaning" away from their dependency.[34] This echoed diagnoses of cocaine or morphine addicts as having "dependent or compulsive" personalities.[35] One author cautioned that those who could become accustomed to smoking would start to be "pulled to tobacco," feeling that it "gives them more strength and stamina."[36] Another referred to the effects of tobacco on mood as a reason for continued smoking, because tobacco can "act in a stimulating manner on the brain, causing a temporary revival of the spirit, improving the state of mind, dispelling melancholy, etc." He attributed this to a rush of blood, which caused "overexcitation of the brain."[37] One researcher proposed that smoking provided "a pleasant feeling of complete relaxation and semiconsciousness," which altered perceptions so that "things begin to change their places, walls to move apart, all around with increasing speed rises above, while the smoker himself precipitously falls below and experiences an extremely pleasant feeling of a sinking heart." After growing accustomed to these effects, a smoker without tobacco experienced "nervousness" and "fussiness," and his work suffered while he waited "impatiently until he [could] again have some tobacco," until the feeling became "so strong and bright" as to be impossible to live through and "habit became necessity."[38]

The perceived benefits from tobacco to strength and stamina, authors argued, were a misperception of neurasthenic symptoms. Tobacco damaged the nervous system, confused perception, and overloaded the brain. One author proposed that tobacco countered the "constant movement" of modern life. The organism requires breaks, and tobacco "artfully lessens the excitation of our nervous system" but ends with the "destruction of the organism."[39] Chronic poisoning with nicotine inflamed the body, resulting in *tabakizmuz* or *nikotinizm*.[40] A doctor suggested that some became "enslaved" and "unable to step away," which unveiled a basic problem in an individual's constitution, and, especially in youth and women, "without dispute, the appearance cannot be called normal."[41] He took a similar stance in his discussions of morphine addicts, where a "predisposition" led to problems. This reference to organic weakness among smokers brought theories of tobacco dependency into line with those of alcohol dependency and neurasthenia generally. [42] Sazhin conceded, though, that even "people apparently with strong wills and self-possession become confused, depressed, and miserable . . . the slaves of nicotine."[43]

Many authors perceived a widespread crisis of the will arising from nervous exhaustion brought on by the political, social, and economic crises of war and civil turmoil. Additionally, the move of many from physical work to office jobs and mental labor and the draining effects of hectic, modern, urban life were considered as leading to the neglect of the body and the creation of a generation without willpower.[44] Discussion of the will increased in Russia in the revolutionary period, and political concerns emerged in degeneracy diagnoses that proposed that capitalism caused neurasthenia.[45] The depletion of the physical and mental force of the population, among youth especially, was evidenced in a wave of neurasthenia and hysteria diagnoses. A railway health investigation of 1924 reported that 7,260 workers had tuberculosis, 12,423 had syphilis, and a stunning 58,065 had hysteria and/or neurasthenia.[46]

Worries over tobacco's role in neurasthenia melded with general concerns over degeneration. Nezlin devoted an entire chapter to the question of how "tobacco weakens the brain and spoils the character." He detailed the similar effects of tobacco and alcohol. Neither of them gave courage or bettered work, but instead alcohol, and to a lesser extent tobacco, "silence[d] the voice of reason." Tobacco provided false relaxation and increased criminality. Citing international examples, he claimed that of one hundred criminals, ninety would be smokers; similarly of one hundred insane, ninety-three would be smokers. Nezlin found most disturbing the ways in which smokers celebrated their habits: "In spite of this, there are men and women who flaunt their smoking even though they should be ashamed. Some even perversely taunt nonsmokers in a group. The great strength of the habit to poor conduct is such that one becomes so accustomed to bad behavior as to consider it beauty."[47]

This crisis of neurasthenia was not a political contortion to distract the population or explain an imagined problem. The massive demographic changes of war, civil war, disease, and famine, which had resulted in an overall loss of some 15–20 million people from a population of only about 140 million, haunted the plans of revolutionaries and the hopes of medical reformers.[48] An additional incentive to fulminate on the will, strength, vitality, and potency of the male population likely came from the imbalances in the ratio of men to women. The census of 1926 found only eighty-three males to every hundred females aged twenty to twenty-nine and only eighty-eight to every hundred over age thirty.[49] Real worries among the ruling elite about the number, stamina, and sexual potential of males provided the context for discussing tobacco dependency.

According to psychiatrists and hygienists, the development of the will coincided with the years of maturation. One doctor baldly stated, "tobacco is the death of youth" and that the unformed organism—in terms of the heart, nerves, digestion, and more psychologically important points of morality and will—was severely damaged by tobacco. He based his conclusions on studies of the mental ability of schoolchildren, young criminals, and delinquents.[50] Another author highlighted a connection among smoking, criminality, and morality.[51] The 1931 movie *The Road to Life* about 1920s street boys depicted smoking as integral to street life, as was criminal activity. It was certainly true that many youths smoked. A Moscow Komsomol group reported that 60–70 percent of members smoked, making it hard to find suitable operatives to go to the countryside.[52] Conversely, propaganda tracts made abstention a healthy and communist choice. Vasilevskii, who had shared his wisdom in pamphlets on hygiene for propagandists and young women, attacked smoking in his widely distributed 1925 *Pioneer Hygiene*, gravely stating that "he who smokes is not a pioneer."[53]

Narkomzdrav's preventative focus and new Soviet institutions fit well with the campaign against youth smoking. Child-care and educational facilities made children readily available for indoctrination, and activists thought children still malleable in terms of habits and consciousness and less warped by the holdovers of the past.[54] True to his social hygiene ethos, Semashko linked childhood smoking to poor environments because "the fragile children's organism is very susceptible to bad outside influences. The brain of the child forms, like soft wax, and takes deep within . . . the effects of daily life." Tobacco's poisonous effects manifested in the countryside, where "children age 8–10 almost openly smoke—getting papirosy and their butts through all means. . . [and] picking up butts presents another means for the horrible threat of syphilis." Semashko continued that teachers, to whom he attributed immense power, should be the first to confront the issue, declaring that if in the past teachers could "overthrow the reason of people with God," then Soviet teachers should be able to fight smoking.[55]

According to Sigal, stopping children from taking their first smoke could save them from a lifetime of regret, as many smokers learned of the danger but then were unable to quit. He concluded: "The first papirosa is the most dangerous. The first inhalation of tobacco smoke is the most terrible, just like the first glass for the future alcoholic."[56] Statistical studies confirmed that youth uptake was prevalent. A 1923–1924 study from Leningrad detailed 46 percent of respondents' age of tobacco uptake was fourteen to nineteen.[57] The observation that after age seventeen the number of new smokers dropped significantly was given as evidence that environmental factors, like bad family examples, were to blame.[58] Others looked to poor examples from other children or even smoking Komsomol members.[59] Sigal's 1927 script for an agitational mock trial, *The Trial of a Smoking Pioneer,* had one child smoking in imitation of adults and another continuing because if he quit, "kids at school would laugh and call me an old woman." The mock trial, a scripted propaganda exercise popular in worker clubs and for pioneer and Komsomol groups, allowed amateur theatrical reenactments of real life issues to be melded with didactic instruction. They often ended with the audience giving a verdict. That smoking would find its own scripted drama bespoke its political, social, and cultural importance.[60] After a set of lectures from other witnesses regarding the dangerous, infectious social diseases transmitted by papirosy butts, the harm to individual health from early smoking, and the provisions of the pioneer oath, the defense laid blame not just on the smoking child but on bad fathers setting poor examples. The children, now chastened, pled for and received leniency.[61]

Social Shaming and Therapeutic Suggestion

For those already smoking, quitting was the cure and propaganda—exhortation through posters, pamphlets, and speeches—the means. One doctor triumphed "knowledge of the danger of smoking" as the first step in fighting it.[62] Another prophesied, "Widespread agitation and propaganda are a threat to tobacco smoking."[63] He advocated a campaign like those against tuberculosis, venereal disease, and malaria.[64] Dr. Nezlin proclaimed that if the truth became known "in books [and] posters, in schools, and from doctors," the information would slowly spread and then people would see tobacco as "a holdover from the past."[65] The faith in the effectiveness of propaganda was strong. As another thundered, "If simple religious arguments could keep a person from smoking, then it is impossible that science could be weaker than religion."[66] Sazhin similarly upheld the effect of scientific reasoning: "They are already the slaves of nicotine. The only thing that can free them from this slavery is strength of will coming from a scientific foundation, *a bright awareness* of the situation."[67]

An entire movement to get children to agitate against adult behaviors, particularly drinking and smoking, became part of the health campaigns in the 1920s.[68] In 1926 a young girl at a conference of school health cells crowed, "We fight smoking in the school and in the family."[69] A few months later, a magazine reported of another school health cell where they put on an anti-tobacco lecture and exhibition.[70] Sholomovich encouraged children to agitate against their parents' smoking by pointing out the dangers of tuberculosis and the rudeness of the habit.[71] As he barked, stopping smoking would come not with laws and decrees but by taking the fight to the "family, school and state institutions, dormitories, and all associations."[72] By attacking what he called the "papirosa infection," a dual goal could be reached—discouraging adult smoking and immunizing children from bad adult examples.[73] Nezlin encouraged pioneers to spread the anti-tobacco message to "fathers and elders."[74]

Sholomovich reported on enlisting children as "active fighters for hygienic lifestyles" and boasted that groups of children in thirty different schools had aligned with the antismoking movement under the rather unwieldy slogan: "We children do not judge the smoker, but we ask of him that he not brag of his bad manners publicly, that he not give children a bad example, and that he not spoil the air that others breathe." The shorter version little improved it: "Smoke where and as much as you want, as long as it disturbs no one. Public smoking we will prosecute." In both, the sting was ameliorated by a promise not to judge or persecute, but the admonishments to not have bad manners, be a poor example, or spoil the air of others all brought with them a great deal of judgment.[75]

Penetrating the walls of the home was essential to a successful fight with tobacco. In a 1925 letter to the magazine *Za novyi byt* an inspired youth wrote of how, after a doctor's lecture at school: "I went home and wrote a slogan with red ink on white paper, 'Smoking is harmful,' and 'smoking is shameful.' Perhaps my father, who smokes a lot, will learn of the danger of papirosy."[76] In 1927 organizers of a pioneer troop boasted, "We often see pioneers who take home the fight against smoking and alcoholism, for cleanliness and fresh air."[77] Another health journal noted how important this fight was even if a cell could achieve little. After all, even though a smoker might be "ashamed to smoke at work, adults forget the danger of tobacco smoke in their own homes."[78] A cartoon in *Krokodil* revealed the campaign's reach. In "The Danger of Smoking" the caption explains that "in the fight with smoking in schools the guilty have their names written on the blackboard." The drawing presents a child watching his father and upends the message. The boy jokes: "Dad, give me a papirosa, or I'll put your name on the blackboard."[79] The light tone and the impishness of the child imply a less than serious attitude toward using state power in pursuit of vice. This ridicule fit within a general pattern of *Krokodil's* coverage of the antismoking campaigns— cessation was an easy laugh.

Children could serve as agents in the family, and other groups targeted single men and women in the factories. The factory brigade or a worker's club circle might convey propaganda, shame, and encouragement for quitting. Some individual work spaces created no-smoking sections and introduced fines.[80] A 1924 article asked for more help for "the healthy minority" to organize smoke-free labor and social spaces.[81] Zolonitskii commended the District Committee of the Moscow Department of Public Health for its fight against smoking in work spaces and the fifty kopeck fines.[82] Some anti-alcohol groups included tobacco abstention in their rules.[83]

In the late 1920s therapeutic cessation, carried out in groups with doctor supervision, became part of dispensary treatment in urban areas. The dispensary system started by serving tuberculosis patients and increased rapidly; by 1928 Moscow alone claimed over three hundred tuberculosis and other dispensaries and reported over seventeen million visitors.[84] A small number of dispensaries were tied to "circles" of motivated smokers at workplaces or through institutions like the Komsomol. Groups at factories reached out to the dispensary for help in organizing cessation challenges and groups. In the 1926 article "Six Months Cessation," a worker reported: "The lads went for the task heatedly, and the results are already evident. Sure, a few men fell off, but the majority stayed, and twenty-five inveterate smokers of tobacco already have not smoked for half a year."[85] A similar campaign at a Moscow mill led to two hundred people quitting.[86] Challenges between groups raised action. The Rogozhsko-Simonovskii District Health Office bragged that in December a group of workers quit smoking together, and "immediately it was easier to work." Although visitors chafed at the restrictions, the group responded, "But without a doubt they must follow it: smoking will not happen among us . . . It is imperative that all health institutions must forbid smoking."[87]

The Soviets used collective shaming in agitational plays, put names of malefactors on factory blackboards to encourage behavioral changes, and employed other more invasive methods. According to advocates, children should instruct family members on the antisocial nature of their habit, encourage them to quit because of the danger they posed to the collective air that all breathed, and make these concerns important to all of society. Another author encouraged mobilizing "public opinion against smokers."[88] Significantly he denounced not the habit (*kurenie*) but the user (*kuril'shchik*) and advocated for the creation of a mass anti-tobacco movement across different groups alongside no-smoking spaces in trams, hospitals, theaters, and schools. He derided those who continued to smoke as "will-less, frivolous, irresponsible, selfish, and egotistical."[89] Sholomovich proposed nothing less than the elevation of the sanitary culture of the entire nation as the essential component to achieving a smoke-free society. He grumbled that posters did nothing if near them "thousands of people continue to smoke."[90]

Social pressure might shame smokers but could form a barrier to quitting. A 1929 pamphlet for Komsomol members declared that the "big obstacle" to quitting was the "loneliness" when coworkers and roommates continued smoking. The author advocated finding a support group.[91] The pamphlet *The Evil Weed (Tobacco Tyranny)* outlined the sensory cues, tempting and revolting, that haunted the days of the former smoker: "You wanted to smoke. Someone else is smoking. You saw an ashtray premium from a tobacco store. You smelled tobacco stench from someone nearby. You saw a butt. You heard a smoker's cough. You saw how disgustingly he spat. You lit up a papirosa. You bought tobacco. You made a papirosa. You are invited to smoke. You see tobacco smoke. You read about a tobacco factory. You feel nauseated from pain in the throat. You see your smoke-stained teeth. You notice an unpleasant odor from the clothing of a smoker or so on and so on."[92] Though each reminder of tobacco was more disgusting than the next, the author pitched these as prompts to desire.

The most comprehensive overview of tobacco cessation methods came in a 1928 essay for *Voprosy narkologii*, where the specialist A. G. Stoiko explained the difficulty of quitting tobacco in a society of smokers: "Tobacco therapy is studied generally with little desire, and the cause of that comes from, of course, its difficulty." The smoker was "surrounded by a whole mass of negative suggestions (spoken in the language of psychology) or conditioned stimuli (in the language of reflexology) that hinder the ability to extinguish an often very lasting, conditioned reflex. They are surrounded by a mass of smokers and involuntarily forced to breathe tobacco smoke, which reinforces conditioned reflex, [as does] the wide reach of tobacco advertisements standing on every corner, and the papirosy sellers everywhere as well."[93] Stoiko set out persuasion, hypnosis, suggestion, targeted therapy, and self-suggestion as promising methods for quitting tobacco. Persuasion, he clarified, meant listening to a doctor's advice on how to live without tobacco. He was more positive about that than hypnosis, which he said was effective in curing susceptible alcoholics but not smokers. The hypnosis patient was "passive," waiting for the doctor to do all the work, and "gives nothing of himself."[94]

Methods came from native and international inspirations. The influence of Lev Markovich Rozenshtein, a psychiatrist of the Moscow school who emphasized therapeutic hypnosis and other psychotherapeutic methods for mental hygiene, came through in these techniques.[95] Bekhterev, a proponent of hypnotherapy, had been active in prerevolutionary alcohol treatment and expanded to tobacco.[96] The German psychotherapist Wladimir G. Eliasberg inspired "targeted therapy," where smokers established a base line of pulse, blood pressure, and other data at a first visit and then by monitoring changes over time appreciated health improvements. Stoiko observed, "The sick by himself, not through a book and not through a doctor's lecture, comes to know the danger of smoking."[97] The method of autosuggestion, in Russian "*Metod sotse*," came from the "optimistic autosuggestion" of the French psychologist and pharmacist Émile Coué de la Châtaigneraie. Coué began as a proponent of hypnosis but became disenchanted with the method because he could not get all patients to sleep. Working instead with conscious patients, Stoiko advanced a modified version of suggestion based on Coué.[98]

The Bolsheviks' vision of psychological science was in a state of flux in the 1920s, but generally the materialists saw mind and body as joined, and a strong materialist psychological movement built on the reflexology of Ivan Pavlov influenced understandings of addiction.[99] The Bolsheviks funded Pavlov more generously than the tsarist state had, and Semashko headed the Pavlov Commission under Narkomzdrav for facilitating the lab's work. Although Pavlov did come into conflict with the Bolsheviks, his theories remained important to understanding smoking.[100] Although tobacco was not considered addictive, the habit came under the influence of the materialist school and Pavlov's ideology, making therapeutics a long process of providing new stimuli and training.[101] The emphasis on the social foundations for behaviors, thoughts, and feelings would increase and was important to tobacco analysis.[102]

Cessation built from psychological theories of alcoholism but varied. Tobacco, according to Stoiko, acted on the body differently than morphine, opium, or even alcohol because it was poison. The complaints of those who quit might be contradictory—from drowsiness to insomnia—and withdrawal from smoking manifested in complaints of "a psychological character," the only commonality of which was a feeling that "something is not right." He finished, anecdotally, that when he himself had quit smoking and deprived himself of the "neurological hammer" of tobacco, his "head worked poorly or got lost somewhere in the rhetoric." From this sensation, he calculated that the least active force in tobacco was the physiological effect on the body.[103]

Stoiko proposed that smokers developed not a bodily need but a conditioned reflex where they grew accustomed to the sensory effects of nicotine and responded to cues for continued consumption. The smoker was constantly reminded of their habit by:

> the attention to the box or port cigar in the pocket, the extraction of the box of matches, the retrieving and lighting of a match, the lighting of a papirosa, etc.... This is a full scene of conditioned reflexes, before which the conditioned stimulus appears in the same moments, in the times when a smoker is accustomed to go get a papirosa: with a full stomach (for those used to smoking after food), mental or physical work, various kinds of emotions (joy or sorrow), and if the smoker says, when they go to get a papirosa, that it calms, then the mechanism of that "calming effect" is keyed into not the physiological effects of nicotine but the analogous action of suckling which calms a child.[104]

Though he did not reference Sigmund Freud directly, the equation of smoking's calming effects with the experience of the suckling child echoed the psychoanalytical interpretation of smoking as an oral fixation. Because Freud was anti-Marxist, Soviet Freudians trod a careful path, attempting to use his techniques without becoming politically suspect.[105]

Further hurdles to cessation were entirely psychological, according to Stoiko. He dismissed smokers' belief that quitting might shock the heart and scoffed at doctors who believed it.[106] From mocking doctors, he went on to cast doubt on self-suggestion, since smokers believed from the moment they started that it would be difficult to quit, they reinforced this defeatism. He noted, "In only one way are they different than people who have quit—they do this easily because they believe in the ease of it."[107]

Stoiko advocated collective psychotherapy, which was the mainstay of the dispensary system and the "most rational" choice because it addressed the "social character" of smoking and allowed one doctor to treat large groups of patients efficiently. Underscoring his commitment to the concepts of Coué, he advised the doctor leading the group to have those in the crowd who had successfully quit detail the ease and benefits of quitting. The first session ideally took twenty to fifty patients chosen from a common social group who attended a week's lectures describing smoking according to psychology, reflexology, prophylaxis, and the physical dangers of poisonous nicotine. Finally, they learned of the social character of smoking. Each lecture ended with a collective suggestion.[108] Smokers were to keep key points in mind through the day, about unpleasantness or bad outcomes, and repeat these for reinforcement. This would build revulsion over the course of a week or maybe a few months.[109] Suggestion therapy was for those who could not summon up alone "the strength of will to quit."[110]

Others advocated for hypnosis with suggestion or suggestion therapy on its own. In answer to readers' letters in 1928, one journal promoted psychotherapy, pointing out it could be found, free for the insured, at facilities on Pisarev Street and Nevsky Prospect.[111] One doctor called hypnosis "one of the more hopeful means for quitting smoking" and pointed to "massive experimentation with this treatment for students and military personnel with good result."[112] Violin supported both for "neglected cases."[113] Others suggested aversion therapy with silver nitrate, glycerin, iodide preparations, salts, and special diets to build revulsion to the taste of tobacco.[114] These matched international recommendations. The Anti-Cigarette League in the US recommended rinsing the mouth with silver nitrate solution, chewing gentian root, or changing the diet to fruits, cereals, milk, and "well-chewed nuts" alongside steam baths to "help relieve the system of the accumulated poisons."[115]

The substitution of a more healthful alternative to smoking or to tobacco became a standard therapy. Zolotnitskii advised: "In place of smoking, one might try eating sunflower seeds or sucking on sweets. Another might try chewing pretzels [suchki], croutons [sukharki]; a third, to mimic smoking, could soak batting in eucalyptus oil, . . . place it in a mouthpiece, and drag on the evaporating oils."[116] Advertisements in Pravda in 1927 promoted a mouthpiece styled on the system "of the German Professor Heintz Gernak." The setup included the "antinicotine" mouthpiece and a glass flask with a preparation of balsam and a glass phial that contained the special "antinicotine elixir." Together, the advertisement assured smokers, these items would reduce by 90 percent the nicotine in a cigarette, or as another advertisement for the product assured, smoking "twenty-five papirosy with the mouthpiece have the same danger as three smoked without it."[117]

Some authorities suggested gradualist therapies with chemical helpmates, leaf substitutes, or safer smoking of higher-grade leaf, but by far the most common proposal was going cold turkey. Sazhin dismissed chemical cures as foolhardy. For those who asked for "drops of some kind" Sazhin countered that "even if medicine found such drops, they would be only a little help." Science would then develop drops "against smoking, against drinking, and against an out-of-control sexual life, etc. etc." He contended that from this slippery slope an explosion of medicine would take over society. People would be taking drops all day and, when they failed, would fall back to the same bad habits. The only solution, he resolved, was for workers to take control of their own health, root out past bad habits, and create a new life.[118] One author dismissed replacing tobacco with "mint, coffee, tree leaves, hops, sage, etc." as inadequate foolishness. He maintained, "An authentically conscious, authentically masculine, and decisive person does not participate in such self-delusion."[119] Another author similarly disputed the healthfulness of moderate smoking or even its possibility as the "passion to stupefying substances can little guarantee moderation."[120] Nezlin advised it was better "to quit immediately and forever," getting over the first few bad days with "candies or something to chew." Visiting a city clinic for treatment with suggestion or going to a tuberculosis sanatorium where smoking was prohibited made it easier to quit.[121] It would not be easy, he explained, as the smoker "will have sadness and disquiet in his psyche (spirit), as if something just does not measure up. The appetite will be imperceptible, and everything will be bland in the mouth. Work will not come together." He warned of the strong desire to smoke and perhaps constipation but promised it would be over in a few weeks and "you will be a new person." For "boredom with work" Nezlin recommended distraction with books, the cinema, and the club and a simple diet with steady labor to aid digestion.[122]

Popular Ridicule and Medical Equivocation

A 1928 satirical essay for *Krokodil* gave a less than glowing review of dispensary-based cessation therapy. Opening and closing with the comment that he smoked "like a horse," the author, B. Samsonov, described his failed therapy. Spurred by a knowledge that his lungs were "national property" and that he would soon be "driven out" for "littering," he smoked two last *Iava* and entered the dispensary for group therapy. Surrounded by a crowd of "gloomy and angry" fellows craving a smoke and staring at "unpleasant pictures," he waited half an hour for the doctor, who then stood at the lectern with "a jar full of gross stuff" and pestered, harassed, and humiliated the group for an hour. The lecture ended with the command to toss out their matches and papirosy right then and "forget about tobacco." Samsonov described the call as effective until he walked out into the hall to the smell of a staff member's smoke and saw him packing up all the surrendered matches and papirosy for himself. Confronted, the staff member cheekily replied that he was not the patient. As Samsonov left the meeting, he met yet another reminder of his habit when he was confronted by a full line of sellers who told him it was the best spot in the city.[123] Resigned, Samsonov bought two packs and groused, "I did not manage to forget even until I made it home, curse it! And thus I smoke again just like a draft horse."

Skepticism over the severity of the problem and derision for clunky, poorly pitched propaganda joined the mocking of the antismoking therapies in a culture not convinced of the problem. Some argued that the Soviet Union had no problem compared to western Europe.[124] Ham-fisted messaging and hyperbolic anecdotes of individuals dying after a few papirosy assured smokers of their individual strengths. A youth-targeted pamphlet from the Moscow District Department of Public Health contained a list of groan-inducing jokes for the cause, including "For whom are papirosy healthy? Tobacco sellers" and "For whom is tobacco not dangerous? Corpses."[125] A 1929 article commended a club at Dnepropetrovsk for using humor to confront smokers since nothing else—not fines nor posters nor lectures—worked.[126] The popular slogan that a capful of nicotine could kill a horse was subject to wide derision and failed to square with the experience of smokers who saw around them thousands who smoked and thrived and lived on. Some wags, like Samsonov, flipped the slogan on its head by pointing out that they must be stronger than a "draft horse" if they were able to keep smoking and keep living. A further knock against poisoning arguments may have come from the popularity of homeopathic remedies that utilized poisons like diluted strychnine.

Portrayals of smoking as humorous undercut antismoking messages. Bulgakov conjured up a short satire on the extraordinary sight of a "Boy in a Million." This child, he told the readers, was spotted not swearing, hawking stuff, yelling, fighting, or smoking. Instead, he was well dressed and carried a math book on his way to school. Bulgakov's amazement, combined with the awe of the rest of the crowd on the street, testified to the rarity of such a boy. Yet the humor, and the list of other missing bad behaviors, suggested that tobacco was on par with cursing or yelling—regrettable but not disastrous offenses against public order and decorum—and to be expected of youth.[127] Insincere advocates similarly hindered the message. A 1928 *Krokodil* cartoon pointed out the hypocrisy of antismoking crusaders. Captioned "Remember, children: smoking brings horrible damage! Tobacco kills the man!" an audience of cherubic, chubby children watched a dissipated, pock-marked, Komsomol speaker with greasy hair and a hunched figure, sucking on tobacco while speaking against it.[128] Even adult party officials mocked or laughed at speeches urging cessation from alcohol and tobacco.[129]

The smoking of medical professionals further undercut cessation messages.[130] One author produced an interesting defense: doctors smoked because when confronted with the stench of corpses during training, they distracted their senses with tobacco, and the habit simply increased with time. He proposed, "Thus doctors smoke not because they are unaware of the dangers of tobacco but under the power of a habit founded on the professional dangers and peculiarities of medical work."[131] Not all were so forgiving of the smoking doctors. A 1924 essay took medical personnel to task for their indulgence, noting that many physicians smoked and did so in public places, meetings, conferences, and even some "are not ashamed to smoke at the bedside of the ill." The author said smoking in health care institutions should not be tolerated.[132]

Doctors' actions sewed confusion and so did their words, because they gave advice in their pamphlets of how smokers might more safely indulge. To smoke safely, one doctor advised readers to choose weaker tobacco, smoke less, not drink while smoking, use a mouthpiece (amber, meerschaum, elderberry, or jasmine being the best), experiment with iron sesquichloride or tannins in the mouthpiece, or use foreign tobacco prepared "in the method of Gerol'd."[133] Others opened the door to so-called safer smoking with a similar list (smoking less of lower-nicotine tobacco). They added a caution that dry tobacco burned more fully, was more healthful than damp tobacco, and with papirosy, more smoke goes into the surrounding air than into the smoker and was safer than pipes. Supposedly dryer tobacco resulted in a colder smoke, which created a better burn and mitigated the nicotine danger.[134] Quick smoking was considered more dangerous, and the setting of smoking could be healthier too—outside rather than inside or not at work or during sport.[135] Another author cautioned against smoking at night or in bed.[136] Sazhin and others recommended holders, dry tobacco, higher grades, and open air, adding that the end of the papirosy contained all the built-up nicotine and should be discarded.[137]

Combining health recommendations with the smoker's dialectical progress, Nezlin focused on the tobacco as the problem, maintaining that "the stronger the tobacco, the more nicotine in it. The most nicotine is from cheap tobacco, such as makhorka."[138] Another gave the percentage of nicotine in makhorka as 4 percent, twice that of higher-grade tobaccos.[139] One clarified that there was more nicotine in Siberian makhorka than in state or cooperative makhorka and that the nicotine in yellow tobacco was about half that. Furthermore, makhorka did not burn as well as yellow tobacco, so that "the lessened combustibility of makhorka leads to quicker smoking . . . and greater nicotine consumption."[140] Since the prevailing opinion was that the nicotine acted as a poison, this focus made sense, but the fact that makhorka was the chosen leaf of the countryside and recently urbanized workers meant it was denigrated as less cultured and civilized. Sazhin hinted at this when he said that it was a blow to conventional wisdom to attack makhorka, because many believed it to contain less nicotine. "Probably users who cannot afford other more expensive tobaccos tell themselves this. But truthfully, the bourgeoisie . . . would smoke makhorka if it was in truth less dangerous."[141] Another doctor complained that the focus on makhorka as being better hid the danger of all tobacco: "Yes, with smoking of makhorka we breathe further into ourselves, into the internals of our organism, more tobacco smoke than with smoking of yellow tobacco. This causes us to say that makhorka is more dangerous than yellow tobacco, but this by no measure means we can consume yellow tobacco or discount its danger."[142]

Industry journals further confused the situation. In 1923 *Vestnik tabachnoi promyshlennosti* presented a case for tobacco's positive effects on health. Although the author recognized some dangers of nicotine, he determined that tobacco was just another of the "stimulating alkaloids [that] humanity needs greatly [for the] stimulation of the organism."[143] Repeating old saws that tobacco increased mental and physical abilities and endurance, the author underscored that tobacco gave a pleasure "that nonsmokers cannot understand or imagine." In the end, this satisfaction was handily won: "It seems that the organism easily and without punishment can withstand small doses of nicotine and other things contained in tobacco for an entire life."[144] The author brought chemistry and the vogue of nutritional science to bear and observed that while nitrogen metamorphosis declined with seven to fifteen papirosy, it stabilized above that point and nutrient assimilation increased. He repeated claims, debunked elsewhere, that smoking served as a disinfectant of the mouth, completely killing cholera, typhoid, and pneumonia, concluding: "In cholera and typhoid epidemics, smoking tobacco may serve as oral hygiene and a prophylactic agent against bacterial lesions."[145] He observed that other items like coffee, tea, and nuts acted similarly to tobacco.[146]

In the same journal, the industry analyst S. Egiz criticized those who said tobacco hurt society or incited immoral thoughts and countered that tobacco served as a helpmate of the man in uniform: "All armies introduced a tobacco ration, and in the Red Army tobacco was handed out more carefully than all other supplies. Tobacco helped weather deprivation on the march. Soldiers asked for papirosy in order to make it out for an operation, on the field of battle, etc." In response to moralizing, Egiz countered that great men—like Isaac Newton and Immanuel Kant—smoked with no detrimental effects on their social or mental functions. He mused, "The most serious foundation for the attack on tobacco production may come from the opinion of agronomists on the danger of tobacco farming for agriculture."[147]

Even though there was no consensus on why people smoked, the pioneering dispensary joined Narkomzdrav's revolutionary anti-tobacco propaganda to create innovative cessation institutions in the 1920s, unmatched by any other country. The therapy—dependent on reflexology and social supports—reflected many Soviet values but drew on international techniques. Popularity outstripped resources, but the clamor for smoking cessation did not extend across all of society. Many continued to smoke, downplayed the danger of tobacco, or ridiculed the system. The depth of antismoking interest was not there. Although pamphlets and articles came out in profusion and the dispensary movement attracted a great deal of interest, international anti-tobacco organizations, such as the Anti-Cigarette League of Chicago, had no affiliates in Russia.[148] This may have been a consequence of international politics, but lack of interest was notable elsewhere. A 1926 guide to propaganda for the railways lamented that tobacco was less visible in health materials than other issues.[149] According to its 1928 guide, the Museum of Hygiene in Leningrad had thirteen separate departments, including exhibitions on tuberculosis, alcoholism, and cremation but nothing on tobacco.[150] At times, the mention of tobacco was more belittling than its omission, such as the 1926 article including smoking alongside a long list of "bad habits" like mouth breathing, spitting, coquetry, or dandyism. A 1928 pamphlet equated the habit of smoking to biting one's nails.[151] Pundits might decry smoking, but club guides emphasized accommodating smoking spaces and making sure to include "sufficient numbers of ashtrays."[152]

Still, propaganda on tobacco's dangers and the need to quit were finding greater resonance. A 1929 poem from the firebrand Maiakovskii made clear that interest in quitting, and the reasons for it, had penetrated society. In "I'm Happy" Maiakovskii crows of his glorious new day, where he could now smell again, would breathe "without one cough or spit," would again be "able to work like a horse." He went on to brag that his head was clear, and he had put on weight. He asked his readers if they wanted the secret and revealed "Today—I quit smoking."[153] Although more than slightly mocking, Maiakovskii repeated nearly every benefit anti-tobacco propaganda attributed to a new, abstemious life.

The message that poisonous nicotine presented the greatest danger from smoking had penetrated through from the propaganda, but the national campaign that Semashko had championed petered out after his removal from office in 1930. Nicotine's status as a poison that created nervous disorders, sexual debility, digestive dysfunction, and mental weakness appeared in a flurry of pamphlets published in 1930, but these polemical tracts perhaps were already in production before the turn in leadership of the Commissariat of Health.[154] Activists lamented that in some cases, the print runs were too small to be effective.[155] The turnover at Narkomzdrav led to downplaying of the problem and the decline of therapeutic options, much as it had curtailed anti-tobacco propaganda. Although health journals continued to feature information periodically on how to quit smoking, the dispensary method faded from view. Even as sanatoriums, vacation homes, children's groups, and schools advanced a nonsmoking message, it was part of a general bundle of information on how to live a "new life" rather than part of a concerted campaign or therapeutic program. Cessation propaganda and therapeutics for adults were effectively abandoned.

UNFULFILLED

Commissar Mikoian and Stalinized Production

In 1931 Anastas Ivanovich Mikoian, the notoriously hands-on head of the People's Commissariat of Food Industry, praised tobacco workers for fueling the Stalinist industrialization drive.[1] He declared, "Papirosy are now a type of weapon in the state's economic policy," and elaborated:

> The worker or the peasant is exhausted by labor and asks, "Give me a little smoke, and I will get back to it" . . . The tractor drivers and the mine workers want to smoke. See, the work is hard. It is not so easy to build. They want to smoke . . . Don't forget, comrades, that tobacco, makhorka, and papirosy—they will decide it . . . The lumber trust directly declares, "You want the trees harvested, give us papirosy." The engineers, going off to a new construction site say, "We'll do it all, just give us papirosy." They announce, "You need us to prepare butter, eggs, and so on—give us papirosy and we will do everything."[2]

Above ground, papirosy incentivized tractor drivers. Below ground, makhorka motivated miners. And Mikoian explained that tobacco workers did so much more, because "every billion papirosy—that is ten million rubles in the state budget."[3] Increased production prevented revenue loss by halting imports, curtailing smuggling, and countering the black-market tobacco that he admitted continued to be a problem.[4]

Mikoian's speech came in the heat of the First Five-Year Plan (1928–1932), which swept away the small-scale capitalism of the NEP years in favor of titanic development built on concerns for a strong Soviet state. The plans hinged, according to Mikoian, on the ability of humble papirosy to push tractor drivers and miners, lumber workers and engineers on to great deeds. The reliance on tobacco would carry through the Second Five-Year Plan (1933–1937) and on to the third (1938–1941), which was cut short by World War II. Preparation for a future war was on Mikoian's mind in 1931 as he concluded, "Without makhorka, it is even impossible to make war. Makhorka is defense. It is, of course, not a cannon or an airplane, but without makhorka the front is difficult. Spirit is not enough for troops. After a good fight, it is necessary to have a good smoke." Here was the end goal. He pled with the workers, "give the country a smoke and the state some money and thereby the men and women of tobacco could revive the spirit [of the fighting man]."[5] Mikoian's militant message echoed Stalin's caution for all industry in the same year: "We are fifty or a hundred years behind the advanced countries. We must make good this distance in ten years. Either we do it, or we shall go under."[6]

In the tobacco industry, "making good the distance" meant expanding harvests, importing machinery, and incentivizing hero workers. Increased output found eager buyers, and the use of ready-made papirosy became more prominent in cities and spread into rural areas. This happened despite the near complete disappearance of marketing, uneven smoke quality, and rudimentary packaging. Even as more tobacco made it out over the 1930s, production failed to meet demand, and complaints on quality, deficits, and wrecking dogged the industry. While manufacturers in the capitalist world battled each other for existing smokers and pushed to expand the habit by seducing new consumers, in the Soviet Union producers struggled to meet the growing demand of a market that already existed, was expanding exponentially, and constantly complained of poor products. Increasingly tobacco availability and quality became an expectation of the new order. As Karl Radek asked in *Izvestiia* in 1931, "What then is this arrival to socialism if among us there is a shortage of not just meat but even of papirosy?"[7]

Mikoian's 1931 call for increased production came on the heels of a decade-long cessation campaign. Perhaps this occasioned the aside to Mikoian's speech, "Even though I have not smoked in six months (having succumbed to Semashko), I understand what it is like for a smoker to not have papirosy."[8] But Mikoian acknowledged the disconnect between the interests of production and health: "We are not doctors, who preach cessation but then smoke themselves to hell. We are practical politicians and economists. When people stop smoking, that will be a different thing, but for now we need tobacco . . . Look, people smoke papirosy, which means we need to give them more."[9] Mikoian was not the only one changing his tobacco tune. Semashko's successors largely abandoned his campaign. With Stalin a well-known smoker, shaming was no longer a viable tactic. Instead, what little cessation material appeared followed state priorities. Fueled by

Stalinism's economic emphasis, cessation works emphasized the costs of smokers as fire hazards or loafers and largely neglected individual dangers except in the case of women and children's smoking. Lenin's anti-tobacco diatribes faded behind the haze from Stalin's pipe.

Increased Production and Increased Revenues

Stalin's "Great Break," a massive campaign for the reorganization of agriculture and colossal investment in industry, came on the tails of his solidification of power in the party and an agricultural crisis that was interpreted as a problem of NEP planning. Stalin launched a two-prong plan for rapid development. For agriculture, collectivization of peasant landholdings into large-scale, mechanized, scientifically managed factory farms would provide larger harvests. Fewer agricultural workers would then produce enough to feed an increased industrial working class, and excess grain would be sold to fund large-scale investment in new machinery to innovate industry. Failure came in multiple forms—poor harvests, global depression, capital loss, incompetent management, popular resistance, and bad planning—and evidenced itself in horrific suffering, famine, and death. Massive social and cultural change accompanied it—from the creation of entire industries, cities, and areas of research and production to the migration of some twenty-three million peasants into cities from 1926 to 1939.[10] Increasing oppression masked and met the problems. Estimates for unnatural deaths from the 1927–1937 period range from four to eleven million.[11]

Tobacco was one of several food stuffs targeted for increased production.[12] Stalin was not shy about using vodka sales to fund development, asking rhetorically what was worse, the "yoke of foreign capital or sale of vodka?"[13] In answer, the state increased alcohol production and moved the money into industry. The state similarly increased tobacco production to reap profit from the population's habit.[14] Yet expanded industry struggled to meet demand. In 1930, the tobacco industry journal put forward that even were they to achieve increased norms, it "would not be enough for the full satisfaction of the popular hunger for smoking products."[15] An industry analyst speculated that the "capacity of the tobacco market was not properly calculated" as increasing numbers of workers meant that "papirosy demand strongly rose in the city and markedly widened in the countryside."[16]

Changes to tobacco cultivation moved forward quickly. According to a history of Georgian-produced tobacco, home to the rich Abkhaziia and Samsun varieties, the harvest per acre more than doubled between 1931 and 1938.[17] Collectivization campaigns in Kazakhstan expanded tobacco growing and other agricultural

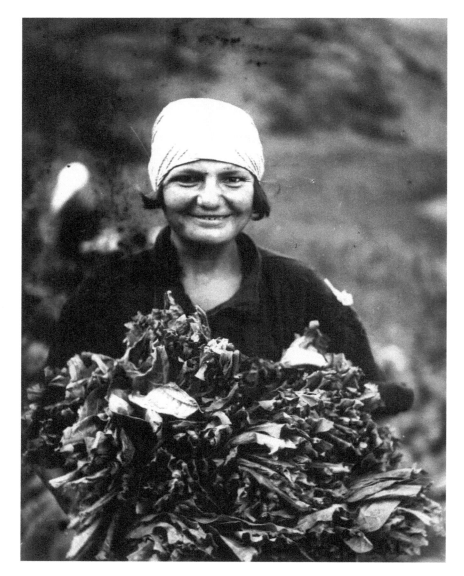

FIGURE 5.1. Photo. Female worker at a Crimean kolkhoz holding harvested tobacco, 1931. RGAKFD, No. 2–81141

development in the region at tremendous human cost.[18] Propaganda of happy agricultural workers included in their midst photographs of happy tobacco and makhorka farmers (Figure 5.1). According to one peasant testimony, life on the tobacco kolkhoz was better than on many others because from tobacco "there was greater profit."[19] The ability to market a bit on the side or get paid in kind was a likely perk, but the fact that millions of peasants fled the countryside for uncertain futures in often brutal industrial conditions indicated the problems in the village. For millions leaving was never an option as the collectivization drive led to forcible removal, executions, or the horrific slow death of man-made famine.[20]

Tobacco factory workers were among the teams of urbanites that went to the countryside to force peasants onto collective farms and kill resisters.[21] Widespread belief that peasants hoarded grain encouraged the participation of workers in the campaign, but so too would their own production pressures. Mikoian argued that tobacco factory workers had a more intimate connection to the countryside because they needed agricultural raw material to meet their own production norms; thus the fight for collectivization was the fight for the needs of the tobacco industry.[22] As a tobacco analyst noted in 1931, "Among other light industries it would be difficult to find one like tobacco which so deeply suffers from shortages in raw materials," and despite agricultural increases, huge demand for papirosy meant more collectivization was pushed.[23]

Against this background of cruelty and death, the 1930s introduced a large amount of land area to tobacco cultivation, greatly increasing tobacco raw materials.[24] In addition, new industry support systems came online. In 1930 there were eight tobacco fermentation points in the Soviet Union, by 1932 there were five more, and by 1941 there were thirty-eight.[25] Entirely new factories, renovated factories, and new machinery all increased production.[26] The innovations affected workforce composition by decreasing the amount of handwork and increasing the need for skilled, trained technicians. This changed tobacco factory dynamics. In tobacco, as in other industries, men were considered more suited to technical tasks and women more dexterous for handwork. One worker recalled that when new German machines were introduced at the Balkan Star Factory in 1929, a woman asked to be trained on them, but the director scoffed, "What can a woman do on a machine?"[27] Still, female participation in tobacco manufacture increased over the 1930s, rivaling the historically feminized textile manufactures. In 1932 women were 57.3 percent of tobacco and makhorka workers, and by 1939 they constituted 65.1 percent.[28]

At first machinery was purchased from abroad but avoiding hard-currency expenditure was preferred. Tobacco industry journals detailed the workings of cigarette machinery, encouraging workplace innovation and repair over requests for new technology.[29] A set of back-and-forth memos from 1939 between the State Planning Commission, tobacco industry planners, and the Commissariat of Food Industry regarding importing machines from Czechoslovakia and the British firm Molins broke down as state planners maintained that there was no need to buy expensive machinery that could be made in country. The exchange ended with a "secret" communication that manufacturers could import one machine

TABLE 11. Tobacco production in tons, 1930–1934

	TOBACCO	MAKHORKA
1930	31,721	73,464
1931	40,848	85,109
1932	45,098	74,611
1933	44,855	77,712
1934	49,582	97,221

Source: G. Bonstedt, "Tabakovodstvo v 1936 godu," *Tabachnaia promyshlennost'*, no. 6 (1935): 12.

and then state planners would copy it and produce five machines for preparation of "papirosy of the American type (i.e., without a mouthpiece)."[30]

With robust cultivation and a push for more mechanization, tobacco and makhorka output jumped, and state revenues from tobacco increased.[31] By 1934 factories began to fulfill plans and increase production, as shown in Table 11.[32] Shortages continued, and *Pravda* reported speculation in Baku, Kiev, and Irkutsk.[33]

New varieties of smoking items appeared, like the "aromatic" papirosa of DGTF—*Novogodnye* (New Year)—that was distinguished by "the scent of violets, fresh apples, etc."[34] Similar products appeared in the west in the nineteenth century.[35] Smell had important implications for taste. Nicotine on its own emits a scent and taste akin to burned rubber, but Soviet manufacturers depended on blends of leaf, rather than additions of sauce with flavorings and scents, to create palatable, smooth-burning smokes. Makhorka was not sauced and oriental leaf, unlike American tobacco, does not take flavors well. Despite this, Russian and Soviet tobacco smokes had sophisticated and well-regarded tastes dependent upon using carefully balanced leaf. The Soviet chemist and agronomist A. A. Schmuk—head of the All-Union Institute of Tobacco and Makhorka Production in the 1920s, director of its chemical sector in the 1930s, and an internationally renowned scientist of tobacco flavor—investigated the chemistry of taste, created methods for improving the flavor of low-grade tobaccos, and experimented with tobacco substitutes such as leaves from trees (poplar, aspen, beech, hazelnut, oak, chestnut, nettles) or inclusion of other items such as hops, hemp, rhubarb, or beets.[36]

Schmuk also attempted to reduce nicotine by stuffing the mouthpieces with glycerin-soaked batting. He held that "the possibility of decreasing the content of nicotine in the smoke will thereby contribute to the preservation of the national health," which was a problem "far exceeding the scope of interests of the tobacco industry alone."[37] Schmuk was not the only tobacco industry insider pursuing healthier smokes. As early as 1930 researchers at Dukat developed a mouthpiece to "influence the composition of tobacco smoke."[38] In Leningrad

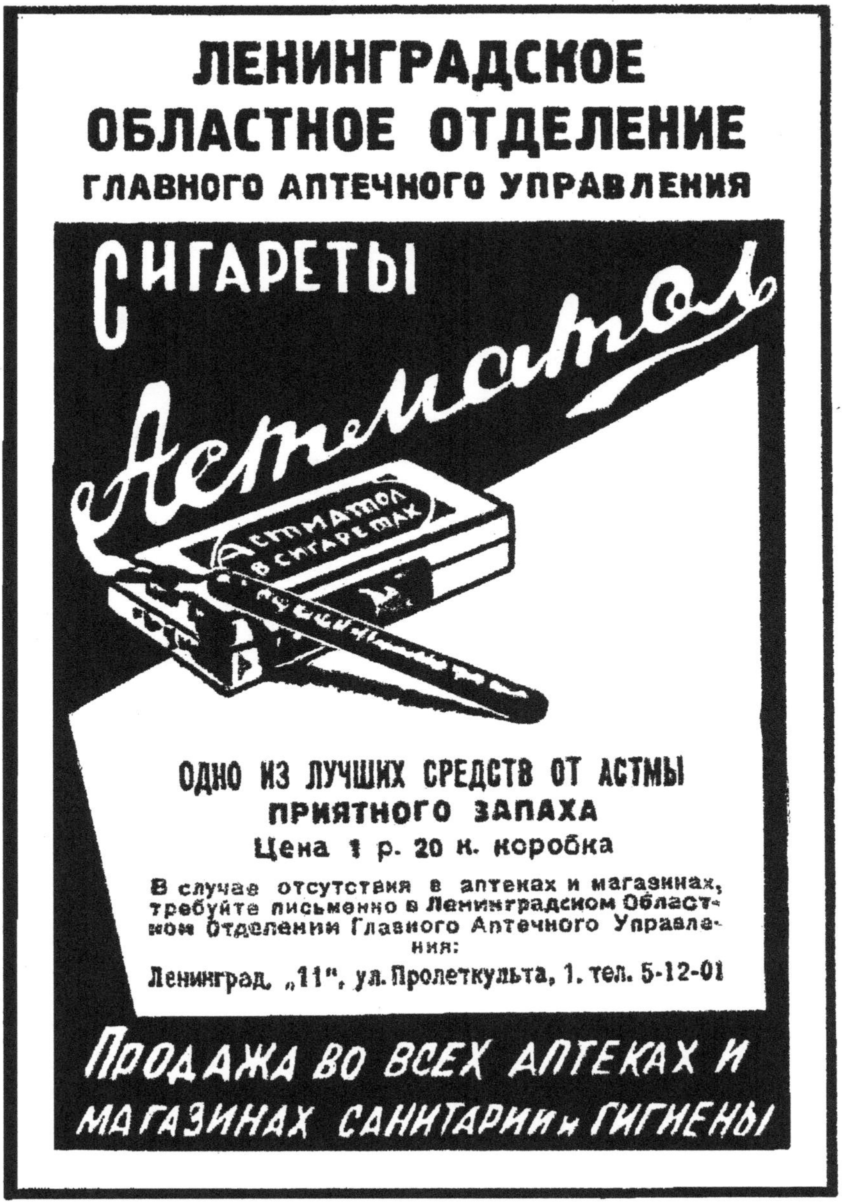

FIGURE 5.2. Poster. "Advertisement for *Astmatol*." *GiZRiKS*, no. 7 (1937): 18. Courtesy Russian State Library.

the pharmaceutical group put out an anti-asthma "cigarette"—*Astmatol*—promoted for its "pleasant scent" (Figure 5.2).[39] Foreign research on filters appeared in industry journals frequently.[40] Soviet health experts dismissed filters as largely ineffective because "they at most stop 10–15 percent of nicotine" and concluded that filters and manipulation were not the best solution as "the only way to stop nicotine danger is to stop smoking."[41] Even the tobacco industry journal reviewed the efforts with a jaundiced eye, concluding that the coal filters of the Iava Factory did not stop "a significant portion of nicotine"; instead these contained roughly "40–45 percent of the nicotine of papirosy without filters." The article noted that the chemical sector had begun researching a filter capable of absorbing 80–90 percent of the nicotine.[42]

Worker life at DGTF, the makers of *Nasha marka*, showed the impact of Stalinist industrialization policies. In 1928 new machinery replaced the prerevolutionary technology. Easier pack production and new leaf processing with less dust sped up production and improved conditions. In 1932 the introduction of seventy-four Katskii-Klimovich and fifty Fel'dman machines eliminated most handwork.[43] Electric stations were added to the factory, allowing rational, less hazardous configuration of the shop floor. Finally, the addition of a telephone line at the same point enabled communication across the floor.[44] More hygienic conditions, less dust, and diminished noise became a focus of factory organization.[45] Social activities for workers encouraged courses after work for basic education and technical training.[46] A kindergarten joined the nursery and summer home for children. An experimental electrotherapy room and dietetic cafeteria served workers.[47] The new electrically lit bathhouse was purportedly not only the best in Rostov-on-Don but even rivaled those of Moscow. A visiting French delegation got to see DGTF's in-house cobbler, beautician, and tailor and may have been treated to the factory's radio program, which broadcast workers' musical requests over eighty-two factory receivers. Additional propaganda and leisure activities came in the form of a choir, orchestra, Komsomol cell, red corner, school, and workers' theater group.[48]

Expectations rose. A cult of overproduction that grew up around the 1935 feats of the coal miner Aleksei Stakhanov reached tobacco workers too. In a much-publicized, carefully staged single work shift, Stakhanov overfulfilled the norm by fourteen times. Newspapers encouraged other workers to follow his example. Tobacco plantations in Georgia claimed agricultural Stakhanovites who overfulfilled norms by 150 or even 300 percent.[49] The Dukat and Klara Tsetkin factories celebrated productive workers with pieces in the industry journal and *Izvestiia*.[50] DGTF produced profiles of the three female and two male Stakhanovites of their factory. All spoke of the incentives such as increased wages.[51] Nina Volkova, a Stakhanovite from Iava, wrote a memoir—*The Limit Has Not Yet Been Reached!*—and recounted meeting Mikoian and hearing Stalin's "novel, precious words."[52] A 1938 profile in *Izvestiia* of the Stakhanovite Iugaber Avetisian claimed a "second birth" for her with the movement.[53] Behind the propaganda, Stakhanovism left a mixed legacy of conflict, competition, and tension on the shop floor and did little to help production as a whole.[54]

In 1935 Mikoian declared tobacco successfully Stalinized. Before, he recalled, miners complained "there's no tobacco, give us papirosy . . . But now . . . We have plenty of makhorka for all, for anyone who needs it. Anyone who wants it can buy it. We also have enough papirosy."[55] Later he promised even more, saying Soviet tobacco "will occupy the second place in the world behind the United States."[56] Before the commissariat he testified that supply problems were over, the price per pack would be lowered, and the amount of higher-quality tobacco would increase, "because just as life has become more joyous, so we must smoke higher-quality, aromatic papirosy (laughter)."[57] Not only Mikoian spoke of the triumph of tobacco. In a 1936 *Pravda* article Ukrainian tobacco producers boasted of the tremendous growth they had achieved. Whereas "in 1913 our tobacco factories produced twenty-seven billion papirosy, now in our factories they produce not twenty-seven but seventy-eight billion papirosy. . . [and we predict] eighty-seven billion papirosy in 1936."[58] By 1938 declarations of plans fulfilled and overfilled packed the newspapers. Dukat, Iava, and DGTF all claimed to have hit half a billion papirosy over plan.[59]

Advertising's Fall and Packaging's Ascendancy

While production exploded in the 1930s, advertising fizzled. By 1932 advertising by private firms was gone, and only state-sponsored advertisement remained. Expenditures on advertising fell by twenty to twenty-five times.[60] In 1936 Mikoian proposed more didactic advertising of consumer products to encourage utilizing items produced in abundance but not consumed. For instance, tomatoes were in surplus, and the population needed to be encouraged to eat them. Advertising could aid this effort.[61] In the same year new advertising sections were established, and in 1937 the first all-union competition for advertising took place.[62] Few papirosy posters appeared in this period, and those that did abandoned the invention of earlier eras in favor of a more direct, if still graphic, introduction of the product with mild hints on cultured usage.

The 1936 poster for *Derbi* (Derby) papirosy traded on the imagery of the city of Leningrad with one of the four horse-tamer statues from Anichkov Bridge (Figure 5.3). The bright cover of the pack provides a burst of color, drawing the eye to the product and more horse imagery. Behind, two papirosy rest in an ashtray, which appears as a base to the horse-tamer statue, perhaps a novelty ashtray. Including the ashtray indicates cultured use meant proper accessories. In this

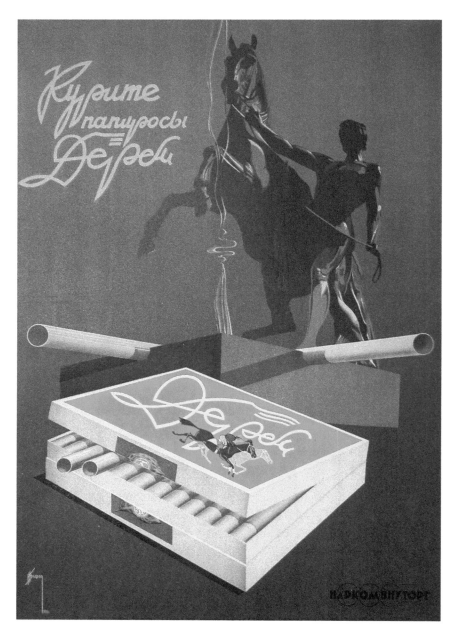

FIGURE 5.3. Poster. "Advertisement for *Derbi*," 1936. Artist Israel Davydovich Bograd. Courtesy Russian State Library.

case, an ashtray allows for disposal of ash and the butt. Further, it implies smoking in a fixed place, like a home or office, rather than while walking in public. The slogan of the poster—"Smoke *Derbi* papirosy"—leaves no room for confusion. The 1936 poster for the many products of the Iava Factory (including *Derbi*, *Kazbek*, *Lux*, etc.) from the same artist brings graphic interest (Figure 5.4). Under the rhyming couplet, "Smokers know the answer/there are no better papirosy" regimented rows of papirosy packs climb dynamically from lower left to upper right as background to another ashtray showing the proper way to rest one's papirosa and dispose of ash. The collage of packs suggests industrial lines and modern simplicity. No user is pictured or implied as with *Derbi*. This makes for a less intimate appeal and less participatory experience for the viewer.

Advertising in posters, magazine, and newspapers may not have been as notable as in the west, but the Soviets did have basic marketing in the form of brand names, pack label designs, special holiday sets, and attention to points of sale. Individual factories produced proprietary brands with unique packaging, blends, and messages to entice consumers to buy their papirosy over those produced in other factories.[63] Special papirosy, at times with exotic flavors, came out for presentation gifts and holidays. For instance, in 1936 in commemoration of the anniversary of the revolution, the Oktiabr'skii Factory produced gift sets of papirosy.[64] New attention to points of sale came out too. Critics in the tobacco industry journal discussed approvingly the innovative, Russian, folk-art-inspired wood display units designed by the artists of Glavtabak (Glavnoe upravlenie tabachnoi promyshlennosti).[65] Many restaurants and cafeterias sold papirosy and other goods alongside food, so that a 1936 report showed only 40 percent of turnover in meals and the rest in sandwiches, papirosy, alcohol, and other goods.[66] Vending machines, around in the US from the 1880s, were introduced in the USSR for matches and tobacco products in 1935.[67] A picture of one such automat in front of the Palace of Soviets metro station in Moscow presented what was undoubtedly an idealized portrait of happy customers and working machinery. With the deficit problems it was unlikely they were well stocked or functioning.[68] A further issue would have been the easy access for minors. A 1937 Moscow city decree forbid sale of papirosy and tobacco products to children under sixteen years, which was to be enforced by city and district trade inspectors.[69]

Even these limited marketing efforts were criticized. A *Pravda* article of 1935 complained that many brands were poorly conceived, such as two new brands with English-language names, which would be "incomprehensible to most of the population."[70] Others complained of shoddy packaging.[71] A lengthy article in the tobacco industry journal addressed the explosion of brands and decried the amateurish implementation as "nonmarketing people, factory people, are making decisions," and they had no expertise in naming products or producing visuals. The author commended "short . . . memorable and sonorous" names for

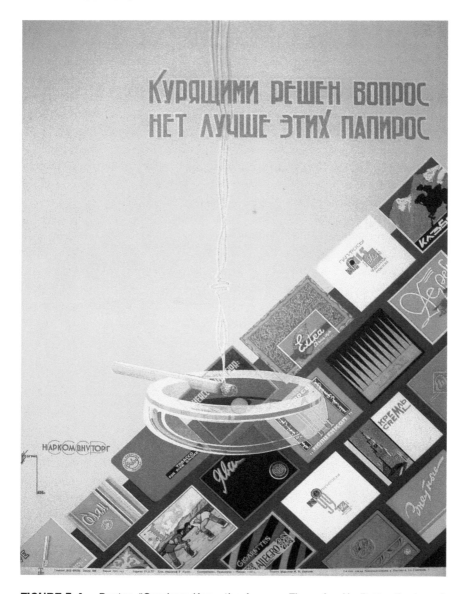

FIGURE 5.4.   Poster. "Smokers Know the Answer: There Are No Better Papirosy,"
1936. Artist Israel Davydovich Bograd. Courtesy Russian State Library.

papirosy. He found the numbered brands of the Iava Factory especially ridicu-
lous because they would be "incomprehensible" to those unacquainted with them
already. He declared even the art inadequate and promoted art that catered to the
tastes of desired users.[72] A 1936 article in *Izvestiia* portrayed the proliferation of
brands—almost two hundred—as ludicrous and unnecessary. The author asked,

"Can all these be to satisfy users?" and pointed out that audits demonstrated that almost half of these brands did not enjoy good sales. In response, brands that were poor sellers were withdrawn and packaging improved.[73] In a *Pravda* editorial, Stalin signaled that concern for consumers should be a consideration for manufacturers of all types.[74] Elsewhere Stalin advocated making the material culture of socialism on a par with that of western capitalist nations as a means of competition with the west and to make more cultured citizens.[75] The interest in consumer experience and increased investment could be seen in packs with better paper, artwork, and quality.

In this burst of creativity and competition, two of the more iconic brands of the Soviet era first appeared—*Belomorkanal* (White Sea Canal) and *Kazbek* (named for the Georgian mountain/dormant volcano) (Figure 5.5). In each case, pack design takes over where poster art had declined. *Belomorkanal* features a

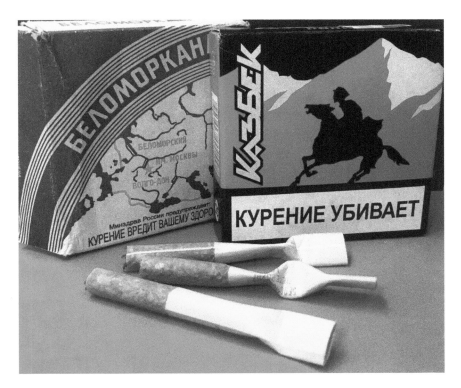

FIGURE 5.5.   Photo. Packs of *Belomorkanal* and *Kazbek*. These are contemporary packs from the author's collection. The path of the canal expanded with time, and the pack changed. These also both feature modern pack warnings along with various pinched presentations for creating crude filters for papirosy.

map on its label celebrating the 141-mile-long canal, which connected the White Sea to the Volga through Lake Onega and was completed in 1933. It joined brands like *Aeroklub* (Aviation Club) or *Bronenosets Potemkin* (Battleship Potemkin) lauding Soviet technology or events. Manliness and the adventure of the Soviet frontier are available for purchase with brands like *Kazbek*, with its rugged background of mountainous landscape contrasted with the silhouette of manly valor on horseback, or *Severnyi polius* (North Pole), released in 1938 as a commemoration of the polar explorations.[76] All allow the valorization of Soviet achievement alongside the inhalation of nicotine, and all employ the iconic Soviet-style pack of thin cardboard without cellophane or lining but incorporating a label with arresting graphics.

Stakhanovskie (Stakhanovites), named for the worker and efficiency crusade launched in 1935, assembles red flag, Soviet emblem, and work ethic with the papirosy for a strong message of communist consumption (Figure 5.6). The saturation of the public sphere with messages about Stakhanovite production and habits would have made this an easily deciphered set of symbols.[77] The embossed crest of the Soviet Union, raised print of the brand name, and metallic accents made this an expensive print job. This was likely a higher-priced gift set.

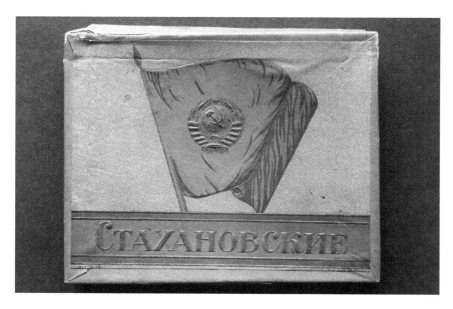

FIGURE 5.6. Photo. Pack of *Stakhanovskie*, 1939. Courtesy of Productive Arts. Russian/Soviet era posters, books, publications, graphics—1920s–1950s, www.productivearts.com.

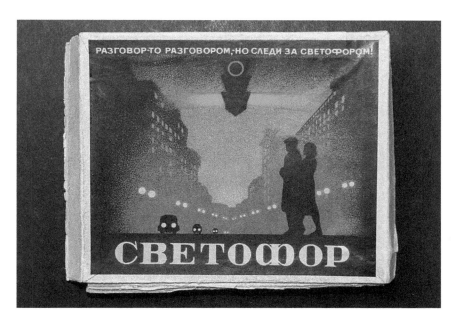

FIGURE 5.7.   Photo. Pack of *Svetofor*, 1941. Courtesy of Productive Arts. Russian/Soviet era posters, books, publications, graphics—1920s–1950s, www.productivearts.com.

Continuing a tendency for striking pack graphics, the 1941 *Svetofor* (Traffic Light) combines an arresting and beautiful visual of a city at night with an appreciation for the aesthetics of the socialist metropolis with its high-rise apartments, wide boulevards, electric lights, and modern automobiles (Figure 5.7). While not overtly political, the red light that shines over this idealized, newly emerging, urban landscape implicates Soviet power in the novel environment. A man and woman in silhouette and arm and arm enjoy this delicately lit scene together. Instead of the political message of *Stakhanovskie*, this pack carried with it a nod to the domestication agenda of the Soviet hygiene and etiquette campaigns. At top, a slogan reads: "Chat away as you like, but remember to mind the light!" This tagline sounds much like one of the many slogans about how to safely navigate the Soviet world—from work to leisure. The slogan takes on multiple meanings as advice for being a good citizen of the city, minding crosswalk safety, and reminding smokers to stop for a "Traffic Light" as part of sociable, modern life.

All too common were complaints over papirosy quality. A 1934 essay in *Pravda* lamented: "There was a time when the whole world praised Russian papirosy, Russian caviar, and Russian vodka.—O-ho—said foreigners drawing on our native papirosy—That's colossal!—Just the same they spoke of our caviar and our vodka." The author promised that these exultations over quality products from Russia and the Soviet Union would return: "It is not long before foreigners with similar ecstasy will respond to our ham, and our cheese, and our candies." Foreign tastes were not the salient issue, because the author concluded, "The most important thing is that our Soviet consumer likes our products."[78] Domestic consumer complaints showed foreigners were not the only ones disappointed. Grumbles over unfilled packs, irregular papirosy, and poor paper appeared throughout the 1930s.[79] In the absence of western ways of understanding consumer behavior through profits or pricing, feedback through complaints served as a valuable tool.[80] A 1935 soldier's letter in *Pravda* whined that because there were no special papers available for rolling tough makhorka and regular papers were too thin, "smokers must then use old magazines, impregnated with typographic ink."[81] When Mikoian remarked in 1936 that "there is so much makhorka on the shelves . . . that manufacturers themselves ask for help in selling it," this may have been a reflection more of poor quality than of satisfied demand.[82] Packaging improved in the 1930s, but the Soviets lagged behind other global tobacco markets in quality and extras such as foil inserts and cellophane wrappers.[83] More industry articles in 1937 and 1938 indicated a sustained interest in quality control.[84]

In the late 1930s complaints of deficits joined laments over quality.[85] In 1938 and 1939 *Izvestiia* ran pieces reporting shortages of salt, sugar, and soap in addition to problems supplying papirosy, makhorka, and matches.[86] Minsk had deficits of sugar, soap, and papirosy, and Moscow lacked flowers, perfume, and "even papirosy."[87] Deficits may have been viewed differently in the center. Another report from Moscow noted it was *Kazbek* that was missing, not all tobacco.[88] Charges of sabotage, wrecking, and misbehavior appeared in the press to explain problems. Theft by workers collaborating with anti-Soviet elements became a scandal for 1935–1936 at Moscow's Dukat, which expanded to critiques of the accounting, security, and management of the factory.[89] A 1935 article recounted the "wild" behavior of a mob that then attacked a tobacco thief before authorities could intervene.[90] Waste connected with slow transport made for a 1937 report from Rostov-on-Don.[91] Multiple stories followed the scandal connected to the head of the tobacco ministry Kravchenko, the director Sanishevskii and the chief of the department of raw materials Gordon, where management was accused of giving out free papirosy, creating a loss of tens of thousands of rubles.[92]

The general downturn in the economy from 1936 to 1940 paralleled an uptick in complaints regarding tobacco quality.[93] A 1937 *Pravda* letter to the editor contained a lengthy list of papirosy problems. The author singled out Dukat and Iava, noting that storage, packing, and counting were poorly done, and the papirosy were of "a bitter taste, too tightly packed, or conversely, very weakly packed."

Packing would affect burn—a crucial component of taste. Of other papirosy he grumbled that despite many different names the taste was virtually the same, so that the only difference between a *Riga* or a *Ialta* was size. The anonymous author identified other problems, including "unqualified women workers" and "patchy" paper. He urged improvements in handling raw materials as "a product requiring very careful storage is dumped in bales straight out in the open air." Additionally, the fact that warehousing was done throughout Moscow meant the leaf mix was "that which they have at hand. Thus the user gets a papirosa of different quality and taste from packs of the same name." The problems of the lowest-sort tobaccos did "not even merit discussion. . . [but] the low prices of these papirosy do not give the factories the right to sell trash."[94] Some papirosy of the same name were produced at different factories, with marked preference shown by users for particular enterprises. To address these issues, the Commissariat of Food Industry advocated labeling to show which factory produced a pack.[95] In 1939 a group of miners protested that the papirosy *Karaganda*, named for the city in Kazakhstan, were of such poor quality as to be "unworthy of the name of this city." Trade representatives promised to rectify this by making sure that *Karaganda* would henceforth be smokes "of the highest sort in beautiful packaging."[96]

Cessation Stalled and Smoking Stalinized

Starting with the turn to industry in 1928, antismoking propaganda posters and agitational materials focused less on the individual danger and more on the societal costs such as fires, work stoppages, and wasted money. The arguments against smoking breaks began in the late 1920s and intensified through the 1930s. A 1928 cover for the magazine *Krokodil* approached the issue with bite, showing a group of men smoking and loitering in what was titled "The Factory 'Club'" but was obviously the bathroom, a classic site for smoking in Soviet workplaces and made clear by the toilet cisterns hovering above the men's heads. A member of the factory committee scolds: "How are you not ashamed, comrades? For eight hours you sit in the lavatory!" To this one of the "loiterers" replies: "Wait a bit. When we move to the seven-hour workday, then we'll only sit here for seven hours." A 1930 *Izvestiia* article listed smoking as one of the many infractions of idlers, where "every lost hour is a crime."[97]

Time loss was more than just a joke. A 1930 *Pravda* article labeled the smoking break an efficiency issue. A 1934 article blamed smokers for wastefulness on the kolkhoz.[98] In the same year, fines for smoking at work were introduced—a return to prerevolutionary policies that had rankled workers.[99] A 1939 article pointed out the time loss from smoking breaks in the aviation industry, where one worker spent twenty-one minutes on six smoking breaks, another wasted an hour and five minutes, and a third a very precise thirty-three minutes.[100] Smoking on the job held the potential for fires, and reports of these, and their costs, regularly appeared in *Pravda*.[101] Material cost received greater attention than loss of life. A 1934 report of a fire from an improperly disposed-of papirosa focused on the damage to the machinery.[102] A horrific 1937 piece in *Izvestiia* recounted how a drunken worker set fire to himself after dropping a match onto his denatured-alcohol-soaked clothing.[103] An even more tragic outcome came when a father set himself and his children ablaze with a match disposed of in a film container.[104]

Maiakovskii penned a series of antifire slogans for industry that became well worn in the Stalinist build up. The warnings—"A small butt is enough to fire up an entire factory" and "A butt/falling from the finger of a drunkard/will stretch to engulf/an entire sleeping house in flames"—continued to appear well after the poet expired.[105] Factories that provided safe smoking areas, such as a Volga factory that put together a smoking area next to fire equipment received praise.[106] In 1930 Narkomzdrav proposed a law forbidding smoking in work areas except during special breaks and forbidding smoking by those under sixteen.[107] Continued complaints make it clear this was neither universal nor well enforced. In 1931 a three-page article supporting such a move appeared in a popular health journal, but an article a year later indicated no progress had been made, lamenting that while there might be a battle with alcohol, "a fight with that habit [smoking] is almost completely not fought."[108]

In newspapers, where wreckers and saboteurs found increasing prominence, the smoker was an easy scapegoat.[109] A 1930 *Krokodil* illustration seemed to both uphold and ridicule the idea. In the image a man sits and smokes on top of boxes labeled flammable and next to a basket that looks to be dry straw and rags. He squints at a copy of *Krokodil*. The large rooster on the cover underscores the danger because "Red Cockerel" was slang for fire. A sign hanging in the back proclaims that "Smoking Is Strictly Forbidden." Mocked under the title of "The Conscious One," the central figure chomps on a papirosa while reading the magazine with a slightly quizzical look and commenting, "I cannot believe that there are such slobs!" The magazine made an interesting choice in deriding its own readers by depicting them as absurd figures incapable of seeing their own hypocrisy and so irresponsible as to smoke on a pile of flammable materials. Missing was a reference to tobacco as dangerous to individuals; instead, tobacco's contribution to industrial problems took center stage.[110]

The arguments of the 1920s that tobacco wasted resources needed for the economy in other ways took on added urgency. Most often the emphasis was on the negative effects, the loss and harm, that tobacco inflicted on the general economy.[111] An intriguing example from *Down with Smoking* (1930) by A. S. Utekhin was the argument that in the paper-scarce Soviet Union, smokers burned up the necessary resources for children's literacy workbooks. As the pamphlet noted, three and a half packs of papirosy contained enough paper from which to make one sixty-kopeck notebook. To put this in helpful perspective, Utekhin calculated that a smoker burned up 204 notebooks a year.[112]

A text-heavy 1930 poster graphically portrays the resources burned up by featuring a papirosa smoldering through a stack of bills on an arresting red background (Figure 5.8). The text bemoans the 122,406,000 rubles "up in smoke" yearly. It was not just loss of money but loss of time, as the text in the yellow box at bottom reminds the viewer that an efficiency study of textile workers found that they spent 14 percent of their worktime in smoking. Oddly, while health is mentioned at the top, not one detail of the poster lists health, and the image does not include a human actor. The cost of tobacco use becomes highly impersonal.[113]

Tobacco's health dangers did not entirely disappear in propaganda. Materials continued to emphasize the role of nicotine, especially as a nerve poison or a danger to sexual function.[114] A poster from 1930—"Smoking Severely Impacts the Normal Function of the Organism"—sums up the major arguments (Figure 5.9). The slogan at bottom right mentions the smokers' susceptibility to tuberculosis, frequency for lip cancers, and difficulty in mental tasks even as the picture shows the connectivity of smoking to problems with salivation, the senses of taste and

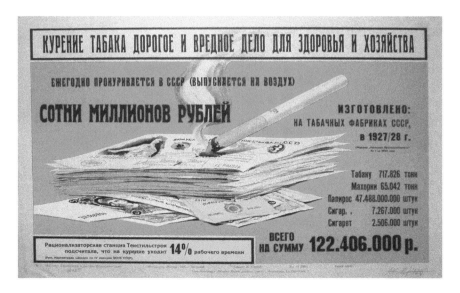

FIGURE 5.8. Poster. "Smoking Is an Expensive and Dangerous Thing for Health and the Economy," 1930. Courtesy Russian State Library.

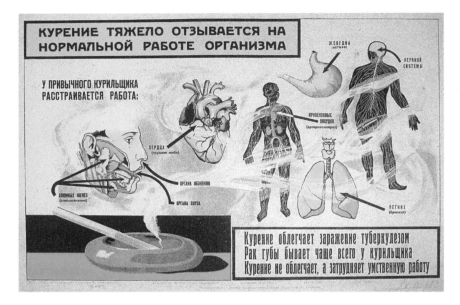

FIGURE 5.9.   Poster. "Smoking Severely Impacts the Normal Function of the Organism," 1930. Courtesy Russian State Library.

smell, heart, arteries, stomach, nervous system, and lungs. The partitioning of the body gives the resulting message a remarkably impersonal feel.

Soviet discussions of cancer, increasingly visible and urgent in the 1930s, did not target smoking beyond the mouth cancers that had long been connected to tobacco, despite emerging research on the carcinogenic effects of tars.[115] The early 1931 publications of studies by the Argentinian A. H. Roffo and America's F. L. Hoffman did not seem to enter into the conversations in Soviet medical health or industry materials.[116] By this point, tobacco discussions had retired from journals and publications almost entirely. Letters to the editor revealed an ongoing interest from the public in smoking's dangers, and especially advice on how to quit, but articles on the subject disappeared.[117] Despite popular interest, commentaries on smoking therapy remained measured. A 1935 story in *Krokodil* mocked the stupidity of doctors and their anti-tobacco therapies even as another story in the same year ridiculed a district attempting to forbid smoking.[118]

A major focus of the little cessation propaganda that appeared in the 1930s was the danger of smoking to women and children.[119] The attacks on female smoking, largely concerned with the ill effects on gestation and nursing, were of a piece with the natalist agenda of the 1936 ban on abortion and emphasis on women's roles as wives and mothers. The Komsomol youth group included anti-tobacco messages—among other advice on an abstemious lifestyle—in its code of conduct.[120] Even the ever-mocking *Krokodil* spoke out against women and children smoking as an evil—full stop.[121] Yet this propaganda conveyed a mixed message. The 1930 poster "Our Ultimatum to Adults!" from the Moscow Department of Health picks up the theme of adults being poor examples as had been part of the 1920s but remains remarkably devoid of commentary on the health dangers (Figure 5.10). The assembled pioneers, as denoted by their red kerchiefs, demand that adults not smoke for the health of the children and so as not to be a bad or hypocritical example, yet says nothing of how it might be a problem for the health of individual adults to smoke. A cover from the next year for the journal *Gigiena i zdorov'e rabochei i krest'ianskoi sem'i* contains a similarly weird message (Figure 5.11). The cover, "Smoking Is Poison—Think of the Children!" shows a child sobbing in the arms of a man. The child cringes away from the smoke, which curls up from the papirosa clenched between the man's teeth. Yet while the child sees danger, the man displays no signs of ill health. He looks young and robust. His hat and clothing indicate his placement as a worker—the lionized class. He is not lounging in a smoke break. He is not broken by ill health or marred by a pale complexion. Holding a child indicates he does not have the problem of sexual dysfunction so warned of elsewhere. The effects of smoking on the healthy adult male had been overcome just as the all-out campaign against smoking was abandoned.

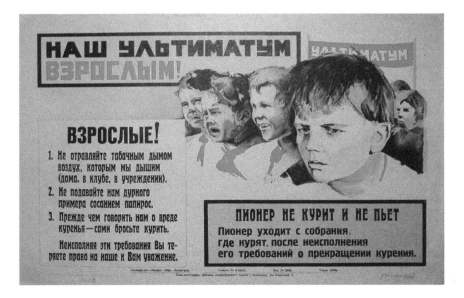

FIGURE 5.10.   Poster. "Our Ultimatum to Adults!," 1930. Courtesy Russian State Library.

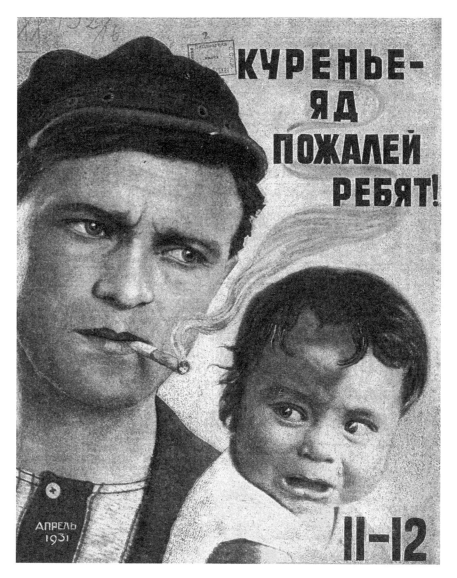

FIGURE 5.11.   Cover. "Smoking Is Poison—Think of the Children!," *GiZRS*, no. 11–12: 1931.

Tobacco emerged as a measure of capitalism's iniquities in comparison to Stalinism's joyous charms. A 1930 piece in *Pravda* lamented the lives of unemployed people in Berlin who received enough each day to purchase only "ten poor papirosy." The author cried, "How can they live on this?"[122] A 1933 article noted how, in the face of economic difficulties brought on by the global financial collapse, the quality of capitalist products had greatly degraded so that to meet demand, German industry moved "from more expensive goods and high-quality sorts to cheaper and lower-quality goods and surrogates: cheaper sorts of papirosy replace the more expensive. Synthetic silk and cotton fabrics replace wool and linen."[123] Yet never far was commentary on the exploitative nature of these industries. A 1932 article in *Pravda* mentioned that profits of American tobacco companies rose from 1928 to 1931 from 93 to 121 million because the companies benefited from the decline in prices for tobacco leaf even as they gouged users with an increase of a cent per pack.[124] American tax increases on tobacco similarly garnered attention from the Soviet press.[125]

Instead of outright attacks on smoking, a new campaign encouraged cultured, socialist use of state-produced items.[126] What and how one smoked were termed indicators of consciousness. For instance, a party man was expected to ask permission before taking a papirosa, while a nonparty, uncultured man might just grab it and leave his butts and ash everywhere.[127] Soviet analysts pointed to the increasing demand for higher sorts of tobacco as a sign of higher consciousness in smokers, returning to the idea that progression from peasant to worker manifested in tobacco preference as the peasant followed a "natural transition from makhorka to lower sorts of papirosy."[128] Communist authorities believed that consumer behavior could express the development of socialist consciousness: as citizens began to consume modern items—be it wine, watches, or phonographs—their views would be transformed from backward political opinions to a socialist consciousness.[129] Members of Stalin's upwardly mobile Soviet intelligentsia could show their rising status through a tobacco dialectic.[130] According to a 1938 *Izvestiia* piece, the desire for higher sorts of tobacco had grown steadily over the course of the decade, and a 1939 report highlighted the growing demand for "American" sorts.[131] Markets were not the only issue for quality tobacco. Measuring output in rubles incentivized production of higher tobacco sorts and meant factories did not always fulfill quotas for low-grade tobacco.[132]

Undoubtedly, the fact that Stalin avidly smoked a pipe led to difficulties in pursuing the same strong anti-tobacco message as under Lenin.[133] Stalin's tobacco preferences were well known—he would break apart the cartridges of *Gertsegovina Flor* (Herzegovina Flower) papirosy produced at Iava Moscow on special, monitored lines, then use the tobacco to fill his pipe.[134] Far from facilitating cessation, the pressure of Stalin's preference even led nonsmokers to take up the habit. According to a biography of Marshal K. E. Voroshilov, although he was an adamant antismoker, he can be seen in a 1930s photo smoking a papirosa alongside Stalin with his pipe. As the biographer concluded, "Evidently, in the presence of the 'people's leader' the marshal happily changed his habits."[135] Masculine models of the 1930s elevated Stalin as a father to all and made smoking a family affair and an admirable habit.[136] This coincided with a general triumphing of masculine behavior as a rejoinder to increasing empowerment of women as workers and wage earners.[137]

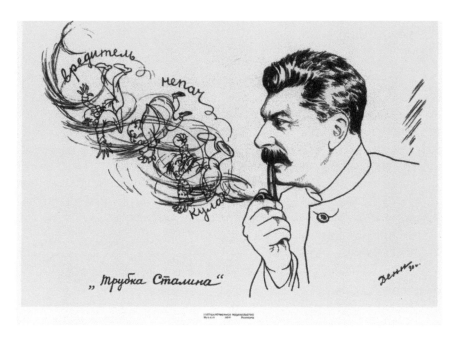

FIGURE 5.12.   Poster. "Stalin's Pipe," 1930. Artist Viktor Deni. Courtesy Russian State Library.

A propaganda poster by the famed artist Viktor Deni titled "Stalin's Pipe" graphically indicates the change in fortunes for smoking. In the striking line drawing, Stalin puffs in profile on his trusted pipe while figures of the kulak, NEP-man, and wrecker tumble out of it (Figure 5.12). Tobacco, far from being antirevolutionary, now becomes the means of cleansing the Soviet Union of its enemies. The smoke makes firm the ideas of Stalin, sweeping away the dangers to the national economy and upending the cessation agenda even as increased production brought in more and more users.[138]

By June 30, 1940, the Iava director Mariia Andreevna Ivanova assured *Pravda* of the strength of the factory, saying that in every eight-hour day the factory produced five million papirosy.[139] The industrial drive of Stalin's five-year plans, which had brought new machinery to tobacco and intensified agricultural production of leaf to fuel the industrial drive through increased taxation and revenues, had come into its own. Not only production expanded. Markets kept growing, so production still had difficulties keeping up with consumers. Deficits troubled the industry and would not be alleviated by the events of the coming years. The industry had recovered just in time for the thundering onslaught of war.

Even as tobacco production and use expanded, the cessation campaign receded from the national spotlight. The production of large-scale, anti-tobacco pamphlet and poster materials decreased after 1930, and cessation advice largely disappeared. This occurred just as foreign researchers were beginning to make concrete connections between tobacco carcinogens and malignant tumors. Instead economic arguments for production took center stage. Mikoian promised at the dawn of the decade that industry would continue to provide tobacco if demand continued, and his argument that production would continue until people decided not to smoke would frame industry attitudes and economic planning for some time to come. If people wanted to smoke, the state would provide. The economic consequences from those decisions would be measured largely not in individual health care costs to the state but in the profit of tobacco. The only loss from smoking came in the form of smoking breaks and fires—not illnesses and death. Arguments against tobacco would become even less visible during the following years of war and struggle. Instead of a danger to health, tobacco would emerge as the helpmeet of warriors on the front and workers in the rear. Cessation had been sacrificed on the altar of steel.

MOBILIZED

Frontline Provision and Factory Evacuations

In the summer of 1944 General A. Khrulev, deputy people's commissar of defense and chief of the Red Army rear, reported in a secret communication to Stalin that a major supply problem for the Fiftieth Army had been solved.[1] Khrulev explained that as the Germans retreated from the area northeast of Kiev, they had left to the Red Army the rich makhorka fields of the Chernigov region. From January 1 to May 1, 1944, Soviet troops harvested the makhorka fields and then, with five DM-300 grain grinders, they crumbled it into 1,856 tons of loose smoking makhorka. Khrulev summed up, with some obvious pride: "The quality obtained from the grain grinder production was completely satisfactory. The soldiers of the First Belorussian Front had no difficulties in reworking the raw material and provisioning themselves with makhorka." The army could now be transferred with the necessary supplies.[2]

Complaints over tobacco provision, or provisioning generally, among the Soviet armed forces should not come as a surprise; munitions, fuel, and even footwear shortages plagued the Red Army alongside problems of food provision and complications of malnutrition like scurvy.[3] But that the troops would take time out at a critical juncture to harvest makhorka and then make from rough-gathered, dried, then inexpertly ground leaf a "completely satisfactory" smoke beggars belief. Yet pictures from the field commemorated happy soldiers from across the operation queuing up to collect their smoking rations (Figure 6.1).

The spring of 1944 appeared to be an inopportune time to divert soldiers' energies toward something as mundane as makhorka. In the same months the Soviets were preparing for Operation Bagration, a massive assault on the

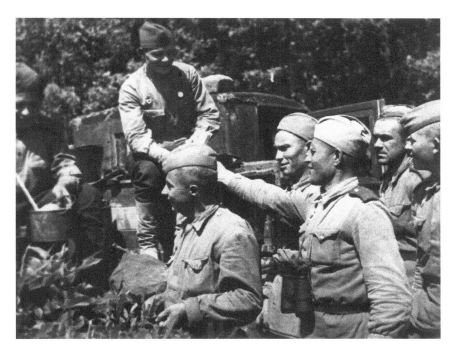

FIGURE 6.1.   Photo. Tobacco ration issue during Operation Bagration, Fifty-second Army, Second Ukrainian Front. Courtesy of the Central Museum of the Armed Forces, Moscow, via Stavka Military Image Research: Specialists in Russian and Eastern European Conflicts, 1900–1945. http://www.stavka.org.uk.

German lines in Belorussia and Ukraine to be coordinated with the allied attacks of D-Day. Named for a general who had pushed back Napoleon over a century before and launched on the three-year anniversary of Hitler's Operation Barbarossa (June 22), the Bagration campaign, one of the largest allied offensives of the war, shoved the Germans back some 450 miles in just five weeks.[4] But instead of using all their energies that spring stocking up on death-dealing armament or calorie-rich foodstuffs, the Red Army's Fiftieth took to the fields to harvest makhorka. And Khrulev seemingly thought that Stalin and the others addressed in the report (Mikoian, V. M. Molotov, L. P. Beriia, and G. M. Malenkov) would find this an appropriate, even laudable, use of Red Army time, energy, and resources.

The Red Army often functioned as "locavores" in the Great Patriotic War, and imperial Russian troops had similarly lived off the land, to greater or lesser success. The Americans and British gave soldiers rations. German troops supplemented their supplies with local foraging. None were as self-reliant as the

Red Army. Throughout the region and over the course of World War II, Soviet soldiers put down rifles to take up plowshares, feeding themselves and their comrades by harvesting at collective farms, slaughtering livestock, and hunting for wild game.[5] Still, the energy expended to gather and prepare makhorka—a consumable without any nutritional benefit—is a surprising allocation of scarce resources and redirection of soldiers' energy. Certainly, tobacco was important in the supplies for the militaries of other combatant nations. As part of the Lend-Lease Agreement, the US provided British and French troops with cigarettes, after first securing smokes for their own soldiers.[6] But US military leaders did not send their soldiers to harvest and prepare tobacco. American tobacco was not pulled from fields recently overrun by enemies or produced with makeshift machinery requisitioned for the purpose. In this, the Soviets were unique.

The Soviets chose to mobilize makhorka for the troops because of a long-established link between the military and tobacco and the importance accorded tobacco by those in command. And they did not just focus on frontline smoking. The tobacco effort began with the industrial evacuation necessitated by Operation Barbarossa and continued through starting up factories in Central Asia and beyond the Urals. Soviet workers made Homeric exertions, moving materials and machines—sometimes by transport, at times on foot—and working through grim conditions. The workers, like those in command, saw this as an essential companion to the effective soldier. According to a machinist of one tobacco factory: "Every papirosa we produce will be a shot at the fascists. A soldier smokes, warms up, and aims better."[7] Military leaders like Khrulev looked for every opportunity to bring the troops tobacco and makhorka. In the spring of 1944 the provisioning officer for the front in Kalinin was flown to Moscow for the express purpose of getting tobacco and ordered not to return without it.[8]

Tobacco was more than a simple ration. At the lines, on the march, in evacuation, and at the rear smoking became a stand-in for feeling full, being rested, or finding comfort. When shared among comrades in arms, smoking became the formative experience for many of the over thirty million mobilized in the Red Army.[9] Tobacco punctuated their breaks between terror and tedium, and its absence could separate the truly terrible times from those that were merely painful. When no tobacco could be found, makhorka shared with friends was flavored by camaraderie. When there was no makhorka, dust, leaves, wool, or bark became a wartime blend that would suffice to remind of the better times that might someday be. Tobacco leaves, smoke, smell, taste, and their meaning made up the texture of Soviet wartime.

Papirosy Weaponized and Tobacco's Evacuation

The earliest stories of papirosy in Russia revolved around the apocryphal tale of a soldier on the front lines forced to wrap tobacco in the fine paper of a gun cartridge to replace a broken pipe. In the Russo-Turkish wars fighting over the lands most associated with production of quality leaf intensified connections among man, military, and tobacco, as did the ready hand of marketers. Brands named for famous generals, advertisements depicting important battles, and romantic portraits of smoking soldiers all wove together in a haze of smoke-soaked, masculine, tobacco bravado.[10] In World War I the Imperial Russian Army was provisioned with tobacco, and this practice continued under Soviet power. This accessibility led to many new smokers who would then carry their habit home, just as tobacco accompanied the military units in other countries of World War I, leading to more smoking after peace. In the US, spurred by tobacco use in the military, per capita consumption of manufactured cigarettes tripled in the period from 1914 to 1919.[11]

In 1931 Mikoian had argued for the necessity of keeping tobacco production going not just for the economy but for soldiers.[12] Advertisements and movies of the 1920s and 1930s backed a vision of the smoking soldier. In the popular film *Chapaev* (1934), the titular hero, a commander of the Russian Civil War, smokes pipe and papirosy and is surrounded by other smokers. Tobacco gifts for the troops became a standard for the ensuing decades. A soldier of the far east recalled a schoolgirl sending "five packs of papirosy, a kilo of candy, a chunk of bath soap, a copy of Maxim Gorky's *Among the People* and six handkerchiefs with red, embroidered, five-pointed stars in the corners."[13] Even enemies provisioned soldiers with tobacco. Soviet newspapers reported from the Spanish Civil War, where a 1937 bomb of German manufacture exploded with a flurry not of shrapnel but papirosy with a letter, "For our Spanish comrades."[14]

After the conclusion of the Molotov-Ribbentrop Pact in August 1939, German troops invaded Poland on September 1 and Soviet troops on September 17. The Soviets deployed tobacco to sow good will in newly occupied territories, and enemies utilized tobacco to try and weaken the Soviets. Reports in Soviet newspapers featured the provision of tobacco as one of the gifts of Soviet power. An October report in *Izvestiia* decried the "prerevolutionary" conditions of an area, detailing how Soviet soldiers now provided the villages with vital materials including 14,300 boxes of makhorka, 10,000 boxes of matches, and 1,500 tons of kerosene.[15] Another article reported how a Polish village was springing back to life with Soviet occupation, including the resurrection of the local furniture businesses, sugar and sausage work, and tobacco factories.[16] In the conflict zones of the Winter War, initiated by the Soviets against the Finns in November 1939 and concluding in March 1940, tobacco proved a point of danger. An *Izvestiia* article lamented that on the ground in Finland, "our soldiers immediately engaged in a method of war dictated by a tough and evil enemy. Caution and vigilance are the firm rules. There are no cigarettes, no papirosy, no candy for our soldiers. All of that might be poisoned."[17]

With the conclusion of the Winter War, the Soviets had a period of calm as Hitler turned his attention to the west. England and France declared war against the Germans with the invasion of Poland in September 1939, and by the summer of 1940 German troops made their way into France and in the fall began the mass bombing campaign against the British. In the summer of 1941, however, Hitler became suspicious of Stalin's intentions, overconfident in the weakness of the Soviet state, and filled with hubris over his own perceived military superiority. On June 22, 1941, over three million German troops surged over the borders between Germany into the USSR, along a nearly two-thousand-mile front and advancing at a blistering pace of at times fifty miles a day. Within a month the Germans were nearing Moscow and had made massive territorial gains. When the effort to take Moscow finally began, in December of a year already experiencing an early winter, German troops were held to the outskirts of the capital. The Germans occupied territory that had been home to some seventy-eight million people or 40 percent of the 1940 population. They held the richest agricultural land and industrial areas responsible for over half of prewar coal and iron ore capacity as well as steel making and rolling. Two-fifths of prewar grain harvests and cattle stocks, 60 percent of prewar pig herds, and all domestic sugar production were compromised.[18] Not just agriculture was threatened. Leningrad— besieged, bombarded, and beleaguered—held millions of noncombatants.

As the German troops advanced, retreating Soviet forces burned, destroyed, or moved that which might help the invaders. Starting in the last months of 1941 and continuing through 1942, the Soviets improvised a massive evacuation of people and materials. In roughly a year an estimated sixteen and a half million people were evacuated to the interior.[19] In total, about twenty-five million would move over the course of the war—two million from Moscow alone.[20] Industrial production, military preparation, and state function took precedence, with party leadership, skilled workers, and potential military recruits evacuated first. Systemic and intentional factors favored urban regions and privileged groups.[21] In addition to people, somewhere between fifteen hundred and twenty-six hundred enterprises were evacuated to the interior along with over twenty commissariats from Moscow and collections of the Hermitage Museum in Leningrad and the Lenin State Library in Moscow.[22] As they were struggling to move mills and factories, people and raw materials, entire scientific institutes, archives, and even Lenin's body, the Soviets were under attack. In July 1941 some 1,470 air raids targeted railways, amounting to an average of fifty attacks a day. Hampered by transport problems, Khrulev reported that animal-drawn transport—be it horses, reindeer, camels, or mules—helped secure the rear.[23]

The fields of war coincided with those of tobacco—almost half of prewar tobacco cultivation lay in areas now under German control.[24] Tobacco production took a big hit. Leningrad contained some of the largest tobacco factories. The evacuation included fifteen to eighteen tobacco factories along with large amounts of their raw materials and workers. They moved into the interior, to places like Shadrinskii, Cheliabinsk, and Gorkii.[25] Although these places were safer, supplying them with raw materials and then returning finished goods entailed thousand-kilometer transfers.[26] Sometimes supplies meant for Omsk ended up in Alma-Ata or Tashkent. Areas of Central Asia saw expansion of existing factories and plantations. Confusion came with the handover of production of particular brands. The evacuation of Leningrad meant the transfer of production of *Kazbek*, *Belomorkanal*, *Katiusha*, and *Sever* to a Saratov factory.[27] Unique difficulties met each factory on relocation. Moscow's Iava Factory was evacuated—along with tobacco, paper, and a few dozen specialists—but the group was split among Kuibyshev, Kazan, and Saratov. Even with the difficulties of relocation, the factory reported that it fulfilled 62 percent of planned papirosy production for 1941 and 139 percent of the loose tobacco plan.[28] Despite the audacity of such reports, overall tobacco production figures were not good. In 1940 Soviet tobacco and makhorka factories made one hundred billion papirosy, but by 1945, even after many factories had come back online, output reached just twenty-five billion.[29]

Another Leningrad tobacco factory evacuated in mid-1941 to the Ural Mountains. In addition to the difficulties of moving people and machinery, the factory switched to working with low-grade leaf because of supply problems, even though it did not have the processing equipment for makhorka. Additionally, the factory began producing artillery shells and hand grenades. It is not clear how many tobacco factories mixed their manufacture in this way, but such crossovers gave rise to a persistent belief that bullets were made at the same diameter as papirosy so that the machinery could easily transfer between the two.[30] This rumor was aided by the slippery, militarized language of the papirosy "cartridges" themselves.

Transfer of factories meant movement of factory specialists and personnel. For all Soviet citizens labor was not an option but an expectation. Many who had never worked (women and children) or had stopped working (the old and infirm) stepped into jobs vacated by recruits. Days off disappeared, and shifts were long.[31] In 1940 the Supreme Soviet made unexcused absences or lateness punishable with fines of up to a quarter of earnings, and in 1941 rules tightened for defense plant workers. Absenteeism could be tried in military courts and result in five- to eight-year prison terms. As the war continued, the state announced it could draft to labor any men and women aged sixteen to forty-five or children above fourteen without parents or supervision. For workers in areas of the German advance, these rules created untenable choices. They were not allowed to leave without permission, but the bureaucracy of evacuation was chaotic. Many faced the difficult decision of evacuation, self-evacuation, or treasonous labor "desertion" as the enemy overran their towns and closed off escape routes. Some workers met the evacuation orders with protest, angered over the way the policy was pursued or worried about the possibility of losing their jobs and access to wages and rations.[32]

A factory history from the workers of DGTF, based in Rostov-on-Don, detailed the harrowing experience of continued work in the shadow of an approaching enemy but gave no hint of the threats from the state that forced such daring actions. One worker recalled how, as the Germans approached in 1941, the city administration organized the evacuation of key factories with important machinery. The tobacco factory was not in the first group, and so its workers were forced to stay and continue producing. As the enemy advanced, the women workers gathered at the Hotel Rostov to get uniforms and organize for the defense of the city. One worker recalled: "my mother said, 'You know, son, if the Germans make it, it will be better to die in the fight.'"[33] While this account concentrated on celebrating the valiant actions of workers, it also told of the cowardice of the director, party secretary, and staff, who secretly left with the factory car for Tbilisi. Such stories of weakness from leadership, many involving theft of money and goods, were regular features of evacuation tales.[34]

Evacuation of DGTF began on November 20, but it was too late.[35] Germans moved in the next day. Volunteers in street fighting units slowed, but did not stop, the advance. The Soviets liberated the city from this first German capture about a week later, but workers recalled there was "not one papirosa left—all had been taken or destroyed by the Germans." Many party members of the factory had been shot—about eighty in total. Even as some five hundred corpses littered the liberated city, the work had to be done. "And so we began to get production going," remembered one worker. The living trained for the jobs of the dead. Another recalled: "Those were hard times. I remember how at night at the factory, wagons and trucks stood waiting for papirosy and tobacco for the front."[36]

Even after the German expulsion and the return to the factory, the situation remained tenuous. Some had collaborated and had to be found. The director who had fled needed to be replaced. Bombardment was unrelenting. Those with children and the elderly evacuated, but the factory machinery stayed, workers remained, and production continued. War duties took up any leisure hours. Fire brigades kept round-the-clock watch on the factory's water tower and electric substation to guard against incendiary bombs. Women workers spent their off hours as nurses. Without steady supplies the factory cafeteria got creative with preparations of nettles, believed to prevent scurvy, and the newspapers published recipes for those wishing to try these culinary delights at home. State cafeterias of the period were notorious for their inventive cuisine, such as dumplings made from grass or creative cutlets.[37]

In the summer of 1942 German troops again threatened the city and evacuation began in earnest even as the factory was hit and damaged extensively. Remaining workers tried to hide what product there was in the hopes that Soviet troops might find it. As the Germans took the town a second time, the workers began a slow retreat that would take them first to Baku and then on to Omsk. Some began in cars and trucks, but military vehicles clogged the roads and the only bridge that spanned the Don. Soon enough, travelers took to their feet. In the early days of evacuation from major urban hubs, train cars of every description— from cattle to freight from subway to suburban—moved people and supplies. For those who evacuated late or from rural regions because of breakdowns, overcrowding, and general inaccessibility, the journey was often on foot.[38] Enduring sun and exhaustion, walking day after day, the workers of DGTF pressed on as feet blistered and then bled. At times, they crossed through rather than over rivers, and when the water became too deep, the "strong, healthy, and tall" would carry the women in their arms. Although in theory workers were evacuated with wages and supplies, and state-organized evacuation centers were supposed to provide food, clothing, and shelter along the way, provisions were wanting, and the 128 evacuation centers set up for the USSR were hopelessly overwhelmed. The DGTF workers foraged in the fields they passed, taking here a watermelon or there corn, which they ate raw. The group reached Armavir by August 1 and then journeyed on to Piatigorsk and finally, Baku, where fellow tobacco workers gave support and provisions of sugar, soap, and tobacco to trade along the road. All told, the journey had been over eight hundred miles by foot and on transport. From there the Rostov-on-Don workers went on to Omsk, which they reached in October.[39]

Wartime Work and Tobacco Shortages

No longer under fire or on the move, evacuees did not find rest. The DGTF workers were not the only newcomers in Omsk, a city some twenty-five hundred kilometers to the east of Moscow. By the end of 1941 evacuees had swelled the city by 42 percent. The mass of exhausted, hungry, louse-infested people overwhelmed housing stocks even as displaced enterprises looked for buildings to handle renewed production. In Omsk and other evacuation cities like Tashkent and Kirov, schools became barracks, prisons transformed into government offices, and in many cases tents, dugouts, or even railroad cars became lodging. City infrastructure was overcome, and the specialists for sewage, water, and electrical supply had gone to the front, so repairs were difficult.[40] When the workers of DGTF arrived in Omsk, they started with an empty two-story industrial building and immediately set to work creating rudimentary stations to crumble leaf and create passable tobacco. Production meant wages and provisions. Crushed for space, they lived in the factory even as they worked. Everything was further complicated by the winter weather, the lack of heat, and their own dearth of warm clothing.[41]

All over the USSR, the workforce had moved and transformed. The percentage of women in the labor force rose from 38 percent in 1940 to 51 percent by 1945. The workers also tended to be young. The percentage of workers under eighteen in the general workforce increased from 6 to 15 percent from 1940 to 1945.[42] Hours stretched, and the work week extended to six or even seven days.[43] In addition to new jobs, women workers took on new tasks outside of work to aid the war effort—donating blood, attending nursing classes, and organizing sales of war bonds.[44] Taking the place of the men, many women vowed to make up the work loss; a group called "Two Hundreders" at DGTF vowed, "to work for myself and my husband" and do no less than 200 percent of the norm.[45]

Without machinery the DGTF workers returned to the hand techniques of the prerevolutionary factory—whether it was hand cutting and crumbling or hand rolling and packing. Once the workers began to produce tobacco, things got better. Pay and rations flowed in, and it was obvious to all, according to one worker, that tobacco was considered "frontline goods." With time, cartridge and packing machines were acquired, although the factory continued to produce loose tobacco for the most part. By the liberation of Rostov-on-Don in February 1943, the Omsk factory had achieved a semblance of normal production with all the hallmarks of Soviet industry—a cafeteria, a union committee, and even party meetings.[46] Just as at DGTF, across the USSR tobacco production rebounded. If in 1940 there had been 26.1 tons of tobacco, in 1941 it dropped to 15.9 and by 1942 was back up higher than before to 40.5; it ended the war at 31.9 tons in 1945.[47]

Conditions in the besieged city of Leningrad differed markedly. The workers of the Uritskii Tobacco Factory (also known as the First State Tobacco Factory or the prerevolutionary Laferm Factory), like two and a half million of their fellow Leningraders, did not get the chance to flee the approaching German forces and instead endured nine hundred days of bombardment, deprivation, and starvation from September 1941 to January 1944. German troops from the west and south, joined by Finnish troops from the north, almost completely encircled Leningrad, cutting off supply lines and escape routes and barraging the city with an estimated seventy-five thousand bombs. In the worst days, food rations were not enough for survival. About half a million would be evacuated by train before the rail lines were cut, some through air lifts in late 1941, and others across Lake Ladoga's ice road after that. Over the ensuing days, into the starvation times of the winter of 1941–1942, the city would see the deaths of some eight hundred thousand civilians.[48]

Despite the siege, the Uritskii Factory continued to put out tobacco products, or at least tobacco-like products, for the city and its defenders.[49] At first, warehoused tobacco allowed manufacture of *Belomorkanal* papirosy, which were then sent to the soldiers defending the city. Tens of thousands of volunteers went to fight, making up about half of the defense force. They received little preparation. Some trained and deployed on the same day. Losses were high.[50] A photo of recruits for the Leningrad defense, sitting next to a railway car in late 1941 or early 1942, memorialized many probably smoking their last papirosy (Figure 6.2). As the supplies of tobacco declined, the blending specialists of the Uritskii Factory created mixes of tobacco dust, leaves (maple burned the best), and hops that one memoirist dryly sniped "reminded smokers of the taste of natural tobacco." In all, some eighty tons of leaves were dried, ground up, and mixed into Leningrad's ersatz tobacco. The resulting musty blend went by the name *Golden Autumn*.[51] The smokestacks of the Laferm Factory were scraped for nicotine residue, nitrobenzene, as a supplement to fight the vitamin deficiency disease pelegra.[52] Leningraders under siege suffered from *alimentarnaia distrofiia*, a peculiarly Soviet condition that medicalized the symptoms of starvation, and the small papirosy produced during the siege were called "dystrophic" (*distroficheskii*)—a grim joke on their content, size, and comparative weakness.[53]

Leningraders produced tobacco and consumed it as a food substitute, folk medicine, and comfort in the face of the increasingly horrific conditions in the city. The daily ration for children and nonworkers from November 21 to December 25 had been a meager 125 grams of bread. Tobacco claimed high prices on the black market. During the miserable winter of 1941–1942 a pack of papirosy could fetch 150 grams of bread.[54] Consumption for all Soviet citizens fell during the war. Food stuffs declined because of the destruction of the initial German advance, the dislocation of evacuation, the chaos in agriculture, and the many factories that moved to produce war goods. By 1942 sown acreage for agricultural production had contracted by 60 percent.[55] Individuals and entire unions organized gardens to fight starvation.[56] Rationing was introduced in July 1941

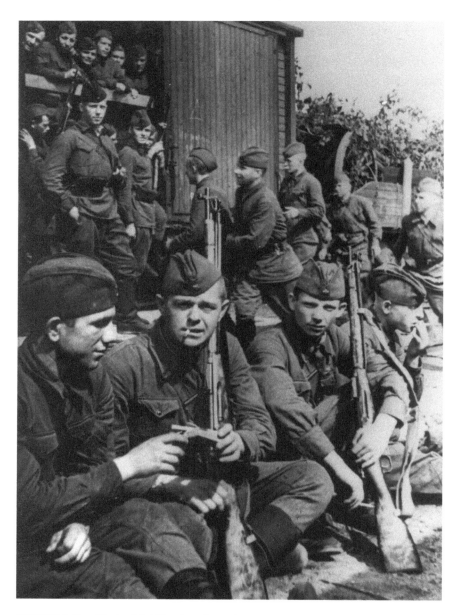

FIGURE 6.2. Photo. Mobilization, June–July 1941, troops leaving Leningrad. From the fonds of the RGAKFD in Krasnogorsk via Stavka Military Image Research: Specialists in Russian and Eastern European Conflicts, 1900–1945. http://www.stavka.org.uk.

and extended as time went on.[57] The priority was for soldiers, then workers, and finally civilians. The caloric consumption for all Soviet citizens dropped from a 1940 average of 3,370 calories to 2,555 calories in 1942. Averages hid the deep disparities between urban and rural areas and between soldiers, workers, and dependents.[58] Even as caloric provision fell, expectations for work increased, contributing to deaths from starvation and complications of malnutrition.[59]

Problems of agriculture and production meant extensive shortages for tobacco too.[60] For the home front, tobacco deficits started early, though ration cards did not include tobacco. In the face of mass food scarcity, the belief that tobacco could stave off hunger resurfaced.[61] Tobacco was part of the special packet of products given out to factory and transport workers as well as educational and scientific personnel. Memos between government departments indicated these were not always filled.[62] In 1942 Muscovites offered a drag on a papirosa on the street for two rubles a puff.[63] Alongside vodka, tobacco was used for exchange.[64] Paper shortages plagued areas of front and rear so that even newspaper became a sought-after commodity for smoking. In the Gulag in 1944 the old newspaper that wrapped a parcel could net an entire dinner in trade because of its use for rolling papers. A copy of *Pravda* or *Izvestiia* would get eight rubles or a coupon for a two-course meal.[65]

Tobacco Rations and the Red Army

Millions served in defense in the Great Fatherland War. Men and women pulled from Central Asia and Leningrad, collective farms and scientific institutes were assailed by confusing situations, unfamiliar faces, and new rules before they even got to the violence of the front lines. Transferred into war, a sensory assault of stench, noise, and physical discomfort threatened to overwhelm the soldier even as adrenaline surges and panic intensified sensitivity.[66] Jostled together in an alienating, confusing, and often terrifying environment, recruits could pull from smoking not just a physical jolt and soothing practice but a set of established cultural meanings, rituals, and images grounded in the over one hundred years that tobacco had been part of Russian and Soviet military life. Papirosy in uniform served as they had before the war. Socially, they opened conversations, cemented status, created communities, and marked barriers. Psychologically, they passed time, signaled relaxation, sparked reverie, invited nostalgia, displayed manliness, and shaped identities. Physically, they created addictions, scented bodies, satisfied withdrawal, and purportedly calmed nerves and satiated hungers.

Provisioning the men and women in arms took precedence over civilian supplies.[67] Soldiers got rations of makhorka and loose tobacco as part of the packet considered "for physical survival" rather than as a luxury, and commanders received a higher amount of better tobacco. Women in uniform earned a supplement of chocolate or coffee if they were nonsmokers, though many preferred tobacco for exchange or sale. As in previous conflicts, the public recognized tobacco as the soldier's helpmate. Care packages regularly included tobacco with other deficit items like "fruit, chocolate, cocoa, butter, papirosy, cologne, soap, pencils and envelopes."[68] A 1942 *Pravda* report recounted the packages of "meat, poultry, butter, eggs, honey, sausage, wine, vodka, beer, and tobacco/papirosy" coming for the Red Army from Kuibyshev oblast.[69] Iava and other Moscow tobacco factories sent packages directly.[70]

Partisan groups, fighters engaged in small-scale, often independent guerilla actions that strained the German forces in occupied territories, also received tobacco provisions.[71] In Bulgaria the large number of Jews in the tobacco industry led to their notable representation in partisan and political prisoner numbers—an estimated 80 percent.[72] Although the percentage of Soviet tobacco workers among the partisans is not clear, Soviet partisans enjoyed a smoke. One Ukrainian partisan included tobacco as part of his carefully crafted image in an artfully staged photo (Figure 6.3). A jaunty straw hat at a rakish slant presents an interesting juxtaposition with the cape for camouflage, but the harmony of fighting élan and smoking pleasure ring out. High command understood the importance of tobacco to partisans and had it delivered to them behind the lines by air on multiple occasions along with supplies of gasoline, spare tank parts, and some food.[73]

Rolling papers continued in short supply. In the summer of 1942 the head of paper production complained to Mikoian that although the group had been charged with producing seventy-one million "smoking books," they had materials for only ten.[74] The books of sheets of five- by eight-centimeter tissue paper made fifty self-rolled papirosy. The Red Army representative chimed in to note the danger this presented to morale: "The lack of smoking papers among soldiers gives the ability of individual anti-Soviet elements to distribute enemy leaflets under the guise of papers for smoking. In addition, with the availability of tobacco the lack of smoking papers creates discontent among soldiers and commanders."[75] Mikoian pledged a monthly production of thirty-five million smoking books by working with paper and newspaper suppliers, but continued complaints suggest he failed.[76] Paper made its way to smokers through other means. A thousand tons of cigarette papers were part of the Lend-Lease Agreement, though there were cutbacks on tobacco because this was considered important for American civilian consumption.[77]

Other supplies for tobacco became standards of soldiers' kits. The bag to hold makhorka, with a bit of cabbage leaf to keep tobacco moist but not wet, alongside

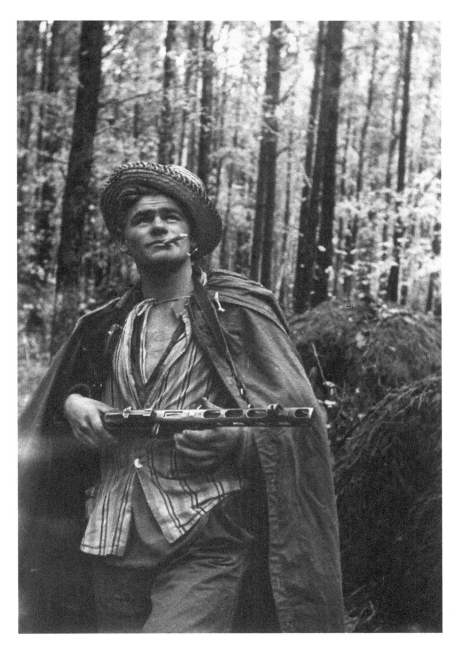

FIGURE 6.3. Photo. A member of Kovpak's Ukrainian partisan unit smoking. From the fonds of the RGAKFD in Krasnogorsk via Stavka Military Image Research: Specialists in Russian and Eastern European Conflicts, 1900–1945. http://www.stavka.org.uk.

some papers or scraps of newspaper, might form a basic bag, but embroidery could elevate this into a keepsake. Time out of battle might be taken up with the sculpting of tins to hold papirosy from spent shell casings or other metal, wood, or even plastic taken as a trophy from the enemy. A craft and remembrance, these often became gifts or reminders of fallen comrades. Invested with memories of not just the tobacco smoked but the people with whom it had been shared, these packs and pouches took on immense meaning. A poem by Vasilii Terkin eulogized a lost tobacco pouch, and from home, perhaps mindful of their importance, anonymously sent tobacco pouches journeyed to the front lines.[78]

Hunger—for paper or tobacco—bedeviled the troops and command. Troops who were not provisioned experienced physically the failures of the government, and the effects on morale were much discussed. As one 1943 article for propagandists observed, "In conversation with the soldiers . . . political officers learned how important hot food, tea, spices, and a smoke could be to men risking their lives in defense of the state."[79] Officers regularly went to Moscow with orders to get smokes.[80] Distribution was a problem. In December General Khrulev received a request for twenty cars to transfer tobacco from behind the lines up to soldiers on the front.[81] The next memo complained that when the previous request had not been filled, the materials had languished at stations and "seriously deteriorated." Under the threat that it would soon be a complete loss, the last telegram in the file asked Moscow for cars to haul the tobacco up to the lines.[82]

Over the course of 1944 even more complaints came to Mikoian regarding military tobacco provision.[83] A long memo from the political department of the Twenty-eighth Army from September 25 protested that when the center could not deliver, they had tried to work with local resources: "Tobacco raw materials were sought on the ground, working it in the field in a primitive way with handmade cutting and crumbling." This had operated as a stopgap measure until the group received a shipment of twenty-eight tons of "Mari Filiche's tobacco from Tbilisi." What looked to be a reprieve, the writer carped, turned out to be a headache: "As soon as the tobacco was given out to the soldiers, a mass number of oral and written complaints about the tobacco's poor quality began to arrive." A commission of several officers detailed the deficiencies. The group concluded that the tobacco was poorly cut, containing stalks and chunks: "The consequence of this is that it is difficult to wrap the tobacco even in dense newsprint." The writers signed their letter with cheerful expressions of patriotism, but only after a strong conclusion: "We understand some difficulties with a lack of tobacco; however, in this case we are talking about the poor quality of tobacco processing."[84]

Even when tobacco could be obtained, the smell and taste of the smoke was notoriously unpleasant. Germans reportedly moved their nonsmokers to the front to sniff out the stink of sweat and makhorka that betrayed hidden Soviet troops.[85] According to one account, Soviet soldiers preferred rolling tobacco in newspaper because they believed it enhanced the taste.[86] The purplish smoke emanating from the Soviet soldiers' papirosy led to them being known as *feliton* (feuilleton—from the French for light news circular and a play on the Soviet tendency toward newsprint).[87] Pages of books would do in a pinch. In 1944 the journal *Krasnaia armiia* published as part of its library for the troops A. P. Chekhov's prerevolutionary one-act vaudeville of a henpecked husband, Markel Ivanovich Niukhin (Snuffer), giving a humorously ineffective anti-tobacco speech. It would be surprising if these pages had not ended up as rolling papers.[88] Some accounts related how soldiers might become so desperate as to roll their identity documents. Even soldiers had trouble getting tobacco. Those without tobacco had been known to smoke the wool of their coats.[89] Some tried leaves from other plants or trees. Antismoking drugs utilizing the alkaloid cytisine can trace their origins to the wartime substitution of golden raintree leaves for scarce tobacco and the accidental discovery of their satisfaction of nicotine cravings.[90]

The front suffered from lack of supply, and records indicated problems getting tobacco to troops in the rear. In February 1944 Khrulev noted the need for tobacco near Tula and other military districts.[91] Similar complaints came to Mikoian.[92] Kiev's military district was in deficit as well.[93] Officials explored importing one thousand tons of tobacco from Bulgaria and moving into a regular relationship with the country for future imports.[94] Another group moaned that they had harvested tobacco, given the raw leaf to a factory, and never received it back.[95] Military schools and engineers complained of supplies.[96] Some couched their appeal in concerns over order, arguing that without makhorka people would steal to get it or the black market would flourish.[97] Improved conditions with provisioning marked the final years of the war. Included in this vision of a new, better wartime was smoking. When an artillery officer in 1945 remembered how conditions had improved, one of the first things he mentioned was "we had enough to smoke."[98]

Images, songs, and memoirs back up the idea that sharing a smoke with fellow soldiers spanned the war and the ranks. According to the director of Iava, during World War II "all the generals" smoked its *Kazbek* brand, and as the factory returned from evacuation "orderlies from marshals and generals" hung about the factory looking for their preferred papirosy.[99] The solidification of the multinational force at Bagration was scented with makhorka. A photograph shows Red Army and Polish soldiers in a comradely exchange of tobacco, perhaps even the same leaf the soldiers of the Fiftieth Army had liberated from the fields of Chernigov (Figure 6.4). A soldier recalled that his bunker smelled differently than those of Germans because it was "filled with the tart fumes of tobacco and the aroma of bread."[100] The photograph of recruits for the Leningrad defense similarly indicates how tobacco scented rituals of bonding and waiting (Figure 6.2).

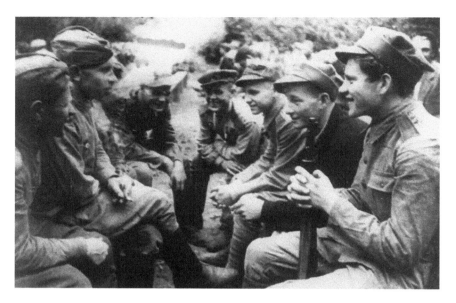

FIGURE 6.4.   Photo. Polish troops sharing a smoke with Russians during Operation Bagration, August 16, 1944. Courtesy of the Central Museum of the Armed Forces, Moscow, via Stavka Military Image Research: Specialists in Russian and Eastern European Conflicts, 1900–1945. http://www.stavka. org.uk.

Other accounts point to the centrality of tobacco to the soldier's life and even the presumed benefit it gave. A Soviet antitank rifleman maintained that smoking was a permitted companion, even in the thick of conflict. Speaking in 1942, he proposed, "'It is permissible to smoke in battle; what is not permissible is to miss your target, miss it just once and you will never light up again.'"[101] Occasionally, as reported in a 1941 *Izvestiia* article "Night on the Front Lines," a commander might prohibit smoking because "there are enemies in the heights."[102] On guard duty, soldiers were not to distract themselves with eating, drinking, singing, or smoking.[103]

Despite its poor quality, but in recognition of its luxury and rarity, shared tobacco became a ritual important to descriptions of rest. Just as mutual hunger could bring together soldiers as they jointly experienced hardship or split a ration collectively, so too could communal makhorka signal becoming part of a group or be a means of exclusion.[104] One report from the Red Army's Political Department detailed how some soldiers refused to distribute tobacco outside of their ethnic group.[105] To secure tobacco for comrades took on broad meanings. Vasily Grossman, reporting from Stalingrad, recalled an anecdote "representative of soldiers' priorities": when two soldiers came in to get supplies for their sur-rounded comrades—ammunition, sugar, and tobacco—they explained "there are two more of our men there, guarding the house, and they need a smoke."[106] Yet the shared tobacco must be of the right kind. One tank commander was reported to meet the offer of captured tobacco derisively: "German! From it you smell human blood!" He countered with a quote from the nineteenth-century Russian poet Fedor Tiutchev, "Better to have our own makhorka: 'The smoke of the fatherland is sweet and pleasant.'"[107]

The 1942 song "Let's Smoke" (Davai zakurim) celebrated the centrality of shared tobacco to the front lines.[108] The chorus called to mind future days when the Germans would be gone but friends could sit around a fire and recall the infan-try, reminisce about their companions, and remember "you, for what you gave me to smoke. Let's smoke comrade, one by one. Let's smoke, my comrade."[109] The desire of Soviet soldiers for a smoke was clear to Americans. Russian-American Music Publishers dedicated its appreciation "of the exemplary heroism of the Peoples of the USSR" by publishing the song "Makhorka" in 1943 for distribu-tion in the US. The lyrics celebrated smoking along the Dnieper, "curling smoke" taking away sorrow, and "grimly" lighting up while taking a stand.[110] Given the mission of the group, it must have been meant to emphasize the commonalities of soldiers' experiences and build sympathy and support for the Soviet fighters.

Tobacco and makhorka had their own story during Soviet wartime that was unique because of the history of use in Russia and the USSR and the Red Army's special relationship with provisioning. Tobacco was seen as important enough to merit movement of entire factories and necessitate breaks from military build-ups to send soldiers out to harvest and prepare it. Soldiers suffered from lack of tobacco and workers struggled through bombings, starvation, and evacuations to get papirosy to them. The resources expended in the preparation, securing, and distribution of tobacco were substantial for a country struggling to feed itself, arm itself, and survive. Yet the Soviet moved, if not mountains, entire industries beyond the mountains to secure it. These priorities for utilizing scarce resources had consequences that extended well after the war. Tobacco shared among com-rades in arms became the formative experience for many of the over eleven mil-lion mobilized in the Red Army for World War II.

The military had inculcated a vast group of new users to the habits, tastes, and understandings of tobacco forged in war, and the ranks of smokers swelled.[111] War deeply entrenched an already widespread habit in the culture of male cama-raderie and masculine display and associated its provision with the bare mini-mum required for life. Every papirosa may have been a shot at the enemy, but it was one that came with tremendous costs for the war's survivors.

RECOVERED

Women's Kingdoms and Manly Habits

In 1949 Iava Tobacco Factory Director Mariia Andreevna Ivanova, sat for a photo. It proved a monumental year for Soviet tobacco, for in 1949, just four years after World War II devasted the industry, Soviet tobacco returned to prewar production levels (Figure 7.1).[1] The abundance of playful packs and Ivanova's casual posture little hint at the difficult times the factory had weathered, but Ivanova, who led Iava from the 1930s, had helped the factory and its personnel endure war, evacuation, and destruction and guided them toward an astonishing rebuilding and reconfiguration.[2] Hers was but one factory of many resurrected. German forces, withdrawing from Soviet lands, had left destroyed tobacco factories and fields in their wake. As part of the general rebuilding associated with the postwar years, the tobacco industry had to be rebuilt—again.

The Soviets sacrificed for tobacco during the war and bringing back production after the conflict required still more sacrifice. The iron will necessary to achieve this rebirth and reinvention is not caught by the black-and-white still, as Ivanova calmly surveys a special gift box of *Osobennye* (Special) papirosy decorated in folk-art style, but by the time of Ivanova's retirement from Iava in 1961, the factory was producing not just esteemed papirosy but also cigarettes and filtered products on western-style machinery. The rows of papirosy and cigarette packs silently salute her achievements. This chapter follows Soviet smoking through its period of recovery after the war until the importation of filter cigarette machinery in 1965. Along the way it outlines the changes on the factory floor, in smoking culture, and the gendered nature of postwar smoking. The death of Stalin in 1953, the Thaw introduced by Nikita Khrushchev, and the

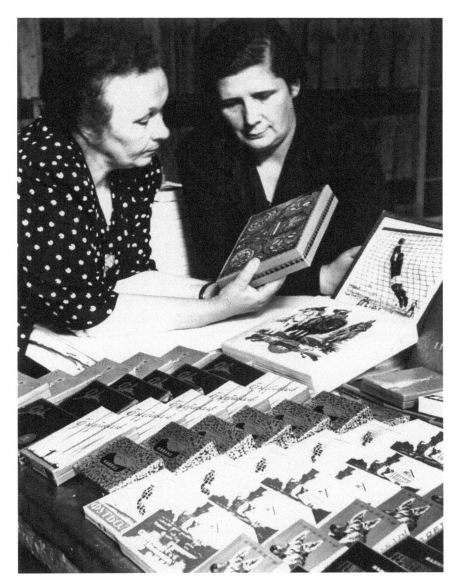

FIGURE 7.1. Photo. Director of the Iava Tobacco Factory Mariia Andreevna
Ivanova (left), overseeing the production of tobacco gift packs, 1949. RGAKFD
0–197125.

transition to Leonid Brezhnev did not lead to intense changes in tobacco culture. Instead, the war provided an ever larger, enduring market of smokers while social and cultural factors influenced the imagery of smoking and industrial developments allowed for product innovation.

Ivanova and her companion were but two of the many who rebuilt Soviet manufacturing after World War II. For the women of Iava, as for women throughout the Soviet Union, there was no chance for a slackening of effort, no moment of reprieve. A new five-year plan, another series of persecutions, a purge of the victors, and recollectivization greeted the peace. And for Soviet women, unlike those in other allied countries, there were further demands. They stayed in the jobs they had taken up during the war, and more women came into the workforce to join them. Pressures for increased birth rates ensured that many women would shoulder a double burden of work and motherhood, and the gender imbalance caused by the war meant many women carried these burdens alone.

Ivanova's photograph showed her frozen in time, but in life there was no stopping. Over the next decade, Ivanova oversaw significant changes at the Iava Factory. The first cigarette machines imported from a vanquished Germany appeared after the war and were used to produce *Prima*, hailed as better than the "strong and to an extent more dangerous papirosa."[3] More machinery was brought in, moving Iava away from handwork. The mass importation, in 1965, of western cigarette machinery accelerated the transition in production and in the workforce. The association of males with machine work, along with the greater mechanization, and the push to hire more males into higher positions, pressured out women. The change was reflected in the leadership as Ivanova was succeeded by male directors and Iava transitioned to male majority employment. By 1970 the female workforce at Iava had fallen to about 40 percent while the male workforce had climbed to about 60 percent.[4]

The shop floor was not the only thing in transition. The change in production saw a move away from papirosy as the preferred smoke to western-style cigarettes. Although it would be some years before filter cigarettes became the main form of consumption, the introduction of Soviet-produced filter brands heralded a new day for consumers. Even as research in the west connected smoking to lung cancer in the 1950s, and the Americans and British introduced restrictions on tobacco in the 1960s, Soviet health authorities continued to emphasize nicotine over tars and resultant cardiovascular problems over cancers.[5] Instead of medical authorities, tobacco industry leaders took up the push for filters and cigarettes over papirosy and makhorka in a call for higher quality and improving consumer tastes. The absence of the Iava-produced *Belomorkanal* from the display was an indication of this development.

Finally the 1949 photo reveals that tobacco manufacture was a "women's kingdom," but the array of brands suggests a male consumer. Surveys indicated increasing numbers of women smokers by the 1970s, but men smoked in overwhelming numbers from the 1950s to 1960s. For many, tobacco had become a habit during the war, a result of the tobacco ration, social pressure, food insecurity, and combat tension. After the war, militancy and masculinity flavored Soviet tobacco products in packaging, cultural display, and the few advertisements that appeared. Images of male bonding through tobacco use showed up in everything from cartoons to high art. Even as smoking prevalence declined in the west because of new health information, Soviet tobacco use, especially by men, grew as quickly as supply could meet it. Social norms and cultural cues conspired to increase smoking among men to alarming rates. The sacrifices made by Ivanova and other women to restore Soviet tobacco would take a toll on Soviet men in failing health and decreased lifespans in the years to follow.

Women's Work and Tobacco's Rebirth

On May 9, 1945, Germany surrendered. Bombings, battle, and violent occupation had reduced Soviet housing and factories to rubble and destroyed about a quarter of prewar fixed assets. Fields left untilled or trampled resulted in severe food shortages until 1949. Human losses remain soul-numbing estimates rather than exact figures. Around twenty-eight million Soviet citizens and soldiers perished. Nearly three million returned disabled from war.[6] Persistent rationing, social discontent, famine from 1946 to 1947, monetary reforms, and the continued existence of informal trade networks indicated that state and economy also suffered.[7] Although offered help from the US, the Soviets refused aid; instead, Stalin meant to prove the superiority of communist planning. The discontinuation of rationing in 1947 was an important political signal of Soviet recovery, but shortages of skilled personnel continued to hamper efforts.[8] The Fourth Five-Year Plan for 1946–1950 tackled the rebuilding of the Soviet Union.[9]

Despite the difficulties, the Soviets renewed their commitment to tobacco production even before opening the front with Japan on August 9, 1945. A page one story in *Izvestiia* on June 9, 1945, called for an increase in tobacco production of over four times that of the previous year, with an emphasis on quality. Noting that although papirosy "during the time of war were put out in the absence of standards," the author contended now was the time for good tobacco. The article acknowledged there would be difficulties, but new schools were training technicians, and although four of the six prewar tobacco paper factories had been destroyed, three had already been rebuilt.[10] Despite the bravado, tobacco agriculture and industry struggled. Caught in the fields of war, sown tobacco had declined nearly fourfold. In 1950 the Soviets returned to prewar levels of sowing, but not until the end of the Fifth Five-Year Plan did harvests reach prewar levels as tobacco plantations expanded outside of traditional strongholds to include Uzbekistan, Azerbaijan, and Armenia.[11]

The story of DGTF typifies the problems tobacco faced. Rostov-on-Don, liberated in February 1943, had seen six months of fighting, and German occupation had destroyed all but 6 of the 274 factories in the city, including what remained of the evacuated DGTF. The factory director returned in March to a city three times smaller than before the war. *Izvestiia* reported that the Germans had carted off what they could steal and burned the rest. Only the warehouse had survived. Holes were patched with wood culled from broken clothing wardrobes. The factory machinery was cobbled together with two tractor transmissions.[12] One memoirist quipped that the factory had gone "po-Asmolovskii" meaning the handwork style used under the prerevolutionary owner, Asmolov. Despite the harsh conditions, optimism accompanied the return to production, and the factory issued its first postwar pack under the name *Pobeda* (Victory).[13] Stories of quick recovery and "lightning" production featured in the DGTF history.[14]

Although there were reports of grand triumphs that exceeded previous norms or surpassed planned outputs, it would be a few years before a full recovery.[15] Other destroyed tobacco factories in Kursk, Odessa, and Kharkov rebuilt and boasted of returning to active production by 1945, though many of these were probably runs of Potemkin papirosy—a symbolic output before closing the factory to retool in earnest.[16] A 1946 report from the Feodosiia Tobacco Factory of Simferopol boasted that the workers had rebuilt the factory and by November had met the plan goal of one billion papirosy.[17] By 1947 the factory in Kharkov was at full capacity.[18] Even factories that had not been destroyed struggled in the aftermath of the war. The Klara Tsetkin Factory of Leningrad reported in 1945 that while the factory had suffered from shelling, it had now been rebuilt, aided by demobilized Red Army soldiers, and returned to operation. By the end of the year they planned to produce more than two hundred million papirosy.[19] The Iaroslavl-based Balkan Star escaped destruction but soon outstripped the capabilities of the machinery it had and would need to retool to increase output.[20] In October 1945 Iava reported raw material shortages, but the effects on production were mitigated because evacuated machinery had not yet returned. Even so, Iava reported producing two billion more papirosy in 1945 than in the previous year.[21] By 1949 prewar tobacco production levels were met, and by 1958 they had increased 2.3 times from 1940 levels with papirosy and cigarette production at 232 billion.[22] An article in *Tabak* in 1950 trumpeted successes by some collective farms in increasing makhorka harvests.[23] As production increased, the prices of tobacco continued to fall, as they had since the 1930s. In 1956 tobacco prices reached the lowest that they would be for the entire Soviet period.[24]

A Soviet news photo from 1959 showcases one postwar expert in the tasting department (Figure 7.2). She is a "Sappho" for the postwar age. She sits back, luxuriating in the taste of tobacco like any nineteenth-century connoisseur and

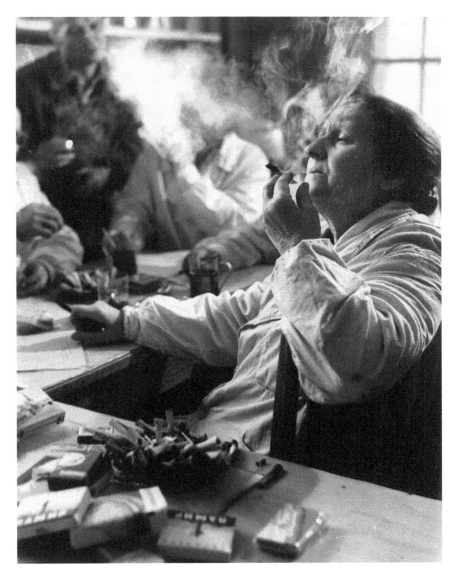

FIGURE 7.2.   Photo. Tasting at the Iava Tobacco Factory, 1959. N. Rakhmanov for TASS. RGAKFD 1–67480.

contemplates what she will write regarding taste—in terms of leaf blend, burn, and mouthfeel—of one of a series of papirosy she has lit up. While the woman is not identified, before her are packs of *Pamir* and other Iava brands. Next to these are glasses of tea with delicate metal holders and spoons sticking out, indicating that sugared tea is part of a palate cleansing between puffs. Compared to the automated units of the big tobacco conglomerates, Iava continued to have a hands-on, even artisanal approach to quality, and for the moment, these hands were women's.

Life in postwar factories was difficult not just because of material problems and the stress of rebuilding. To meet production quotas, factories often put on three shifts to work machinery day and night. Because of a 1944 law focused on the health of working mothers, the night shift could not go to a pregnant or nursing mother, and this left further burdens on the remaining workers.[25] As tobacco was a female-heavy industry, this is likely to have led to increased work for other women. Even into the 1960s tobacco factories depended on intensification, working three shifts, alternating days and nights, six days a week. According to one employee of the time: "papirosy lines worked almost without break twenty-four hours a day. The lines did not stop."[26]

Despite the amped-up production, demand for tobacco products was not being met, and protests over quality continued. A 1948 *Pravda* piece reported on the problems of *Belomorkanal*: "In a random pack you will find empty or ripped cartridges with dirty, sprawling print on the mouthpiece. Papirosy that according to the opinion of smokers are completely inadequate." The author further criticized the "disgusting taste."[27] A 1953 *Izvestiia* criticism from the vice-chairman of the Executive Committee of the Kologrivskii district similarly called for greater attention to *Belomorkanal* quality.[28] Cartoons and asides in *Krokodil* indicated continued discontent. One 1950 piece mocked the leadership of the Dukat Factory for inadequate responses to smoker complaints and urged readers to make their disappointment known.[29] Another piece joked of how the management of the L'vov factories that produced *Kazbek* and *Katush* were doing their best to help smokers quit. The papirosy from the factory were so bad that "the stores won't take them and the smokers won't smoke them because the papirosy have trash mixed in with their tobacco."[30]

Much of the work being criticized and much of the labor rebuilding fell to women. Men made up over three-quarters of the war dead, and imbalance characterized the adult population. Huge losses of able-bodied males meant that the women who had entered the workforce during the war were not turned out of their positions, as in other countries. Sixty percent of the population over sixteen was female, and if in 1940 women had been 38 percent of workers, by 1945 they were 55 percent. Even with the influx of women, the labor force after the war only met about half of the demand.[31] State campaigns urged women to take up more, do more, and produce more. Joyous portraits of female Stakhanovites featured in the press along with calls for women to enter leadership positions.

Statistical celebrations of renewed production hid difficulties. Although Soviet citizens recognized that it would take work to rebuild, by 1947/1948 the public became increasingly impatient for an end to sacrifice. Women and even children who had entered the workforce during the war never returned to the home. Men who had survived, unable to have rest and relaxation during the war, now integrated directly into the workforce upon demobilization. Additionally, living conditions continued to be grim. In Novgorod in 1947, about a third of the population (nine thousand of twenty-nine thousand) sheltered in temporary barracks, basements, or dugouts. A 1956 Union-wide survey found that tens of thousands still, a decade after victory, lived in temporary housing. Shortages of basics like soap and butter dominated daily life.[32]

The state called women to work and have children all while handling these shortages of goods and housing, and even as support services were recognized as inadequate.[33] Many women struggled without help. If in 1940 there were 37.6 million women and 34.8 million men aged twenty to forty-four, by 1946 the number of women had stayed about the same, but the number of men had dropped by ten million.[34] Even so, the state pushed higher birth rates through new policies. The 1944 Family Code included incentives for increased child bearing and penalties for those without children. It also reduced burdens on men who fathered children outside of marriage and kept the abortion ban, while expanding supports for unmarried mothers.[35] Increasing numbers of women had children outside of marriage. In 1947, 747,000 children were born to unmarried women, and by 1949 the number reached 985,000. It declined somewhat by 1952 to 849,000, but there were large numbers of women managing parenthood on their own while maintaining full-time employment.[36] Additionally, large numbers of women who had been widowed by the war and others who had divorced fell under the rubric of "single mother."[37] The women rebuilding tobacco struggled under many burdens.

Cultured Smoking and Filtered Cigarettes

For the Soviet Union in the postwar era, a general increase in the standard of living and provision of consumer goods indicated recovery and the march forward.[38] People expected a reprieve from sacrifices and scarcity. After the breakneck pace to recovery immediately following the war, and over the next decades, meat consumption rose as did ownership of televisions and refrigerators.[39]

Automobile ownership increased.[40] A boom in construction meant more individual apartments.[41] In 1961 Khrushchev announced that communism would be attained by 1980, and the measure of it would be in production and consumption. Khrushchev argued for attention to consumer goods as important to the achievement of communism and made material comfort central to the Third Party Program, which was adopted in 1961.[42] Although not all of Khrushchev's reforms were sustained, gradual improvements in living standards followed over the next several decades, and Soviet citizens did increasingly see product provision as essential to state legitimacy. Under Brezhnev consumer markets developed further, as in exchange for compliance, the population gained some economic freedoms.[43] This "little deal" echoed the Stalinist 1930s, when in exchange for support of the state, the population enjoyed material comfort, and even luxury, in an abandonment of the most ascetic and egalitarian aspects of 1920s revolutionary ideology.[44]

Even though consumer goods were more evident, attitudes toward consumption remained tempered.[45] Attention to consumer goods quality, and even luxury, started in the 1930s as part of a Soviet campaign for progress, and coincided with a belief that if the state could instill better taste in citizens, then the cultural level of the population could be raised, and there would be a subsequent achievement for all of society.[46] Such attention to quality and consumption did not conflict with the antiwestern campaigns of the 1930s and postwar era. Instead, after the war attention to consumer goods again occupied planners intensifying after Stalin's death in 1953 and with Khrushchev's de-Stalinization campaigns, which included a rebuke to the perceived neglect of aesthetic qualities and a new emphasis on industrial design along western lines.[47]

Planners explored options for better packaging with a modern, pared-down aesthetic that challenged the heavy opulence of Stalinist style.[48] For tobacco manufacturers, paper quality was a major concern.[49] Never far away were the voices of consumers and their complaints. A 1953 article in *Tabak* exposed problems at several factories. One smoker complained that *Raketa* papirosy were "hard as nails." Another joked, "They should be sold with a hammer so they can be softened before smoking." A third letter reported grass in the tobacco and another pointed to paper fragments. One factory was accused of "being well known—well known for being bad."[50] Iava faced paper and cardboard deficits, uneven processes, overstuffed smokes, poorly made copies of western machinery, and electrical supply troubles. At regional factories, dense packing disrupted burn and created a bitter taste, while "the paper filter quickly dampened in the mouth and fell apart." The aesthetics similarly disappointed with, even on the most up-to-date packaging, "faded colors on the labels, poor, wrinkled cellophane on the packs, [and] slipped tape and slanted foil."[51]

American propagandists of the postwar period similarly focused on consumer culture, but to contrast the American "good life" with that offered by communist systems in an attempt to undermine Soviet power and global influence.[52] Tobacco was a crucial component of these visions as US tobacco firms advanced into Europe and the bloc to offload surplus leaf while spreading a taste for American cigarettes. The 1948 Marshall Plan included, in its estimated thirteen billion in aid, a full one billion for tobacco—a third of the included "food" aid.[53] American tobacco slowly trickled east, so that by 1960 American flue-cured tobacco entered Poland, and other soft-power moves included tobacco. Americans sent exhibitions abroad to the Eastern Bloc of an idealized, capitalist life touting the supposed superiority of American homes and the easy availability of consumer goods like cigarettes.[54] Eisenhower invited Soviet delegations to the US to showcase the differences between the world systems. Exhibitions of US products, including tobacco, became a regular feature of postwar Europe. The most famous of these efforts, the American National Exhibition in Moscow in the summer of 1959, brought nearly three million Soviets to a six-week exhibition in Sokolniki Park to view the wonders of American kitchens and drink samples of Pepsi-Cola.[55]

The filter cigarette served as a prop in these visions of capitalist domestic life punctuated by leisure, consumption, and ease.[56] At the 1966 Leipzig Trade Fair a two-room exhibit regaled viewers on the benefits of American tobacco.[57] Internationally, filtered cigarettes increased in production and popularity after the war. In the wake of medical developments in the 1950s and 1960s, they were marketed as not just milder in taste but healthier for the body.[58] Although the Americans had introduced filtered cigarettes with Brown and Williamson's *Viceroy* in the 1930s, the launch of brands like *Winston* (1954) owed much to health scares after epidemiological studies connecting lung cancer and smoking. In 1950 less than 1 percent of smokes in the US were filtered, but by 1960 that number had reached 50 percent. Western marketers claimed filters trapped tar and other dangers, while filtered and lower tar cigarettes reassured smokers.

Filters did not make smoking any safer. Capitalist tobacco manufacturers manipulated filter construction and tobacco additives to maintain high dosages of addictive nicotine. Many filter components were dangerous, such as *Kent*'s asbestos filters in the early 1950s. At the time, these issues were incompletely understood or willfully obfuscated. It was not until the 1980s that the fraudulent claims that filters lowered risk became clear. In 2001 studies showed that filtration actually reduced particle size and allowed deeper penetration of lung tissue.[59] Filters did lower manufacturing costs, kept small tobacco pieces from escaping the packing and troubling the mouths of smokers, and lured consumers away from other brands.

In addition to being a marker of western luxury, after years of scarcity tobacco availability was an important sign for Soviet smokers of the return to normalcy and part of the general rise in consumption and labor productivity after the war.[60] Tobacco use climbed. If in 1913 per capita use was 143 papirosy, by 1960 it had reached 1,296, and by 1970 it increased to 1,580. This scale was well below the 2,700 per capita in the same year in the US but increasing yearly.[61] And more was not enough. It had to be better.

During the Khrushchev era Leonid Andreevich Sinel'nikov first entered the Iava Factory, where he served from the 1960s to the 1990s as engineer, then head engineer, and eventually director and architect of its transition into the post-Soviet era. In his memoir and personal correspondence, Sinel'nikov recalled the move of the Soviet elite to smoking imported filtered cigarettes purchased at closed shops even as the general population smoked papirosy or unfiltered cigarettes. Moving to international standards, in 1947 Iava introduced the filtered cigarette *Prima*.[62] Iava was one of the few factories to produce cigarettes, and even so, 85 percent of production was in papirosy, many of which were made on prerevolutionary machines still in use. Tobacco improvement required state commitments in hard currency. According to Sinel'nikov, to close the gap, the decision was made "at the highest level" to purchase foreign equipment, and "this was the first purchase of western technology for food production in the USSR and a token of the relationship of the state to smoking."[63]

The move to filtered cigarettes in the 1950s and 1960s fit within the general campaign by the Soviets to instill better "taste" in the population.[64] The effects of this transition were especially profound in terms of design and sensory experience. As Sinel'nikov explained, moving Soviet smokers required rethinking nicotine delivery: "It was very important to giving the strength, which is the most important factory in the formulation of habit. Our smokers were used to strong products, but the acetate filter lowered the nicotine content." Iava specialists did not simply take a papirosa and apply a filter but looked for ways to retain the nicotine intake despite the filter. Sinel'nikov continued, "The main specialists of the factory were put on this question. We predicted that smokers of papirosy would move to cigarettes with filters. We just needed to increase the attractions of the new products, providing for this an increase of taste, quality, and strength."[65]

Soviet cigarette engineers looked not just to gustatory experience. When, in 1965, Brezhnev authorized an infusion of cash into tobacco machinery, the Soviets brought in fifty Molins cigarette machines for some five million pounds. For the Iava Tobacco Factory this meant moving away from the older machinery or poor copies.[66] The machinery was distributed to multiple factories and resulted, according to Sinel'nikov, in a tobacco revolution: "Practically, these became the first consumer goods produced in the country answering to international standards."[67] He noted that this was a total redesign of cigarette and packaging. Finnish partners, as part of a broad trade agreement, helped the Soviets with the transition and particularly with paper. As Sinel'nikov remarked, "The Soviet Union provided forests and Finland, as a more technologically developed country, provided paper . . . and experience." Finnish graphic designers guided the construction of the new look and feel of Iava filtered cigarettes, which according to Sinel'nikov, became a "long-time leader of tobacco production [and] a beloved cigarette for smokers."[68] The product was so anticipated that Sinel'nikov did not recall needing any advertising. Indeed, Sinel'nikov did not remember any advertising for tobacco products from Iava until after 1991.[69] He noted further that the management of the factory did not concern itself with increasing markets as "New production was done not in order to increase sales."[70] He was not the only one who noted a lack of advertising. In internal memos representatives of the foreign tobacco giant Liggett and Myers marveled in 1968 that in the USSR 50 percent smoking among high school students could be "achieved without advertising."[71]

Still, cigarettes with filters were quite expensive, and the mass of smokers stayed with stronger, unfiltered cigarettes, which fit tastes and budgets better. For the government this was fine. Despite the campaigns for "taste," producing more filtered cigarettes required too much hard currency.[72]

The tobacco taste hierarchy of makhorka to papirosa to cigarette was inflected by packaging. For Iava filtered there were two choices—hard or soft pack. They differed in their graphic design so that it would be clear to casual observers which grade of tobacco was nestled inside. The hard pack had a white background with blue stripe and gold script. For the soft pack, the blue was replaced by a red circle with gold lettering (Figure 7.3). The look and feel of the packaging echoed a western style. The transition was seismic. As Sinel'nikov rhapsodized, "The cigarettes were truly of a high quality. Modern new equipment. Imported materials. Color packaging printed in Finland. In comparison to our traditional production, it was as they say the difference of heaven and earth."[73] The new packaging design trickled out into other products creating a Soviet semiotics of cigarette packaging. As Sinel'nikov recounted, "Cigarettes with hard packs were more expensive and positioned as elite products. Cigarettes in soft packs were more democratic for lovers of strong cigarettes. Therefore, we decided to use an improved mix of *Kazbek* for cigarette production in hard packs and *Belomor* for soft packs to retain the accustomed strength of the product but markedly increase the taste, quality, and aroma."[74] Even the Soviet-era factory history recalled the differentiation in customers as these higher-mark smokes became the choice of middle-income groups of the population.[75]

The western move toward filtered products came in the wake of worries over carcinogens, but for Soviet smokers belief in the mitigating effects

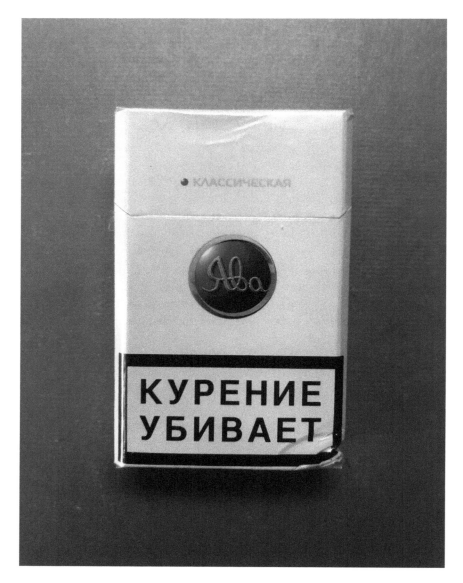

FIGURE 7.3.   Photo. Pack of *Iava*. Modern manufacture of classic Soviet brand. Author's collection.

of filters conformed to long-held concepts that the primary danger of smoking came from toxic nicotine, which could be filtered by water, cotton batting, or even distance (using long holders). Medical authorities created a health hierarchy of tobacco with high-nicotine makhorka at the bottom followed by traditional Russian papirosy with oriental tobacco, then filtered cigarettes, and finally pipes.[76] Research on carcinogenic tars and filters was not a breakthrough for the Russians—just an addition to already established narratives of the chemical dangers of tobacco and the benefits of filtering. Soviet tobacco manufacturers, state planners, and medical authorities advocated for filtered tobacco as safer, just like their western manufacturing counterparts, but they had been saying it for far longer. Since the prerevolutionary era brands had employed cotton batting in the tubes of papirosy.

Bolstered by a belief in the healthfulness of filtered cigarettes and interested in providing higher-quality products to Soviet smokers, Soviet planners anticipated the production of 140 billion cigarettes, with 50 billion of these filtered, by 1970, an increase of thirteenfold in just five years.[77] Outside of Iava, there were few options for producing these new-style cigarettes, which required imported machinery.[78] Shortages continued for preferred products, and raw material deficits—along with the cost of imported paper, filters, foil, and cellophane—impeded output.[79] Sinel'nikov confessed that even at Iava "stable quality was not possible," and because foreign machinery required higher-skilled mechanics who had often to make do without replacement parts, the process remained idiosyncratic and different personnel could completely change output.[80] Sinel'nikov remembered that producing boxes to transport finished papirosy and cigarettes to the stores could be such a problem that goods just piled on the floors waiting for enough boxes to be scrounged together to arrange transfer. Once the goods finally made it to stores, "products were sold practically on the day they hit the floor."[81] Production increased over the next decade, as did research in filter technology and better leaf blends.[82]

Demand far exceeded output. To fill the gap, the Soviets imported from their partners in the bloc. From 1960 to 1975 Bulgarian cigarette imports to the Soviet Union rose from 10 to 71.4 billion sticks, and Bulgaria became the world's largest exporter of cigarettes by 1966. They retained this title until 1988 because of their provision of tobacco to the Soviets. A full 90 percent of their tobacco exports went to the USSR. Soviet smokers snapped up *Vega* and *Rodopi*. The Bulgarians employed more advanced filter technologies, American blends, higher-nicotine leaf, and western-style packaging. American specialists came to Bulgaria in the period to guide them on how to cultivate Virginia and Burley tobaccos.[83] It was an end run around barriers to trade in the USSR.

Historians of addiction tie the rise of filtered cigarettes in the west to aggressive advertising of misleading health claims, but the complicated relationship of the Soviets with the "bourgeois capitalistic excrescence" of advertising had fully soured after the war, according to a report from US marketers. Aside from some general event notifications or consumer guidance to new products and how to use them (soy, for instance), few promotional materials appeared in Soviet cities.[84] After the war, paid advertisements began in newspapers, and by 1947

Radio Moscow broadcast three eight-minute blocks of advertising per day, and some foreign firms began to buy advertisements in Soviet media. For the most part, little was promoted. Chronic shortages lessened the need for marketing, but so too did the standardizing of the market. As one Soviet marketing authority contended, "When a consumer buys canned goods or cigarettes, the necessity of selecting a can or package out of the general (undifferentiated) mass does not arise."[85] According to one observer, "Mass media advertisements are short, tiny, and unostentatious. Like a timid guest at a party who sits tucked away in a corner and tries hard not to attract attention, advertisements tend to be crowded together and are limited in most newspapers to less than one column."[86]

Tobacco product advertising, at least for foreign products, was available, according to a report of the *Times of London*. One foreign firm had placed advertisements for cigarettes into the *Moscow News*, described as "a Russian paper . . . which is published daily in English and French."[87] The Soviet press reported tobacco advertising was "discontinued" in the late 1960s, implying there had been some before.[88] A 1971 article in *Literaturnaia gazeta* crowed over the advertising ban as a sign of the strength of the Soviet system over that of the west, "because among us in this country, where there are not cigar 'kings' or 'pipe' princes, . . . we hear of the machinations of a tobacco monopoly only in the newspaper."[89] According to Sinel'nikov, however, this must have been largely symbolic, because he recalled no such restrictions. Even if there had been, Iava did not have to do any advertising to sell products. There was absolutely no need.[90] Elaborate window displays and stacks of tobacco packs made to look like a ship or building, for instance, formed the most prominent source of goods promotion.[91] Although by 1961 Soviet advertising authorities claimed they had improved their work and the quality of their graphics with new attention and oversight, the last tobacco advertisements in the State Library collection came from well before this point, in 1950.[92]

Largely independent of the influence of advertisers, Soviet smokers constructed their own meanings for tobacco. Display of a cigarette—in its smoking, its presentation, its packaging, its sharing, its gifting—all held power as a signifier of status or aspirational status, gender, and even locality. With every puff, smokers exhaled a complex language articulated through type of smoke, place of production, and scarcity of brand. Display of western fashion, including cigarettes, became an important sign of cultural sophistication in the postwar Soviet Union.[93] Many Soviet men remembered their encounters with western goods and cigarettes in Central Europe during the offensive of 1944–1945.[94] In areas of Eastern Europe, fashionable youth of the 1950s would take American pack labels and pin them to everyday ties.[95] Fashionable young men would smoke *Lucky Strikes* or *Camels* to distinguish their western clothing and hairstyles and stand out further from the norm.[96] The availability of western cigarettes within the closed stores of the party elite made having them a sign of status and connections and an entrée into the life of the west. Such an idealization of western goods held true for large segments of society, not just among the fashion forward.[97] Youth generally preferred cigarettes and were often caricatured with them.[98] A slovenly manner and chain-smoking of poor tobacco distinguished the hooligan.[99]

For those who did not have access to foreign stores or the money for imported goods, there was still a desire for filtered cigarettes over papirosy, hard packs over soft packs. Certain factories were considered better at producing certain brands than others. Although Brezhnev smoked Dukat's *Novosti* brand, in Leningrad the local Uritskii-made *Belomorkanal* papirosy did well. Among domestic brands, *Iava miagkaia* stood at the top in Moscow because Iava always got the best-quality materials, since they provided for many of the elite. When the Dukat Factory began to produce runs of *Iava miagkaia*, dedicated smokers took to calling the authentic Moscow produced ones *Iavskaia*.[100]

Postwar Smoking and Male Sociability

The line of tobacco boxes in front of Mariia Andreevna in 1949 indicated that Iava produced for a primarily male smoking public. It may not be clear for whom *Osobennye* (Special) was made, but the other two gift sets for *Futbol* (Soccer) and *Bogatyri* (Heroes) featured males prominently on their packs. Packs on the table from left to right are *Sovetskii soiuz* (Soviet Union), *Iava*, *Festival*, *Kavkaz*, *Futbol*, *Severnaia Pal'mira* (Northern Palmira, a pet name for St. Petersburg), *Drug* (Friend—a newly produced cigarette), and Stalin's preferred *Gertsegovina Flor*. Most labels show manly pursuits like military battles, hunting, or sports or invoke male role models like the heroic bogatyr or Stalin.

The culture of smoking after World War II and the messages it had for men extended beyond the pack labels and into visual culture and the cinema. After World War II, the image of the Soviet male underwent a significant transition, and he was accompanied by cigarettes. While militarism had been intrinsic to the creation of the New Soviet Man in the 1920s and 1930s, the experience of war and devastation transformed the image of the ideal Soviet male. Visions of the super-soldier of the 1920s and 1930s became problematic, as the heroic veteran exemplified an alternative power. The strength of this myth was partially neutralized with the pause of Victory Day celebrations from 1947 until 1965, the Purge of the Victors, and a more romanticized vision of the soldier outside of combat and danger.[101] In addition to this fluctuating vision of military masculinity, the meaning of smoking was influenced by the campaign to inculcate better taste into the population with a turn against the makhorka smoker, who was always depicted as male.

The last two advertising posters in the collection of the Russian State Library conveyed the postwar possibilities for smokers (Figures 7.4 and 7.5). Both come from Glavtabak and advertise cigarettes. Both feature men. The first is for a nameless brand of unfiltered cigarette; note the bulge of the cigarette holder around the butt. The smoker, dressed in a sharp suit and with a tight, Stalin-like coiffure, smiles at the viewer in an invitation to social acceptance. The warmth of his skin, illuminated by the glowing match in his hand, calls to mind nineteenth-century portraiture's reliance on glowing candles, fires, and papirosy to bring forth healthy, shining skin tones.[102] The casual, cheery pose assumes a return to normality, but demobilization was not complete. Shortages remained, and cigarettes of any kind were a relative impossibility, given the barely launched Iava *Prima* of 1947. Matches were in deficit too, for that matter. Yet here is a vision of a life made normal and peaceful.

The second poster, also from 1950, copies the tropes of postwar military art in the late Stalin period. The sailor, like many military men of the imagery from the era, is pictured well away from the scene of battle, as evidenced by his relaxed smile and casual smoke.[103] It is again a cigarette, with all the attendant problems of accessibility. Finally, the name of the cigarette—*Avrora*—calls to mind the famous ship that fired the first shot of the October Revolution and whose guns were later used in the defense of Leningrad. The ship was made a monument to the revolution in the wake of the war, occupying a point of pride on the banks of the Neva. In a return to normality and a vision of peaceful service tinged with red fervor, the new smoking possibilities reprise earlier ideas but with a postwar flair.

Smoking occupied a space in other constructions of the memory of war. Nostalgia for the war figured heavily in the decades following the peace and was a constant, if contested, theme in literature and the visual and cinematic arts.[104] While the men changed—from collective to individualistic and from stalwart to tormented—the papirosa exercised a near omnipresence, moving adeptly from conveying satisfaction to signaling turmoil to showing shared affection. Tobacco took on added meanings because of the legacies of World War II and the perceived place of tobacco in male bonding on the front lines. In visual culture, the New Soviet Man's image transitioned from the late Stalinist to the Khrushchev and then early Brezhnev periods, and tobacco remained important in visual and cinematic depictions throughout.

The 1951 Iurii Neprintsev painting *Rest after Battle* showed a scene pulled from the popular wartime poem *Vasilii Terkin: A Book about a Soldier*. The poem captured a view of wartime that soldiers found authentic, and in the artistic rendering by Neprintsev, smoking occupied center stage. Terkin holds the attention

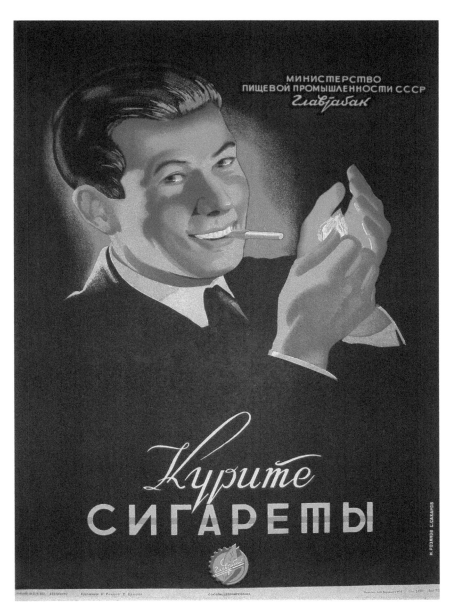

FIGURE 7.4. Poster. "Smoke Cigarettes," 1950. Courtesy Russian State Library.

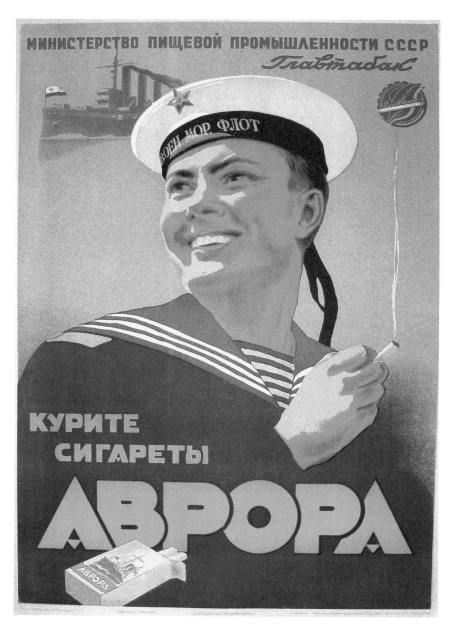

FIGURE 7.5. Poster. "Smoke *Avrora* Cigarettes," 1950. Courtesy Russian State Library.

of his group of resting soldiers even as he pulls closed his tobacco bag in preparation for finishing up his self-rolled smoke. Several others of the group smoke even as others laugh and attend to the story. The sensual logic of the painting—crisp-smelling snow and warm friendship, pungent smoke and ringing laughter—creates a full tangle of sights and smells and feelings to unpack as part of the postwar vision of wartime life. Boris Fedorov's *Morning of the Tank Drivers* (1952–1954) similarly places tobacco smoke in the center of male bonding rituals. Here it accents the morning ablutions of a group of laughing young men as they hack through the ice to clean up before heading back to their tank in the background.[105]

Soviet movies made after 1945 use smoking to set the scenes of war experience, indicate collective bonds and misery, and delineate the times of waiting. The 1949 *Fall of Berlin* features Stalin with pipe and papirosy. *Ballad of a Soldier* (1959) depicts soldiers on a train to the front divvying up a newspaper for rolling smokes. The collective nature of the act and the shared conversation that invariably accompanied such activities reflected descriptions and imagery of smoking from during the war. Smoking is part of the fabric of wartime in the director Andrei Tarkovsky's 1962 *Ivan's Childhood*, despite the desire of the youthful hero that his compatriots not smoke, perhaps a nod to the director's own fight with tobacco. Tarkovsky died of lung cancer in 1986. The 1964 *Father of a Soldier* similarly depicts wartime bonding over tobacco, but here a peasant searching for his hospitalized soldier son shares his tobacco with a group of travelers. A fine tobacco (probably oriental leaf) from his Soviet Georgia home, the smoke does not satisfy the legless, former navy man who drives the cart. After a few puffs, he complains it had "taste but no strength" and hands the rest back on the peasant. The wounded navy man grumbles that he has smoked makhorka for so long that good tobacco makes him cough.

The association of smoking with the transition to male adulthood continued in the postwar world and took on added significance. The 1951 painting *Big Surprise* by Adolf Gugel' and Raisa Kudrevich constructs a narrative around smoking and the postwar family. In the composition, three children of declining ages from teen to teddy-bear-hugging schoolgirl surround a table in an apartment living room. The oldest of the three, in a coat with fur cap and collar, purses his lips to blow smoke rings while his companion turns a startled face to the door as Mother returns to the scene. Noticeably absent is a father figure, indicating the marginal place of males in the postwar family.[106] Although certain to cause trouble with the entering mother, the smoking could be an indication of the boy's place in the family. Other hints as to the boy's status as the eldest and now male head of household come from his oversized coat and dress shoes that he must be growing into. As "man of the house" the boy is taking on the trappings of adulthood with his clothing and smoking. The transition from boy to man is still not complete, as the litter of spent matches and crumpled papirosy on the floor indicates a few attempts to get inhalation right and the half-complete smoke rings show still-imperfect technique. The painting's story indicates that even for those males not directly involved in the war, the long shadow of combat and tobacco's meaning for manliness would continue into the lives of the next generation.

After the devastation of war both the personnel and production of tobacco needed a recovery, but there would be no pause. Women who had entered the factory earlier remained, and more joined them. Conditions stayed hard. Hours stretched long. Demand remained high and grew, and investment from the state assured tobacco would come back. Tobacco's recovery was necessary as part of Cold War comparison of Soviet power to that of the capitalists. Western cigarettes trickling in from the east, imitated by Bulgarian trade partners, or fleetingly experienced through closed store windows gave the Soviet smoker a point of comparison and may have highlighted the problems of Soviet products. Although still falling short of western standards, Soviet manufacturers proudly reported of the reduction in makhorka. A 1967 essay in the industry journal *Tabak* noted that if in 1913 makhorka had accounted for nearly 80 percent of tobacco products, by 1966 it had fallen to only about 10 percent, which spoke to "the large growth in the cultural level of the population not just in European Russia but throughout the entire Soviet Union."[107]

Government investment in machinery and a push to raise the tastes of the population manifested in the increased filtered cigarette production and use. This changed the factory balances to more male workers, and the market for the new products was largely male. Smoking flavored by the wartime experience became a male behavior in visual and cinematic culture even as mechanization transformed tobacco factories into spaces for men, not women. With the dawn of filter cigarette manufacture, the women's kingdom was no more.

PARTNERED

Space Cigarettes and Soviet *Marlboros*

In 1964, the same year the US Surgeon General released the landmark *Smoking and Health*, the tobacco giant Philip Morris (hereafter PM) began what would become a more than ten-year campaign to invade the Soviet ruble market. Through negotiations in the 1950s and 1960s with Bulgarian, Polish, and Yugoslav manufacturers, PM gained a soft entry. In efforts dubbed "Mission to Moscow" and "Operation Red Carpet" they engaged the Soviets directly. Over the course of years of meetings, exhibitions, and symposiums, PM cultivated personal relationships with Soviet ministers and manufacturers. Finally, in 1975 they negotiated an agreement for the joint production of a US/USSR cigarette called *Apollo-Soyuz* (or from the Soviet side *Soiuz-Apollon*) to commemorate the linkup of the Soviet and American space programs.

For PM this was one play of a long game. Designed jointly, manufactured in the Soviet Union, and sold in both countries, the Soviets saw *Soiuz-Apollon* as a recognition of their international competitiveness. PM officials projected *Apollo-Soyuz* would have trouble selling and would probably be a loss globally. No matter. Their goal was to get their top seller, *Marlboro*, onto the ruble market. In 1976 they made it. The Soviets purchased licensing for production of *Marlboro* cigarettes for domestic distribution. After over ten years of negotiations and building relationships, after swallowing a loss on their joint-produced cigarette, PM attained its end. The company anticipated that from this beachhead, it would steadily build market share.

The Soviets were not just patsies to PM's game. From the other side of the Iron Curtain, Leonid Sinel'nikov, a longtime engineer and then director at Moscow's

Iava Factory, remembered how his industry struggled to meet demand, stumbled along with older machinery, fought for every square foot of space in crowded works, and wrestled to compete with international standards without the leaf, papers, or even glues to do so. Paper, acetate filters, cellophane, foil—almost all came from abroad and fluctuated in supply. Sinel'nikov recalled the *Soiuz-Apollon* process as a learning experience, a warm cooperation, and a complete public-relations triumph—a Soviet cigarette sold in the US.[1]

For Sinel'nikov, if the 1975 *Soiuz-Apollon* was a blue ribbon, then the 1976 *Marlboro* licensing agreement was a world title. Being allowed to produce *Marlboros* proved Soviet production could meet international standards. It signaled something new, as Sinel'nikov enthused: "The production of *Marlboro* cigarettes was not just a big achievement for the Soviet tobacco industry but also a significant event in the social life of the country. It is mistakenly considered that the first project in the USSR symbolizing the American way of life was the noisier 1990 opening of the McDonald's restaurant on Moscow's Pushkin Square. In reality it happened much earlier, when production began of *Marlboro* cigarettes along with Philip Morris."[2] Although the partnership ruptured in the 1980s, the *Marlboro* Man cast a long shadow across the red frontier, influencing tastes, inspiring longing, and inviting comparisons.[3]

What Sinel'nikov termed the introduction to "the American way of life" also proved a crash course in the western ways of addiction. The Soviets produced to meet demand.[4] PM designed cigarettes to create it. *Marlboro* was a juggernaut globally; the world's top seller from 1972 on. Even without massive advertising campaigns, *Marlboro* was a symbol for Soviets of the good life and luxury and had tremendous brand recognition. *Marlboro* was blended to entice the palate, engineered to give the quickest dose of nicotine, packaged to seduce the senses, and marketed to excite desire. The contrast between western and Soviet-produced cigarettes and papirosy, in terms of psychosocial factors of addiction and bioavailability of nicotine, help explain somewhat the allure of western tobacco brands in the late Soviet and post-Soviet periods. The scarcity of first *Soiuz-Apollon* and then *Marlboro* added further charm. The experience of consumer products provided yet another front for the Cold War, with the *Marlboro* Man at the barricades.

PM's introduction of first *Apollo-Soyuz* and then *Marlboro* exposed inadequacies in Soviet agricultural productivity and industrial standards in an easily consumed, but not always readily available, commodity. When and if Soviet smokers finally got hold of a pack, they could not just see but physically experience the western difference. Joint production tangibly, physically, and pungently showed the distance between US and Soviet manufacturers in cigarette quality, packaging, and marketing, even as the regime promised abundance and quality somewhere in the future.[5] The concept of using a seemingly growing number of Soviet consumers interested in tasteful items as a point for Cold War competition had been a stock of western analyses of the Soviet public since the 1950s. The *Marlboro* seemed an ideal weapon.[6] PM's techniques for wooing the Soviets, through third parties and with high risk, illuminated the lengths to which they would go. The lack of discussion about tars, cancers, or disease in any of the materials indicated that health was not of concern. Finally, this early history of PM with the Soviets laid the foundation for the post-1991 mutual interest and cooperation between Russian and transnational tobacco companies.

As PM executives began their campaign, social discontent might have convinced the Soviets to forge an agreement. Cigarette shortages were not new for the Soviets but by the 1970s reached higher visibility because of a less patient public. In 1972 at the Dukat Factory, an official from Glavtabak praised the importation and installation of new machinery as "of paramount importance" in light of the general dearth of tobacco products.[7] In 1976 disturbances broke out in Kuzbass, and a letter from a miner's wife sent to the Central Committee of the Communist Party of the Soviet Union identified tobacco shortages as the point of ignition. The woman complained: "My husband returns from his shift in a foul mood. He sends me out for cigarettes. He wakes in the morning, and if there are no cigarettes, fights start in the house. I understand that there is not enough meat and butter . . . we are used to that. But it cannot be that it is impossible to provide cigarettes."[8] Sinel'nikov recalled that leadership in the party and the Ministry of Food Industry paid attention and worried over popular anger over other deficits. Faced with a "tobacco crisis" planners were forced "to allocate resources for the development of the tobacco industry."[9] Funds went to upgrade facilities, increase production of at least nonfilter cigarettes, and come to agreements with Molins and others to buy new machinery with precious hard currency. From 1977 to 1979 over two hundred new cigarette lines were imported, and Sinel'nikov reported that this "eased the position of tobacco factories in the USSR."[10] Some of these machines came to Iava for free "as a type of advertisement."[11] Some of them were provided by PM.

Détente and the Mission to Moscow

Soviet planners of the 1950s and 1960s looked to bolster production and increase imports while struggling to fill market demand. Desire for quality tobacco rose as options for imports fell, production capabilities remained nearly stagnant, equipment aged, and there was little money for new.[12] Meanwhile, American growers had been interested in opening Europe to leaf exports for decades. Leaf surplus had led to depressed returns for farmers and government at home. The US government stepped in with programs to manage tobacco cultivation and sales to aid growers in their uneven exchanges with manufacturers, but farmers tried to help themselves by actively pursuing market expansion.[13] The tobacco-hungry lands of the Eastern Bloc seemed ideal for offloading leaf surplus. As a US government spokesman argued in 1964, "It is in the national interest to sell all the tobacco we can to the Soviet bloc countries." Because of severe droughts, the Soviets were looking for around 150 million pounds of leaf.[14] Further, in the US increased worry over the health effects of tobacco caused dips in tobacco use. The unsteady nature of the market and increasing pressure from anti-tobacco groups had US farmers and manufacturers looking abroad.[15] Spurred by their own decreasing demand and trying to find a soft-entry point to feed the seemingly insatiable market of the Soviet Union, US tobacco producers explored sending raw materials to Bulgaria.[16] It was not until 1975, however, that Bulgaria signed licensing agreements with R. J. Reynolds (hereafter RJR) for production of *Winston* and PM for *Marlboro*.[17] The Americans also initiated relationships with Yugoslavia and Poland as gateways to the Soviet market.[18]

PM had struggled more with sales declines than other companies and monitored Soviet supply problems eagerly.[19] After a 1964 visit to the USSR, Justus Heymans, senior vice-president at PM-Overseas, left a detailed account, pointing to current Soviet consumption trends, production capabilities, and areas that PM might exploit. He said very little smoking was evident on the streets and that about 80 percent of the market was still in papirosy, but he noted with satisfaction the great amount of importation by the Soviets, especially from Bulgaria. After a tour of Dukat and a celebratory, and boozy, lunch, Heymans seemed thoroughly enchanted and gushed: "I never had such a hearty, jovial and fine reception." Bemoaning the fact that the Italians were well ahead in cooperative agreements and hoping to provide PM cigarettes for tourists, Heymans finished his report optimistic for the future: "I consider my visit to USSR most fruitful. If any business can be done for later, *WE ARE PRESENTLY IN* . . . The USSR is fully alive, progressive and active. They will have financial foreign exchange problems, but they will get there in time. LET'S BE *IN!*"[20]

PM documents recount the trade fortunes of the Soviets and note the increasing demand in the Soviet market for raw tobacco and finished, especially filtered, western-style smokes. Consumption in the Soviet Union and Eastern Bloc was growing even as that in the US slowed, but because the Soviets did not allow the ruble to be freely converted to other currencies, Americans were finding it difficult to get direct entry into the market and entered surreptitiously through Bulgaria or Poland.[21] The Soviets introduced some cigarettes from the US and Western Europe starting in the late 1960s, but only for sale to foreigners. Imported for up to ten cents a pack and sold at up to ten times that price, these brought in hard currency in specialized stores for foreign visitors.[22]

Although Heymans was hopeful, insistent even, and PM and the Tobacco Institute were keeping an eye on the Soviet market, getting "in" would take time.[23] Tastes among eastern smokers tended to favor oriental tobaccos rather than American blends, and previously foreign firms had stuck to providing the Soviets with machinery. But PM wanted more.[24] There were risks, as the US experience with trade in leaf to Yugoslavia in 1965 and the domestic brouhaha raised by the Miami-based, snappily titled Committee to Warn of the Arrival of Communist Merchandise on the Local Business Scene made clear.[25] The international situation was dicey. The 1968 Soviet invasion of Czechoslovakia fanned tensions. Soviet diplomatic ties with the Chinese and the US affected trade. The Soviet Union was compelled to look outward as environmental crises and problems with molds led to declines in leaf production.

The warming of relations changed possibilities for industrial, technological, and scientific exchange. Nixon journeyed to Moscow in 1972—the first US president to do so—and Brezhnev went to Washington in 1973. Nixon's trip "cleared the way for normalization of trade between the countries," according to a report from the US Department of Commerce in PM records. The report highlighted the "prospects for sales of certain consumer products and equipment for light industry to the U.S.S.R." and the new organizations established to facilitate trade. The US Embassy in Moscow would provide "a wide range of services to U.S. Businessmen," including briefing materials, commercial counseling, and even typing and copies. The department gave advice and addresses for American businessmen corresponding with Soviet organizations, recommending direct, personal relationships as most efficacious.[26]

PM officials outlined their strategy in a confidential document of June 1973 titled "Mission to Moscow."[27] Eventually to span into multiple international meetings and an entire second operation—Project Red Carpet—the venture would go far more smoothly, quickly, and successfully than PM initially anticipated.[28] For June 1973, executives just wanted to coordinate a 1974 symposium with the Soviets to focus on PM's strengths. Meetings with representatives of Soviet technical, food, and trade groups exceeded expectations. The Soviets eagerly told the PM representatives of the "popularity of cigarettes" in their country and their desire for more filtered products. They also "immediately picked up on the suggestion" of a co-produced US-Soviet cigarette and trade of Soviet-grown oriental tobacco for American leaf. The Soviets considered this "most appealing" because it would allow them to trade in kind rather than use hard currency. The Soviets even made the first move, suggesting "an exchange of cigarettes, with Philip Morris becoming an agent in third countries (normally, but not necessarily, this means other

Socialist countries) for the sale of USSR produced American type cigarettes." The hunger from the Soviet export official, for not just any smoke but especially the premier PM brand, was clear when he sighed: "Marlboro is the cigarette which is first sold-out" at the closed foreign stores.[29]

R. Thompson, president of PM-Europe, got a glowing report. The goal for the symposium, to acquaint the Soviets with PM as an industry leader, was "accomplished" without the event even having taken place.[30] Overall the initial meetings gave great hope: "It is clear that direct sales . . . can be developed in the Soviet Union, and that there is a possibility of developing a joint venture for the production of American-type smokes in the Soviet Union. The result of this would be to upgrade the Soviet market to the U.S. type of cigarette." The report observed not just that this could happen but that it could happen speedily: "The Soviets have advanced the discussions more quickly than could have been expected." Speed brought pressure, because "if Philip Morris does not pursue this activity, the Soviets will inevitably follow up with other companies. Even with a prompt follow-up, competition from other sources may well enter into the picture." Although PM corporate leaders felt they had a foot in the door, they knew that this was not enough, especially given the difficulties in creating an equitable settlement. The report ended with the caution: "Negotiations can be long, tedious and involve hard bargaining. Success can only be achieved by constant and persistent follow up and initiative by Philip Morris."[31]

Worries over competitors, especially RJR, animated PM responses.[32] Almost immediately upon return, meetings began at PM-International in New York to plan the symposium for early 1974 with a clear understanding that the goal was to offer the Soviets technology in exchange for market access.[33] As planning progressed, members of the Industrial Research Institute, the Department of Agriculture, and the Tobacco Institute, Inc., became involved.[34] Helmut Wakeham (vice-president of research, PM-USA) wrote to PM-Europe offices asking for a background file on tobacco production in the USSR.[35] The report that "even though the U.S.S.R. is a major producer of tobacco, the domestic production is not sufficient to meet requirements" could not but increase the desire of PM to proceed with all haste.[36] Wakeham remained integral to future meetings and strategizing.

Not even waiting for the symposium plans to be finalized, PM undertook a second "Mission to Moscow" in September 1973, the ostensible purpose of which was to hand-deliver a letter to the Committee for Science and Technology. In Moscow, Nobel M. Melencamp, the economic and commercial officer of the US Embassy, advised PM executives on how to proceed using Don Kendall of Pepsi-Cola and his bottling plant in Novorossiisk as an example.[37] After much discussion, the symposium was scheduled for March, and expert visits were to proceed starting in November.[38] In these early stages of negotiation, embassy staff, according to confidential reports, were extremely helpful to the PM executives, even promising to keep an eye on any outgoing cables involving PM and other companies approaching the Soviets.[39]

PM-Europe executives explored barter to overcome hard-currency issues. While the Soviets considered trade of raw tobacco ideal, PM analysts considered no Soviet tobaccos "appropriate." These difficulties did not seem crippling as PM moved forward and assigned more personnel to the campaign.[40] In December representatives of PM tobacco, tobacco packaging, and brewing traveled to the USSR.[41] The tobacco representatives reported in over thirty detailed pages the mood of the Soviet delegation, its questions, the possibilities for further investment, and trepidation over the dangers of the Soviets backing out without a deal since they had been known to reverse-engineer machinery and goods without compensating developers.[42] PM decided to tempt the Soviets with "small amounts of information" to create deeper relationships. The Soviets seemed eager and were full of questions regarding mechanization of harvesting, growing low-nicotine leaf, and bettering production, though "quality seemed of secondary interest."[43]

The Americans and Soviets agreed to the "Mission to Moscow" symposium in the spring, with a Soviet-suggested agenda heavy on construction, technology, production, equipment, and filters. The Americans suggested presentations on lower tar and nicotine products. The word "health" did not appear in any of the proposed or approved agendas.[44] In December PM-International drafted an "Agreement on Scientific and Technical Cooperation between the State Committee of the Council of Ministers of the USSR for Science and Technology and Philip Morris Incorporated (USA)" to be signed at the symposium the following year. The agreement promised regular visits and exchanges of information, did not preclude work with another group, and would continue for five years (but could be unilaterally cancelled).[45] Executives for PM, led by PM-International President Cullman, traveled to Moscow to sign the protocol in March.[46] In introductory remarks, Cullman thanked the Soviets for their hospitality and boasted of the size of PM and the reach of their prime brand—*Marlboro*—"the largest selling cigarette in the world having total sales of approximately 119 billion in 1973."[47] The Soviets seemed won over.

Apollo-Soyuz and Space Cigarettes

The March symposium resulted in an agreement for the joint production of a commemorative cigarette for the 1975 joint Apollo-Soyuz Mission.[48] According to

PM, Glavtabak was "aggressively" seeking "good relations." This tobacco détente coincided with the "ultimate objective" for PM of either importing and selling blended cigarettes in the USSR or "developing and producing" same with the Soviets. The main problem was Soviet reluctance because they could not produce the required tobaccos. To overcome this, PM would need to assist agriculturally, which would develop a Soviet taste for American-style smokes to eventually begin "Marlboro sales in the USSR ruble market."[49] The first meeting about the joint-produced cigarette was scheduled for May 13, 1974, and was guided by the idea that this would be a "first step" cigarette with US and Soviet tobacco.[50] PM executives did not consider this an even exchange; it was about future possibilities. The goal was to sell *Marlboros*. It was clear to PM analysts that "consumption of cigarettes [in the USSR] is growing faster than the population. . . [and] as the economy improves, smoking increases."[51]

PM did not publicize its success because of worries over the possible reaction in the US. In a memo on the "U.S.S.R. Strategy" hand-labeled "Private" Cullman reiterated that the long-term goal was to get *Marlboro* or another cigarette "manufactured under license in the U.S.S.R." He worried this might antagonize US farmers and others and could create "adverse reaction, particularly by Jewish and other student groups and parts of the trade and customers generally." Given the perceived problems, Cullman insisted on top-level corporate review and approval.[52]

In May the Americans finalized a deal to help the Soviets in joint production of a cigarette, growing American-type tobaccos, increasing efficiency, and helping in factory design. In an "urgent" memo to Cullman, A. G. Buzzi, vice-president of PM-International, excitedly gave the details of the "friendly and fruitful discussion" between PM and the State Committee for Science and Technology of the Council of Ministers. The plan was that Soviet oriental tobacco would make up 30 percent of the blend, and their payment would be either in dollars or in tobacco to PM. To meet the "quality and technical standards of Philip Morris," PM would provide filters and all design and printing.[53]

Buzzi tempered any thoughts of great sales, listing "customs barriers, prohibitive introductory advertising, monopoly situations preventing short term cigarette sales, lack of producer control of distribution, the general impossibility of insuring substantial sales on the international market even with tens of millions of dollars of advertising investment and other characteristics of the international cigarette market." He called *Apollo-Soyuz* a "symbol of mutual cooperation and only an initial step." Buzzi advised that the "long term manufacture and substantial sales of one of its brands of cigarettes in the Soviet Union" animated the PM partnership.[54] In pursuit of this, PM promised to provide "technology, know-how, and training of GLAVTABAK personnel" for efficient production with fewer workers and decreased material loss. The agreement was signed in English and in Russian.[55]

"Inter-Office Correspondence" at PM-USA in September 1974 was very upbeat for future business possibilities, noting that the Soviets even hoped that PM might open an office in Moscow. The possibility of a Moscow branch surprised the people at PM "since many U.S. companies who have requested permission to do so have been turned down by the Soviets." In further positive news, the *Soiuz-Apollon* production run had been increased from three hundred million to five hundred million cigarettes.[56] Still, the focus at PM was long term. As a PM-International Inter-Office Correspondence of April 1974 resolved, "Our ultimate objective . . . is a long-term contract . . . to produce Marlboro in the U.S.S.R. in the initial quantity of 4 billion units per year (1% of the market) . . . to be scaled up over time."[57]

In the USSR, production began for a July release. The plan was for five hundred million with fifty million going to the US. According to Sinel'nikov, when PM executives visited to start preparation, "much of what they saw was, to put it mildly, astonishing," and they declared the task "impossible." He chalked this up to their naivete: "They were simply not aware of the peculiarities of our realities." He celebrated Iava's technicians, who were able "to adapt and make do." PM engineers sent specialized tools and spare parts, and Iava's workers were delighted with the equipment.[58] In their own documents, PM executives diagnosed storage and supply problems at Iava but considered the factory better suited than any other Soviet manufacturer.[59]

Some issues, however, could not be overcome with new tools or enthusiastic workers. Sinel'nikov remembered that PM decided to import the fully prepared tobacco directly from Richmond rather than using 30 percent Soviet tobacco because of quality concerns. Two hundred kilogram blocks of tobacco packed in polyethelene and then heavy cardboard arrived at the Moscow factory. According to Sinel'nikov, the quality was stunning: "We would open the box, and there was the beautiful golden color, with a dark shimmer. It was tobacco worked with a special sauce and releasing a sumptuous scent. It was simply fantastic."[60] He enthused that the taste put smokers in "ecstasy" and "I have not encountered a more aromatic and tasty cigarette since. Of course, there was the technology of Philip Morris and the highest-quality tobacco and materials, but the labor was all us, and that means a lot."[61]

The packaging was luxurious. The most sought after were the commemorative cartons, which featured a vibrant painting by the cosmonaut Alexei Leonov. Leonov, the first man to complete a spacewalk on the 1965 Voskhod-2 mission and twice named a Hero of the Soviet Union, also painted, and his space scenes made it into the State Tretiakov Gallery and onto postage stamps.[62] In the carton image, the joining of the two crafts in the first international cooperative space mission is framed against an earth covered in swirling clouds and partially obscuring a crimson sun. The optimism of the painting shines through in the joyous coloring and lovingly detailed spacecraft. The ten packs arrayed flat within the carton display a blue sphere on a white background against which the docking crafts are framed (Figure 8.1). In block, sans serif lettering *Soiuz-Apollon* or *Apollo-Soyuz*

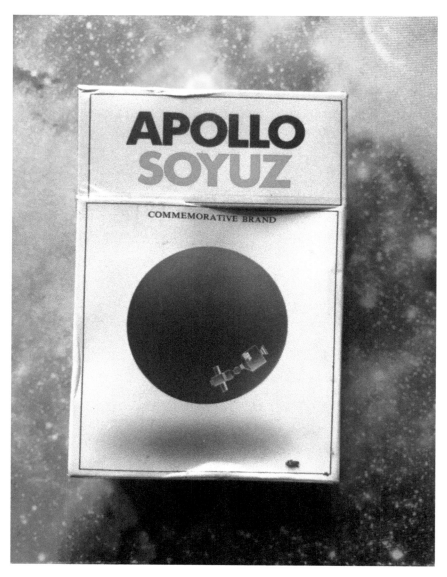

FIGURE 8.1.   Photo. Pack of *Apollo-Soyuz*, 1975. Author's collection.

adorned the top of the pack in red and blue with Russian on one side and English the other. The cigarette itself had American-made cellulose acetate filters with cork tipping and blue lettering on brilliant white cigarette paper.[63]

The feel of the packaging was as pleasing and modern as the look. Silver foil lined the inside of the box. A six-millimeter red tape could remove the covering cellophane while also popping out the first smoke. Compared to American products, the cigarettes were a bit heavier with lower nicotine (1.2 mg), higher sugar, and twenty mg of tar. According to PM testing, the "smoke panel judged the smoke taste to be of medium impact and slightly sweet with spicy notes. In general, the panel liked the taste of the product."[64] The ease of opening, attention to design, and execution of the packaging were singular for Soviet cigarettes. The only thing close was *Iava*, which had been co-designed with the Finns. Sinel'nikov recalled that Soiuz-Apollon were "the first consumer product in the country answering to international standards."[65] The pack was in marked contrast to the much rougher look of traditional papirosy in coarse cardboard without an easily closed top or foil or cellophane to keep the tobacco reliably moist but not too damp. The bright white of the cigarettes themselves along with the smooth quality of the paper would have stood out to Soviet smokers, felt slicker in the hands and on the lips, and burned differently for a unique mouth feel.

As production hummed along in the Soviet Union, PM sent a confidential update to the US Department of State and to the National Aeronautics and Space Administration (NASA). The letter outlined the history of the scientific-technical agreement, the details of the production and distribution, and even the package design and pricing. Noting that it was the "first American-type cigarette manufactured in the U.S.S.R. and the first American-type cigarette available for purchase with Soviet currency," the letter asked for confidentiality as the Soviets awaited an official announcement. Unlike previous comments on the project, this statement was the first to baldly admit that American sales were "*not expected to yield any profit to Philip Morris and will probably result in a loss*." Still, the sale of the same product in the American market was, according to the note, "*extremely important*" to the Soviets.[66] For its part, NASA responded that they had "no legal objections to the proposed cigarette" but would offer no "letter approving the matter, because this might somehow or sometime be construed as consent by NASA to an effort by Philip Morris to register the 'Apollo Soyuz' name as a trademark." Les Gaver of the Public Information Office at NASA did express a desire for a few cartons, especially one of the presentation packages with the Leonov painting.

Excitement on the Soviet side was widespread. The first samples immediately went to the minister of food industry. According to Sinel'nikov the production had exceeded expectations, and many wanted to be caught in the reflected glory, because "the Soviet tobacco industry had produced a cigarette of international quality together with a leading international company—Philip Morris. This major event must be maximally used—all the more so because Leonid Brezhnev was an avid smoker."[67] The finished cigarettes were to be distributed through the Ministry of Trade and priced at an obtainable sixty kopecks a pack. Few made it to sale, and they were "high deficit" items.[68] Soviet sales started on July 17 and American sales on July 28. Outside of the Soviet Union, reception was mixed.[69] In the US, the vice-president of PM, James C. Bowling, sent packs to John Mills of the Tobacco Institute, hoping he would get them to the president. Mills sent a note of thanks but said that while he had "distributed the packs to key people in the White House as souvenirs," he did not intend to present them to the president.[70] Sales in Britain fell apart because of requirements for a health warning and because the flavor did not market well.[71] PM promised distributors to buy back unsold cigarettes.[72]

By the fall of 1975 PM-Europe had moved on from *Soiuz-Apollon* to next steps for the Soviet program: licensing, growing programs in Moldavia, and continuing cooperation. The Soviets were not quite ready to abandon the joint venture and asked to produce another three hundred million *Soiuz-Apollon* in 1976. As it stood, the Soviets were going to have to buy, for the foreseeable future, American tobacco for production. Even though both sides wanted to have as much as possible come from internal sources, and the Soviets were loath to part with hard currency, the cigarettes proved too important for these things to stand in the way. Despite progress in cooperation on manufacturing, difficulties remained. The Soviets confessed that they would need more tobacco for this second batch to account for losses—an extra 5–6 percent. The Americans advocated for a box, but the Soviets could only produce soft packs.[73]

In 1976 PM finally achieved its goal. The Corporate Products Committee Meeting at PM-USA approved, according to a confidential memo, a one-year license for the Soviets to manufacture *Marlboro*.[74] According to the *Philip Morris News*, an industry publication, this was "the first agreement involving the Soviet tobacco industry and a foreign company," and production would begin within the year.[75] Unlike the previous deal, the news was made available fairly quickly. The *Wall Street Journal* carried a piece in January 1977, remarking that advertising would be "thin" so "there won't be much call for the brand's hero, the Marlboro man." Still there would be a cigarette with "largely U.S. flue-cured and burley tobaccos," with maybe a bit of "Soviet-grown oriental leaf," if there was success with the "experimental program to produce flue-cured and burley tobacco in the Moldavian Republic."[76] This time, production would take place in not just the Moscow Iava Factory but also in Leningrad, Kishinev, Baku, and

Sukhumi.[77] In 1981 new discussions began for production of an American-style cigarette in Kishinev to the tune of two hundred million sticks.[78]

The *Marlboro* Muzhik and the Communist Frontier

While gaining know-how on smoother mass production, the Soviets were actively abetting transnational tobacco companies in the transition of the Soviet market to the engineered-for-addiction American-style cigarette. For Soviet smokers accustomed to an old-school papirosa like *Belomorkanal,* with uneven burn, leaf mixture, and taste quality in a rough cardboard pack with loose tobacco shifting in the bottom of the pack or escaping into the mouth while smoked, the cellophane-wrapped, foil-covered, well-balanced, reliably burning, and consistent-tasting *Soiuz-Apollon* or *Marlboro* was a revelation. Even those familiar with *Iava* must have noticed a difference. Sinel'nikov was very clear about the improvements in production brought by PM, and from the other side, records show the lack of consistent quality of Soviet leaf and manufacture had been particularly worrisome to PM in the run-up to *Soiuz-Apollon*.[79] PM had not test-marketed their wares on Soviet smokers, but they had labored intensively to develop their brand, and marketers had investigated how to hook consumers around the world on not just the nicotine and flavor but also the feel of the packaging, the look of the logo, the image of the user in the marketing, and the luxury of the design.[80] The *Marlboro* promised a world-class, American cigarette, and the smoking experience held more than just the allure of packaging. It promised innovations in drug delivery. The introduction of the relatively unsophisticated Soviet tobacco market to some of the most carefully engineered cigarettes in the world may have held importance in the creation of a more biologically addictive, psychologically compelling, socially pressuring smoking experience in terms of nicotine delivery and taste, packaging and imagery, and luxury and design.

Soiuz-Apollon promised western packaging, but the leaf blend catered to eastern flavors (and hence sales problems elsewhere), but with *Marlboro* Soviet smokers experienced a unique, new taste. The Soviet papirosy and cigarettes that had been pushed over makhorka utilized largely oriental tobacco leaf blended by experts to produce distinctive flavors.[81] Although there had been some menthol cigarettes produced in the 1950s, the flavor and smell of Soviet tobacco was largely the natural odors of the leaf. While often considered more luxurious because of its intrinsic aroma and strength, oriental tobacco does not take saucing like American tobaccos and is lower in nicotine. American Burley tobacco acquired flavors very well, allowing for the introduction of sweet and savory complexities of tasty fruits, exotic spices, flowery aromas, woody scents, and more sugar in the saucing process.[82] Iava had produced the only "sauced" cigarettes in the Soviet Union—*Zolotoe runo* (Golden Fleece), which flavored the tobacco with black cherry, honey, and walnut.[83]

The leaf for *Marlboro*, engineered for the American-blend market, had been expertly sauced. The taste was sweeter and less spicy than conventional Soviet blends. The smell was less acrid than makhorka and less pungent than oriental. Western tobacco companies created cigarettes that delivered the fastest dose of their already higher-nicotine leaf while also activating desire for sugars. *Marlboro* was designed for dependency.[84] The transition was not instantaneous. Prices and availability would limit the impact of flue-cured American leaf. The effect that American leaf had through the Marshall Plan, when availability was not a problem, is instructive. There informal surveys showed that 85–90 percent of West Germans preferred American flue-cured over oriental blends by 1949.[85] Soviet youth had gravitated toward filtered cigarettes and lighter tastes from their introduction, but there were older smokers for whom these were either too expensive or not to their taste. They wanted a stronger smoke.[86] Bulgaria provided American blends that had high nicotine doses, but the Soviet market continued to prefer domestic styles of smoke as late as 1985.[87]

Iava might not have been accustomed to advertising, but that did not mean that the *Soiuz-Apollon* and *Marlboro* were without a set of incentivizing images and tie-ins. Although seemingly an accident of dynamic personalities, diplomatic developments, and scientific advancement, the tie-in of the first American-blend, joint-produced cigarette with the Soviet space program could not have been a more advantageous launch for the PM venture. The state directed propaganda campaigns for cosmonauts, and the population expressed enthusiasm for the programs. A culture of kitsch—from pins and stamps to music boxes and cigarette packs—accompanied Soviet space exploration.[88] The Soviets had produced their own tobacco brands for the space program in the 1960s.[89] *Sputnik,* named for the October 1957 launch of the artificial satellite, features a pack with a deep blue swath of space punctuated by stars and the vision of the satellite itself, streaking through the sky. The pack came in either rough cardboard or higher-quality packaging, presumably for export (Figures 8.2 and 8.3). The *Laika* pack features an image of the space dog against a stylized vision of her 1957 ship sailing through a beautiful cerulean sky. Laika had her own propaganda campaigns that idealized her as man's faithful companion, a role the cigarette often took on as well.[90] *Kosmos* traded on the image of later rocket programs, appearing in a flip-top box with a more stylized and modern image. With each brand, however, it was a link of tobacco products with the heights of Soviet technology and

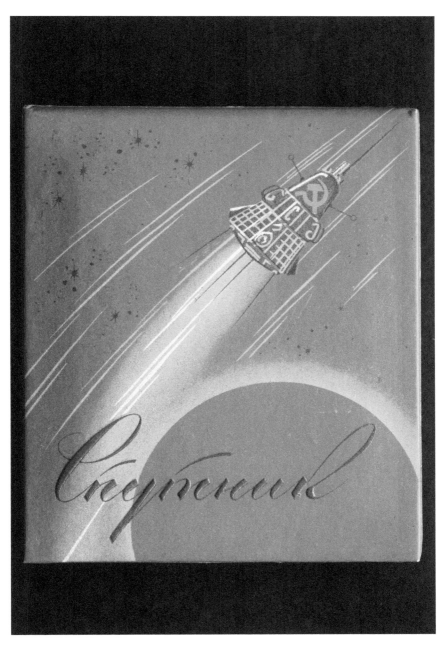

FIGURE 8.2. Photo. Pack of *Sputnik* for export (labeled on the back in both English and Russian). Courtesy of Productive Arts. Russian/Soviet era posters, books, publications, graphics—1920s–1950s. www.productivearts.com.

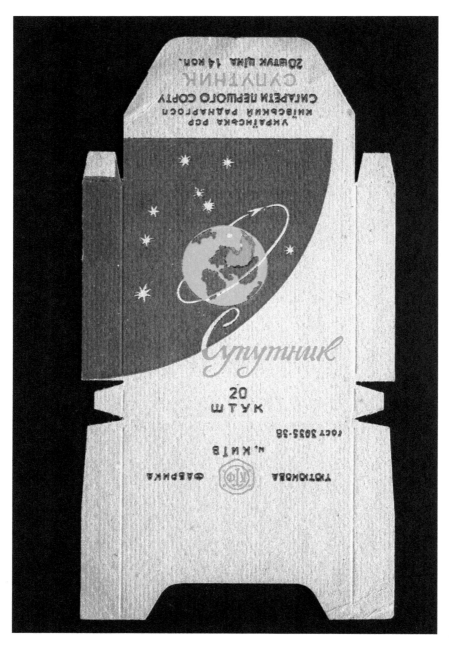

FIGURE 8.3. Photo. Pack of *Sputnik* for domestic market. Kiev manufacture. Courtesy of Productive Arts. Russian/Soviet era posters, books, publications, graphics—1920s–1950s. www.productivearts.com.

achievement. To open a pack of *Kosmos*, to light up a *Laika*, to smoke a *Sputnik* was to join physically with the great Soviet achievements.[91]

With Iurii Gagarin's 1961 orbital flight, the space program became party to a reinvigoration of the masculine within Soviet culture. Although there was one female within the group of cosmonauts—Valentina Tereshkova—it was the males whose imagery coincided with a general campaign to create a new "New Soviet Man" who could carry the country forward to communism.[92] The masculine thrust of the propaganda on the space program coincided with an established association of men and smoking to emerge in venues like the popular 1963 song, "Fourteen Minutes to Liftoff" that originally featured the astonishing lyric of a cosmonaut lighting up in the capsule prior to blast off. As it began:

> The space maps have been stowed.
> The navigator has verified the route one last time.
> Before the countdown lads, let's have a smoke,
> We still have fourteen minutes to liftoff.[93]

A quick smoke before liftoff was nothing compared to the claim that the Soviets had the first man to smoke (and drink vodka) in space—Valerii Riamin.[94] Of course, space was only the first step—a satirical poem in *Krokodil* claimed that the Soviets were going to send a man up to smoke on the moon.[95]

PM could not market in the Soviet Union, but its products tapped readily into imagery of tobacco as masculine, modern, and luxurious in addition to space kitsch. In Eastern Europe, a popular sense of "the luxury and fashionable nature of American cigarettes" had been around since after the war, according to a Bulgarian tobacco executive, and this same imagery appeared in the Soviet Union.[96] Tobacco was an expected accessory for the fashionable and the young.[97] Two Soviet blockbusters of the 1970s expected an audience already acquainted with the status and quality of *Marlboro*. In the 1973 comedy *Ivan the Terrible Changes Professions*, a character sings of longing. He then turns suddenly to the camera to reveal a pack of *Marlboros* just as the song turns into an upbeat assessment of how life has become "like a fairy tale." Clearly the good life came with a good smoke. In the 1977 *Office Romance* the unctuous but connected foil to the romantic couple ingratiates himself with the spunky secretary using a carton of *Marlboros*. She immediately drops everything and takes care of his appointment. Contemplating the exchange later while talking on the phone, she dreamily blows out smoke and languidly asks: "Guess what I'm smoking right now? *Marlboro*." The hierarchy of Soviet smokes becomes clear in the blockbuster *Sportloto-82,* where the rogue and profiteer San Sanych Murashko lights a *Marlboro* for the camera but, when asked for a smoke by his companion, hands over, to comic effect, a Soviet-made *Prima*. The smoking of luxury cigarettes like *Marlboro* joined an already tobacco-soaked cinematic realm where now even women smoked elegantly in films like *The Diamond Arm* (1969) and *The Irony of Fate* (1975) or for comic effect as in *The Twelve Chairs* (1971) and the female doctor in *The Pokrovsky Gate* (1983).

Unconventional promotion crept in for other areas of the Eastern Bloc where marketing was off-limits. Bulgarian producers regularly traveled with product displays and free samples, including to Moscow.[98] In 1979 British American Tobacco (BAT) contracted with a Moscow sociological agency to conduct a survey of product preference in Uzbekistan. It promised forty-five thousand dollars for two thousand in-home interviews with smokers and one thousand with nonsmokers at nine urban centers.[99] For the 1980 Olympics the Soviets wished to showcase their best brands and imported cigarettes for foreigners. Kiosks throughout Moscow were stocked with expensive *Marlboro*, *Kent*, *Camel*, and *Salem* cigarettes, which awaited crowds that never materialized after the American-led boycott. Eventually, though, these packs made it out to the public as gifts, bribes, and inducements.[100] In 1989 Poland PM succeeded in involving Lech Wałęsa in advertising campaigns, which in theory celebrated the Bill of Rights but in practice showed PM sponsorship and tied tobacco to American freedoms.[101] This foundation of cultural capital for *Marlboro*, laid during the period of communist markets, would pay off big in the 1990s.[102]

A further aid to the image of American flue-cured tobacco outside the normal western brand launch was scarcity. Through production hikes and imports, the Soviets met most smoker demands, but desire was a different issue. As with most Soviet consumer goods, poorly designed or produced items might sit unbought and unused on shelves, but there were shortages of preferred goods.[103] Soviet *Marlboros* retailed at one ruble a pack, but they did not make it into stores, remaining an item of extreme deficit that many hunted for but few possessed. At the factory the worries over theft for first *Apollo-Soyuz* and then *Marlboro* required the creation of special "crystal rooms" to keep track of worker movements.[104] Tobacco had long been part of irregular exchange, the black market, and the culture of the bribe in the Soviet Union, and as travelers in the 1970s and 1980s could attest, a pack of cigarettes or a carton could open many doors.[105]

It is likely that the mystique that accompanied scarce commodities made *Marlboro* taste even sweeter. Sinel'nikov argued, "If the cigarettes had come out in general sale, I think they would have drawn lines no less than McDonald's." For those who did manage to score a pack, the *Marlboro* had symbolic power. Smokers showed off the packaging as they flamboyantly puffed away. Many would restock an empty *Marlboro* pack with local cigarettes just to show off the label. Tobacco was a preferred gift in an economy run on them.[106] Even nonsmokers valued *Marlboros*—a carton might be given and gifted over and over, never being opened, just serving as a sign of respect.[107] Soviet consumers were sophisticated in their estimations of foreign goods. Imported *Marlboros* topped domestically made ones, and rumors that Soviet *Marlboros* were filled with Moldavian, not western, tobacco led to careful assessments of labeling and production information.[108] This was a publicity that PM could not buy.

A picture from the last days of the Soviet Union captured a little of the mystique of the American symbols of McDonald's and *Marlboro* (Figure 8.4). A family of five poses for a photograph in front of the newly opened Pushkin Square McDonald's (1990). Commemorating their day in the Soviet capital, they have chosen a distinctive prop, though the pack is more main character with the family as frame. Four of the five have their eyes closed. Only the mother and the *Marlboro* pack are directly addressing the viewer. The pack—roughened up, filthy, and

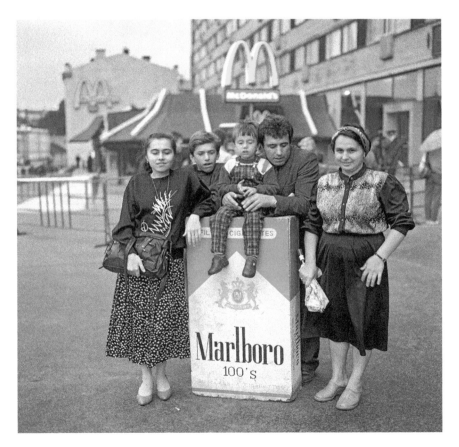

FIGURE 8.4.   Photo of *Marlboro* and McDonald's. Courtesy of David Hlynsky. *Window-Shopping through the Iron Curtain* (London: Thames and Hudson, 2015).

worn on the edges—is the dominant figure for this portrait at the twilight of the regime. To be in the modern city was to have fast food and fast nicotine.

Under Mikhail Gorbachev, the agreement between the Soviet Union and PM for the licensing of *Marlboro* faltered. Sinel'nikov recalled that Gorbachev's move into power changed the personnel for agreements and "the style of work and the procedures for reaching decisions." The changeover in ministries for production, the movement of personnel who had brokered deals, and the personal animus of Gorbachev toward smoking all led to the collapse of the agreement, along with the deficit of hard currency and the economic decline of the Soviet Union.[109] But *Marlboro* and others remained available in the Gorbachev era—bought in foreigner-only stores, exchanged by travelers who gained increasing access to the former Soviet Union, or smuggled.

Despite the collapse of the agreement PM had gained its foothold in the Soviet market Heymans had wanted "in," and through the successive introduction of *Soiuz-Apollon* and then *Marlboro* it happened. For the personnel of Iava it was a learning experience, technological boon, and complete triumph. For PM the short-term loss was a long-term win. For Soviet smokers, now prey to the world's most popular brand of cigarette and perhaps most sophisticated product design tobacco had to offer, it was a massive loss.

Even as PM agreements broke down, the hoped-for transition in tastes from Russian-style papirosy to western-style cigarettes trundled forward. The advertisers' arguments for filters that aided the tobacco industry recovery in the US and Britain found a ready audience in the USSR. With just a slight modification of target from nicotine to tars, the western-filtered cigarette fit right into an established role as the safer smoking alternative. Hiding behind this message of healthful smoking was the greater addictive potential from higher sugar content and engineered nicotine delivery, seductive packaging, and the allure of scarcity that cloaked western-manufactured cigarettes. It was not just the taste of the tobacco that attracted smokers but the display of taste that it allowed. Showing off packs, presenting them to others, and even donning labels as a fashion accessory became a way to perform sophistication and show distinction. The status of a *Marlboro* was such that in 1990 a pack could pay for a taxi across Leningrad. Cartons of western cigarettes became the standard accompaniment to foreigners requesting paperwork or bureaucratic assistance. Even without the ability to aggressively market their products, western manufacturers could depend on the scarcity, desire, and mystique of the *Marlboro* or *Winston* to carry them through Soviet cities and society.

PRESSURED

Demographic Crisis and Popular Discontent

In 1968 one of the more admired journals for serious commentary, *Literaturnaia gazeta*, published an essay by the Soviet economist and demographer Boris Urlanis. Urlanis opened by pointing out that the so-called "weaker" sex was outliving the "stronger" by eight years as men died at an average age of sixty-six and women at seventy-four. This was not just the legacy of the war. Urlanis worried: "Already at the age of 15–19 years the death coefficient for boys is twice that of girls of the same age . . . at age 25–29 men have a death coefficient 2.5 times higher than that of women!"[1] Urlanis blamed the differential on "lifestyle" illnesses—alcohol abuse, tobacco use, and accidents.[2] He noted that alcohol sales were rising at a higher rate than that of the population, occasioning alcohol poisoning, cirrhosis, heart troubles, and social problems like divorce. And tobacco sales had reached a pack a day for every adult male in the USSR, leading to increasing lung cancer and "substantial damage to the male organism."[3] Urlanis wed the two, declaring the combination of accidents, alcohol, and tobacco a public health crisis that required society-wide action. As the headline cried out, it was time to "Save the Men!"

A flood of letters, essays, commentaries, cartoons, and even two romantic comedies (1981's *Save the Women!* and 1982's *Save the Men!*) answered Urlanis's call.[4] *Literaturnaia gazeta* showcased reader letters that indicated the popular upheaval. The engineer M. Barovich proposed that Urlanis had correctly seen the health problem but thought urbanization was the root cause. Vladimir Zharko, a pilot, attributed the higher male mortality to dangerous professions, and he rumbled that feminizing men "to hang around the kitchen" would not solve the issue; besides, Marx's wife "did not demand that her husband rearrange his life to completely revolve around the house. And humanity has only benefited from this."[5] Since Urlanis had mentioned nothing of men retiring from the public sphere or taking up domestic work, Zharko's protestations exposed a great deal about the drinking, smoking, and danger expected of Soviet men. Perhaps years of antismoking propaganda focused on women and children had undercut this same message being turned on men.[6]

The eruption of social critique after the publication of "Save the Men!" revealed male health as a divisive issue and part of a more widespread anxiety over social collapse.[7] The massive loss of men in the war, Stalin's death, and the Thaw's challenge to reform the system intensified worries that men were softening, and even feminized, while women grew harder and more masculine.[8] Calls for men to be more authoritative in families and more present as fathers in the postwar era and into the 1960s implied that the men who were around were seen as inadequate in strength and number.[9] Adding to the gender trouble, women would be the ones to "Save the Men!" because of their overwhelming presence in the medical profession. Feminization of the medical force had begun in the 1920s, and by the late 1960s four-fifths of Soviet doctors were female.[10]

Smoking took on a strong resonance in this commentary on male authority, social decline, and Soviet power. It was the manliest of habits, widespread and popular, yet being unable to quit was a symptom of weakness. Cessation propaganda—which increased in the same period, spurred not just by demographic concerns but by international example and increasing tobacco usage—played on these two contradictory themes of strength and weakness. Health poster production rose, starting from an almost standstill and surging in the last years of the 1960s. Pamphlets increased in number of titles and size of print runs, boosted by the popular scientific society Znaniia. Some limited attention spread to methods of tobacco usage beyond smoking, such as Central Asia's *nas* tobacco (a powdered tobacco similar to dip).[11] More stories ran in the pages of mass-readership publications such as *Literaturnaia gazeta*, *Krokodil*, and *Izvestiia*. This propaganda—prompted by worries over demographic decline and attendant to western research on tobacco danger—was more than simply a commentary on a health habit. It was a message tempered by a socio-cultural crisis, fueled by concerns about declining male authority, and powered by anxiety over the status of the entire country.

Unlike in earlier eras, the antismoking message found purchase. In surveys and letters, it became apparent Soviet men were interested in being saved or many wanted to save them. Soviet citizens called out medical and state personnel for inaction, and journals like *Literaturnaia gazeta* magnified their complaints.[12] This popular discontent, channeled by editors who asked for answers and called for action, pushed cessation into the national conversation. Medical and state authorities followed in proposing measures and eventually, finally, fulfilling them in the 1970s. Soviet tobacco condemnation joined an already strong international discussion. The Royal College of Physicians issued its condemnation of tobacco in 1962, and the US Surgeon General's report came out in 1964.[13] The Soviets quickly reported these moves but did not take action immediately on their own programs.[14] New cessation propaganda was reinvigorating the antismoking movement, but further moves were not forthcoming. The reasons for slow action on tobacco in the USSR (disinterest and medical recalcitrance) differed from the impediments in Britain and the US (industry obfuscation and lobbying).[15] For its part, the Soviet tobacco industry did not actively undermine the propaganda, did not resist warnings, and tried to amplify "safer" smoking by increasing production of filtered cigarettes, searching for lower-nicotine products, and working on lowering carcinogens.[16] Tobacco manufacturers debuted warning labels voluntarily but to dubious effect. The state had seemingly little, if any, resistance from industry, trade, or agricultural groups when it finally put forward anti-tobacco policies. They only argued that consumer demand had to be lessened before output was decreased but demand skyrocketed even as industry struggled. New cessation action launched in the 1980s, but for a society in turmoil and a government in rapid decline, saving the men would have to wait.

Demographic Concerns and a New Cessation

From the revolution forward, policies to increase birth rates, be it birth incentives or abortion bans, had largely targeted women, but anxiety over the number of men and their neurasthenic decline haunted these initiatives.[17] In 1944, when the new family law loosened obligations for fathers of children born outside marriage and increased supports for single mothers, it was a acknowledgment of the declining proportion of males in the population. Legalization of abortion in 1955 and a new family law in 1968 recognized the rising numbers of single mothers and the difficulties of their lives. The capitulation on abortion, an officially discouraged procedure, revealed not a softening on women's right to bodily autonomy but increased anxiety over demographic decline and fragile masculine health.[18]

Urlanis was not the only one concerned for Soviet public health in the 1960s and the perceived and real increases, in crime, suicides, abortions, drug abuse, and infant mortality.[19] With Khrushchev's removal and Brezhnev's ascendancy statistical reporting on public health became much more fragmentary, but foreign researchers estimated infant mortality in the USSR went up by more than a third in the 1970s.[20] Increased availability and consumption of alcohol and tobacco were connected to declining health.[21] Per capita alcohol consumption skyrocketed by over 300 percent between 1950 and 1970.[22] By 1960 vodka production sat at double the prewar levels, and beer production had quadrupled.[23] Tobacco boomed. Measured from 1913 to 1956, tobacco production increased by 810 percent.[24] A drive for even more began in 1962. By 1975 the Soviets were third in the world in production of tobacco, and they could not meet demand.[25] Consumer complaints indicated that the Soviets could not supply tobacco products of high enough quality and quantity to satisfy their growing market, even as western manufacturers competed heavily to hook and retain a dwindling number of smokers.[26]

Surveys were fragmentary, but the number of Soviet smokers was comparable to those in the US and less than in Britain, even if production did not provide a similar number of smokes per individual. Works from the late 1960s estimated about seventy million Soviet smokers (a little over 34 percent of the 1970 population), with male smoking rates of 13–45 percent.[27] For comparison, in 1964 smoking in the US had reached slightly over half of men and a third of women.[28] British smoking was much higher, peaking in 1948 at 82 percent of men; women's smoking fluctuated in the low forties.[29] Individual surveys found high regional variation. A small (3,226 respondents) survey from Minzdrav's Institute of Sanitary Enlightenment in the 1960s found that over 60 percent of men and 26 percent of women had smoked by age eighteen. Male smokers tended to be workers and female smokers, engineers. The cost in work hours was steep—seventy-seven million workdays per year. Of these, 88 million were spent in bed, and 306 million days at lessened strength. For men aged forty-five to sixty-four, tobacco was responsible for 28 percent of their illnesses. Compared to nonsmokers, they suffered from chest pain thirteen times more often, heart attack twelve times more often, and stomach ulcers ten times more often.[30] A 1965 survey of Gorkii reported that 50 percent of men and 2 percent of women smoked, whereas a Kiev oblast hospital survey found a general smoking rate of 43.1 percent (63.3 percent of males and 16.9 percent of females). Of these, 79.9 percent smoked a pack a day.[31] A 1980 report in *Sovetskoe zdravookhranenie* emerged as an outlier by estimating overall Soviet smoking rates of 45 percent of males and 26.3 percent of females in the 1960s and posting growth in the 1970s to 56.9 percent of males and 49.1 percent of females.[32] This increase in female smoking differs from regional estimates and numbers extrapolated from longitudinal surveys of the 1990s. Even if inflated, these numbers contribute to the perception of an increasing problem of women's tobacco use.[33]

Soviet smoking rates were high in the 1960s, but the connections to health concerns being made in the west were not being made by Soviet authorities.

The number of cancers and reasons for them were debated. Just as the science in the west was not yet settled, so too was there debate in the USSR. In 1962 the researcher A. N. Novikov argued in the premier medical journal *Sovetskoe zdravookhranenie* that the Soviets were at the forefront of cancer research, prevention, and early detection with, therefore, lower risk than in the west. Novikov argued that if a survey of ten thousand in the US revealed three to four hundred with signs of cancer, a similar study of Soviet citizens would reveal only eleven to seventeen.[34] Surveys of cancers in the USSR from the 1950s and 1960s presented deaths from lung cancer as 15.7 percent of all cancer deaths and attributed the problem to pollution, industrial exposure, and preexisting conditions (tuberculosis or pleurisy), as well as smoking.[35] Pollution, especially, became a focus for lung cancer rates.[36] At the Moscow Cancer Congress of 1962, Soviet medical authorities argued further that Soviet tobacco was different from American, had fewer carcinogens, and did not cause lung cancer.[37] A general study of lung cancer from 1967 gave no mention of smoking as a precipitating factor, instead arguing that the disproportionate numbers of cancers of the respiratory organs in southern Ukraine indicated that a "southern factor" such as "climactic influence" or "an especially large dirtying of the atmosphere with natural (*prirodyni*) dust" was at fault.[38] In the same year an essay by the leading oncologist Vladimir Nikolaevich Demin pointed out that lung cancer rates between city and countryside belied smoking as a singular cause of lung cancer, as did the number of dogs and cats with lung cancer, because "as we know, animals do not smoke."[39] Even as later Soviet antismoking materials incorporated cancer, the larger focus remained on cardiovascular disease. For example, a 1980 essay in *Sovetskaia meditsina* emphasized smoking's role in cardiovascular disease, giving cancer only a brief mention on the last page.[40] This aligned with the most prevalent causes of death for Soviet citizens, as estimated by US analyst Murray Feshbach. If in 1960 heart disease accounted for 34.7 percent of Soviet deaths and cancer 16.2 percent, by 1980 it was 52.5 percent heart disease and 13.6 percent cancer.[41]

Starting in the 1960s, Soviet smokers also remained unconvinced of tobacco danger. A 1960 Gorkii Psycho-neurological Institute survey of five thousand smokers showed that older anti-tobacco messages were well understood. Ninety-eight percent of those surveyed knew that smoking endangered their health and reported complaints of breathing difficulty or nervous and digestive problems.[42] Most did not understand smoking's connections to cancer and cardiovascular disease, even though research from 1930s Germany and British and American work from the 1950s had entered into Soviet anti-tobacco publications.[43] A 1959 handbook for lectures from the Institute of Sanitary Enlightenment included up-to-date information on the chemical composition of tobacco smoke and the many dangers from it, including cancers, vascular problems, bronchitis, gastritis, and ulcers. The author encouraged lecturers to point out comorbidity—that is, the ways in which alcohol and tobacco worked together to endanger health. But more propaganda was not necessarily going to be effective. Many anti-tobacco appeals appeared unsophisticated and outdated.[44] For instance, a 1959 lecture series burrowed all the way back to Tolstoy, Chekhov, Pavlov, Bekhterev, and Lenin.[45]

Sanitary enlightenment workers in the state apparatus, however, renewed the attack on smoking. Many international public health activists believed that Soviet cessation propaganda would work because of the established health service, high literacy rates, central control of media, and cheap access to the means of distribution.[46] In the west, advertising's emphasis on smoking and glamour, outdoor activities, and youth led antismoking forces to utilize the same vocabulary in cessation. Advertisements featured celebrity testimonials, pristine natural settings, or unsullied beauty.[47] Without advertising to counter, Soviet health consultants encouraged artists to produce clear medical messages. Many of the established tropes of the 1920s—tobacco as poison, the communal danger of individual habits, and the arresting graphic styles associated with constructivism—reemerged. This resurrection of 1920s anti-tobacco messages may not indicate a paucity of new ideas so much as the popularity of past appeals.[48] New media joined the campaign for health, including films like *Two Habits (Alcohol and Smoking)* in 1970; *The Business of Tobacco* (1972); *The Danger of Smoking* (1975); *Smoking Leads to . . .* (1978); *Don't Smoke* (1978); and *Passive Smoking* (1978).[49]

A new emphasis on communal response and attacks on connections of smoking and manliness joined older themes, as in the stunning 1964 poster "Cosmonauts Don't Smoke!" (Figure 9.1). Here smoke charts the rise and decline of civilization, where the smoke of the rocket, in white and on an upward trajectory, contrasts with the dark smoke of the papirosa emitted by the next generation. Wafting aloft, the crossing lines of smoke and their shading indicate the progress of one and the fall of the other. The poster turned the frenzy of interest in Cold War space exploration, the manliness connected to cosmonauts, and rising concern about a crisis of masculinity against child smoking. Many other posters of the 1960s spouted a similar message aimed at youth of smoking as debilitating, such as the 1967 "Which Do You Want to Be?" In this before-and-after poster the weakling lifts a pack of papirosy while the healthy boy holds a barbell. In a similarly themed 1969 poster a young man smoking in a mirror can see the shadow of his debilitated future self.[50] When songs of cosmonauts boasted of their prelaunch smoking, Brezhnev gulped down tobacco avidly, and even the roguish wolf character of the beloved children's cartoon series, *Well, Just You Wait,* chainsmoked away from its beginnings in 1969, the effect of antismoking propaganda was probably outweighed by the many other cultural signals for children to take

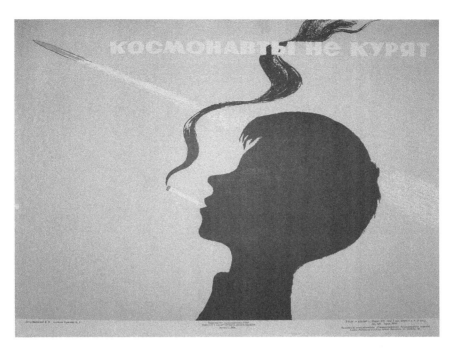

FIGURE 9.1.   Poster. "Cosmonauts Don't Smoke," 1964. Courtesy Russian State Library.

up the habit. For boys, the connection between smoking and the passage to adulthood likely outweighed such warnings. Surveys of uptake by youth indicated vast numbers continued to light up.[51]

The 1964 poster "Quit Your Smokin'/Papirosy Are Poison!" juxtaposed old slogans with bold graphics (Figure 9.2). The warning is the same 1920s Maiakovskii verse, and the writhing snake conjures a century-old appeal against alcohol as the "green serpent." The "gray serpent," an occasional name for tobacco that never quite caught on, rears up to threaten the heart with its poison-tipped fangs. The blood red of the end of the papirosa and the heart make clear attack and target. Although the poster advises smokers to quit, it does not offer any suggestions on how to do so or even a caveat about consulting a physician. No posters archived for the period conveyed this type of concrete information on therapy or an advance in understandings of dependency. How to quit remained little discussed.

A skull revealing papirosy in place of yellowed teeth gives a similar greeting from death in the 1968 poster "Papirosy Are Poison!" (Figure 9.3). Here Maiakovskii's verse is abbreviated, as it has become so familiar. The message is old, but the design is inventive, with the slogan cleverly forming the spine of the appeal

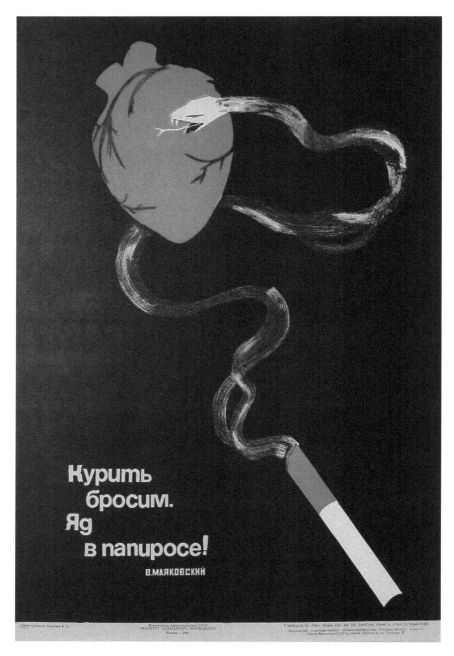

FIGURE 9.2. Poster. "Quit Your Smoking," 1964. Courtesy Russian State Library.

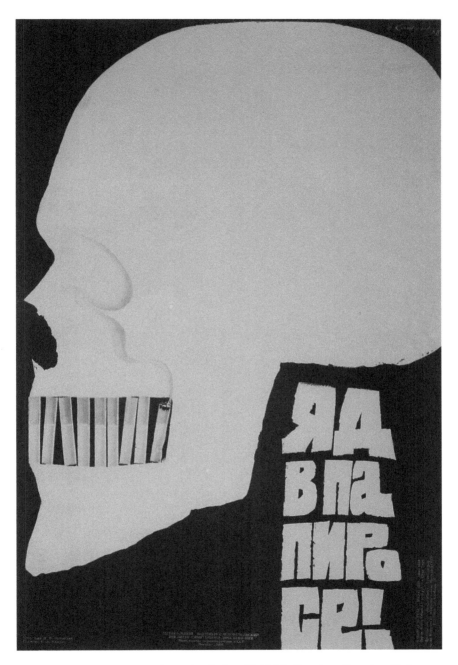

FIGURE 9.3. Poster. "Papirosy Are Poison!" 1968. Courtesy Russian State Library.

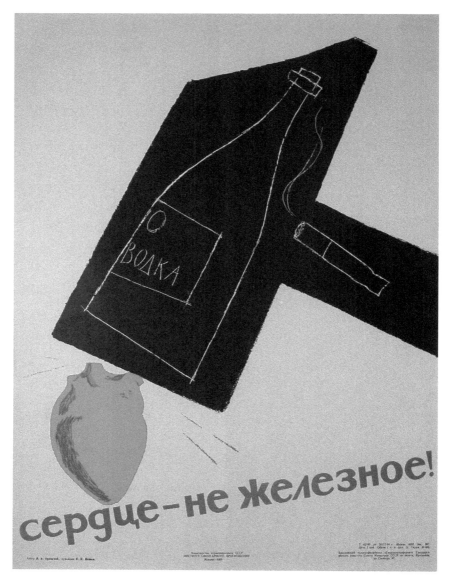

FIGURE 9.4. Poster. "Your Heart Is Not Made of Iron!" 1965. Courtesy Russian State Library.

and body. The second half of the slogan asking smokers to quit is omitted, leaving just the scare. Frightening messages are standard. The yellowed teeth, presented as papirosy, evoke not just the danger of tobacco but the revolting aftereffects of soured breath and a dingy smile. One of the teeth is even dislodged, a hint to smoking's toll on vigor and links to premature aging.

New also to this wave of propaganda was attention to comorbidities—the ways in which alcohol and tobacco worked together to endanger health. Chronic alcohol use hardens arteries and tobacco overworks them, leading to increased risk of cardiovascular disease, stroke, and death. The graphically arresting "Your Heart Is Not Made of Iron!" conveys a sense of the devastating cardiovascular effects of tobacco and alcohol together (Figure 9.4). The striking visual and brutal chromatic palate utilize an interesting mix of a more realistic heart with modern block graphics and the crude chalk drawings of the bottle and papirosa. The pinching of the mouthpiece and the short cartridge mean this is a papirosa, perhaps allowing viewers to believe that a filtered cigarette was not as danger- ous. Pamphlet literature pointed to the mistake in such assumptions, but the simple graphics of posters allowed no nuance and played on popular wisdom. The striking 1969 poster "Alcohol and Smoking Destroy the Organism" brings together alcohol, tobacco, and danger to heart and lungs (Figure 9.5). The verb employed—*razrushat'*—can mean destroy, ruin, or shatter. A man in silhou- ette, not identifiable as an individual, is pierced by a vodka bottle to his very core, where only three crumpled papirosy reside. The decimated, fractured body becomes an ashtray. The minimal color palate draws the eye to the touches of hazardous red and the combined dangers of tobacco and alcohol.

Dark humor simmered at the edges of these frightening messages. A 1969 poster with a funeral wreath "For the Smoker" implicates papirosy, cigarettes, and makhorka (Figure 9.6). If a laurel of victory could greet the successful athlete or cosmonaut, the smoker instead merited the stylings of death. The colorful wreath on an austere black background is festooned with funereal white. A simi- larly grim tone echoes in the 1967 poster "Kuril Kurilych Kurilkin" (Figure 9.7). The martyrdom of this smoker has curiously religious overtones for the secu- lar state. His cross sits atop a bare Golgotha, like the "hill of skulls" on which Christ was crucified, an iconic image. The Orthodox cross that marks his grave is constructed of papirosy, and his name, Kuril, means "smoker" and plays off the popular male name of Kiril.[52] Kuril's name implies he follows in the steps of others, because his middle and last names indicate he came from a family of smokers. The poster hints that smokers pass on a deadly legacy.

In the late 1960s, although older, more established arguments about nico- tine as a poison continued, these were joined by information on carcinogens like polonium.[53] The 1969 pamphlet *Bad Habits and Cancer* displayed this increasing emphasis. The cover had an artistic image of lungs blackened by papirosy, and the last pages contained a survey of global literature that argued for "the strong connection between smoking and lung cancer."[54]

Lungs began to appear frequently in pamphlets and posters, but new ideas on how to quit were lacking. For example, the 1969 poster "Now That's a Picture," illustrates the consequences of smoking but gives no exit (Figure 9.8). Cool hues

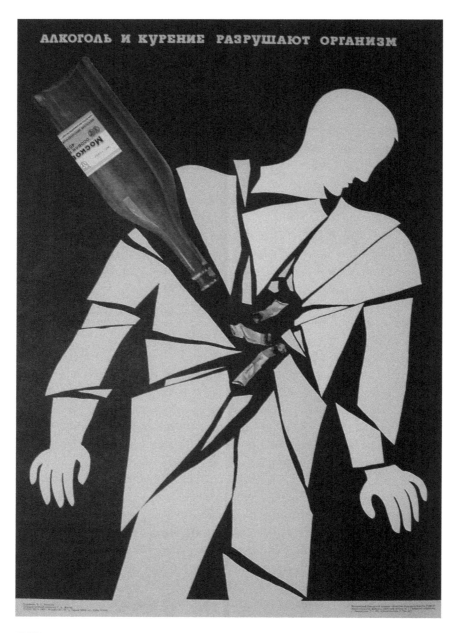

FIGURE 9.5. Poster. "Alcohol and Smoking Destroy the Organism," 1969. Courtesy Russian State Library.

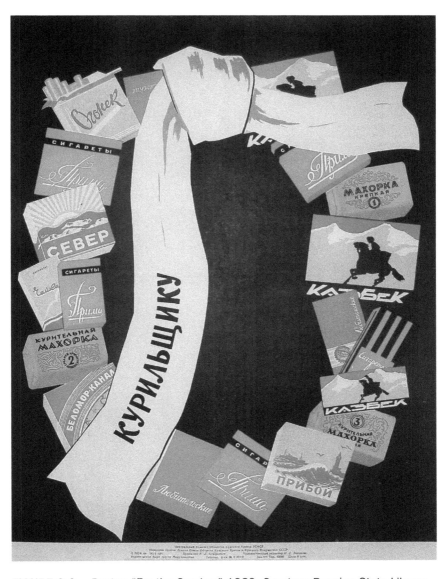

FIGURE 9.6. Poster. "For the Smoker," 1969. Courtesy Russian State Library.

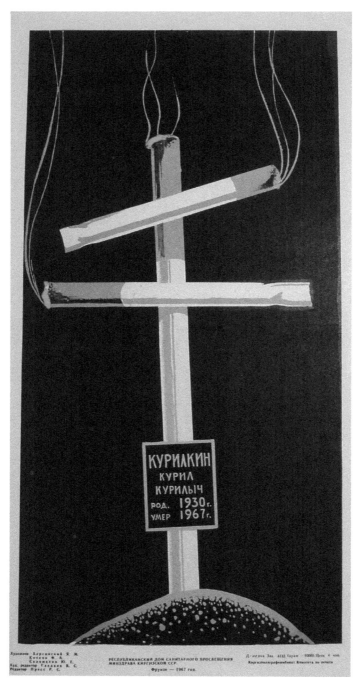

FIGURE 9.7. Poster. "Kuril Kurilych Kurilkin," 1967. Courtesy Russian State Library.

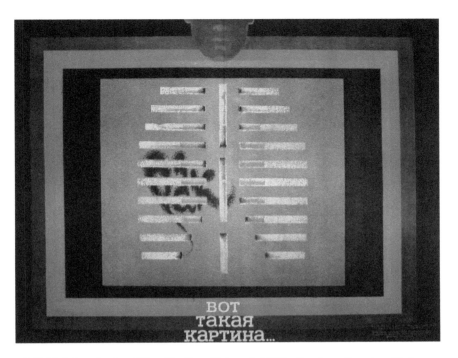

FIGURE 9.8.   Poster. "Now That's a Picture," 1969. Courtesy Russian State Library.

and a screen like framing imitate a lung X-ray, clouded by the smoky specter of the word "cancer." Caged in, the smoker has become his habit, his very bones now made up of the many papirosy he has consumed over the years.

In the 1971 poster "Smoking Leads to the Loss of Health" different ailments take up the spaces where the names would appear on packs easily identified as popular brands like *Belomorkanal* and *Prima* (Figure 9.9). The poster turns advertising on its head to promote the diseases, not the habit. The cleverest is the remake of the popular Iava as *iazva* (ulcer) in the same font and red bull's-eye. Not only have the packs been repurposed as vehicles for health risks—heart attack, lung and throat cancer—but the poster's smudged, darkened outlines take the otherwise clean design to connote the dirty aftermath of smoking, perhaps even calling to mind tarry, carcinogenic residues.

Many Soviet anti-tobacco posters featured smoking, rather than smokers. Disembodied hearts, skulls, or lungs mingled with featureless, usually masculine, silhouettes or dead seen only through their funereal trappings. Smoking was a problem of every man, but these were not men important enough to stand out.

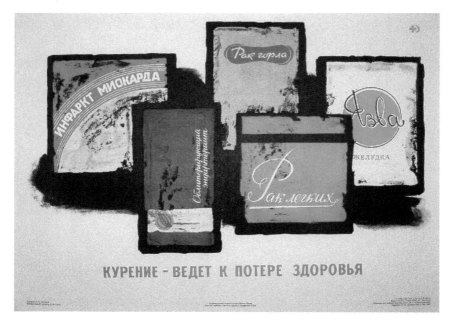

FIGURE 9.9. Poster. "Smoking Leads to Loss of Health," 1971. Courtesy Russian State Library.

Some propaganda wiped out the smoker almost entirely to focus on the victims of their actions. A piece in *Krokodil* condemned the "glad uncles" who readily gave over tobacco to underage smokers.[55] Calls to remove tobacco vending machines and limit smoking in public spaces like schools and medical facilities were often couched as protecting youth.[56] A 1960 cartoon in *Zdorov'e* draws the automat as the beginning of addiction for a youth—the end was a heart attack.[57] A central feature of earlier Soviet cessation, communal danger, appeared now as calls for smoke-free social spaces, as in the 1960 pamphlet *Quit Smoking*.[58] A 1961 poem in the journal *Zdorov'e* advised nonsmokers to confront coworkers who bothered them and was accompanied by a picture where the smoker becomes a huge papirosa, puffing out a vile cloud as coworkers struggled to breathe.[59] A 1969 pamphlet proclaimed smoking "a social evil . . . a holdover, which has no place in our socialist society."[60] A 1971 film, *Two Habits*, features smokers and drinkers inconveniencing a group of nursing mothers, passengers on a train, and others in a bid to shame them.[61] Equivocation remained: another *Krokodil* vignette played smoking for laughs when a story of a schoolboy in trouble for smoking ends with the father upset that the child smoked *Priboi* and not *Belomorkanal*.[62]

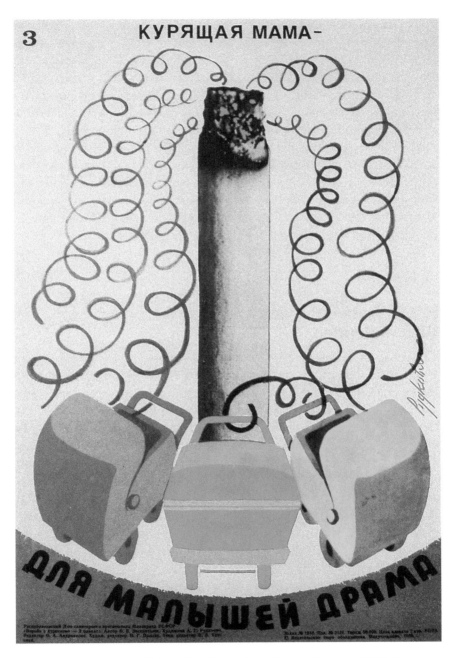

FIGURE 9.10. Poster. "A Smoking Mama for a Baby Is Drama," 1988. Courtesy Russian State Library.

Smoking by women received less emphasis, despite the growing numbers. The lone poster for the period in the Russian State Library addressing women's smoking is the 1988 "A Smoking Mama for a Baby Is Drama," which connects women's smoking and children's health (Figure 9.10). Tendrils of smoke snake out from an oversized, overpowering cigarette, and the curling wisps snag the assembled blue, pink, and yellow prams. Tobacco subverts the salvific pram ride in the fresh air into a poisonous pastime. Not just posters conveyed the message. A 1960 *Zdorov'e* article presented information on the dangers of smoking by breastfeeding mothers.[63] A 1965 sanitary enlightenment lecture guide advocated informing smoking mothers of the dangers of low birth weight and antenatal complications from nicotine in breast milk. The guide emphasized the need for different messages centered on appearances because, the male author argued, women started smoking to lose weight but might be worried over pallid, wrinkled skin, yellow teeth, or repulsive breath.[64]

Public Reception and Therapeutic Dissatisfaction

Public reaction to antismoking materials in the 1960s and 1970s indicated that a shift in attitudes had begun. Essays like "Save the Men!" occasioned calls for greater regulation. Thousands of letters from concerned readers suggested that antismoking policy was popular. An exchange between readers and *Zdorov'e* editors began in 1971 with the publication of a letter from Galina Serikova, a deputy of the Supreme Soviet, and Darikha Khodzhikova, a doctor from Kazakhstan. Their letter titled "A Question to Readers: Is It Not High Time to Limit Smokers?" proposed that everyone knew and had known for some time that tobacco was dangerous and that smokers continued out of selfishness. Complaining that smokers fouled the air of restaurants, airplanes, and building entryways, the authors argued for a change in attitude: "Smokers need to be taught respect for those around them and their health. Smoking in social spaces must be seen as a break in norms of behavior, with all the consequences that entails." They proposed less attractive packaging, a ban on advertisements, and pack warnings. They asked readers to weigh in.[65] Since advertising was reportedly banned in the late 1960s, this was an interesting inclusion.

In 1973 the magazine editors returned to the question, having received "thousands of responses." The replies ran a gamut from attacks on "ineffective" sanitary enlightenment work to demanding smoke-free workplaces, transportation, and theaters. One letter asked that passengers in taxis not smoke. A chauffeur lamented: "Not long ago the [traffic police] watched that no one smoked behind the wheel while moving. Now for some reason this good rule is not enforced." Some respondents proposed restricting access to vacation homes and spas, since smokers consciously destroyed their health. More radical proposals included having doctors refuse to treat smokers, minimizing papirosy production, reducing tobacco agriculture, and restricting sales. One reader suggested grisly warnings.[66] Many advocated forbidding sales of papirosy, cigarettes, and tobacco to those under age sixteen, fining those who sold tobacco to youth, and shaming owners of press kiosks that sold magazines like *Zdorov'e* alongside papirosy. Readers called for more gum production.[67]

The next issue of the journal followed up with heads of the aviation, health, transport, and trade ministries on how and if to put limitations on smoking. The first, and longest, response came from the minister of health, who pointed out the already "well-known" strictures against smoking in transport vehicles, theaters, clubs, schools, and health facilities. He reiterated that it was forbidden to sell tobacco to children and pointed to newer measures, including the 1961 change to the military tobacco ration that allowed those who did not want the tobacco to get compensation. The complaints from readers indicated few if any of these provisions were being carried out. Minzdrav listed the sanitary enlightenment measures underway and those in development, noting that anti-tobacco materials were already part of school curricula, more were being planned, and a group of one hundred government officials was developing a plan for health betterment.[68] The minister of trade responded that certain cafes allowed no smoking and that there was no smoking at lunch breaks at food product factories. Representatives of transport and aviation pointed to regulation of smoking on long-haul buses (travel time over one hour) and on flights (travel times over one hour and a half and in designated spaces).[69] In a follow-up article, the minister of aviation touted smoking prohibitions on flights up to three hours.[70]

In 1974, *Krokodil* joined the fray with a full issue devoted entirely to the dangers of tobacco. On the cover, a bald man sits at table his head down and eyes closed. In his hands, a box of *Prima,* with one smoke extended takes on the image of a gun, his finger cocked on the pack. The message of slow suicide from tobacco continued through the entire issue with articles, cartoons, poems, and even an antismoking song with music for children.[71] Moving forward *Krokodil* increasingly featured information on the dangers of tobacco. A short piece in 1976 publicized the many ways that people could quit, including *Tabeks* tablets.[72] The flippant attitude toward antismoking messaging had fallen to the wayside.

Having already caused waves with "Save the Men!" on April 2, 1975, *Literaturnaia gazeta* published V. Mikhailov's "Tobacco Death." The article heralded a new era after the "banal . . . threadbare, endless repetition of slogans." Mikhailov insisted that things were changing: "The time of the joke about a caplet of nicotine is ending . . . The time has come for alarm and disgust, the time of serious research on the problem, and the time of societal awareness of all the significance and dangers." Mikhailov condemned not just the poison nicotine but the many other chemicals and tars in cigarettes. He also stepped away from earlier equivocations made about lung cancer and reported that lung cancers had doubled in five years, 95 percent were caused by smoking, and there was only a 3 percent survival rate. Noting that some 70 percent of Soviet males smoked, and in areas of Siberia smoking among women reached 80 percent prevalence, he argued the time to do something had come.[73]

After outlining the many dangers, Mikhailov turned to theories of why people smoked. He ranted against the prevalence of what he derisively termed the "psychological" theory, which dismissed smoking as "mischief, dissipation, evidence of poor inclinations, and weak will. . . [from] boredom, imitation, fashion, habit, aspirations to self-destruction, easing social interaction, psychological displacement from unpleasantness, and the like."[74] Mikhailov's depiction of a tyranny of moral/psychological explanations for smoking is borne out by the offerings in newspapers that dismissed smokers for following fashion or addressed only children's smoking, discounting later smoking as an irrational choice, not a compulsion.[75] A 1974 *Pravda* article contained the typical mashup of scare tactics, little advice on how to quit, and dismissal of why people smoked. For women the author helpfully advised, "Step back, girls! This is not like the desire for a miniskirt or platform shoes."[76] The majority of another column was taken up with terrifying propaganda, a dismissive tone, and only a short paragraph on the need for unspecified "medical assistance" for quitting.[77]

In "Tobacco Death," Mikhailov admitted he smoked and found the psychological approach wrong-headed, arguing it did not explain why so many could not find the strength to quit: "Frighten us—we get frightened, but we don't quit in any greater numbers." Displaying a nuanced understanding of dependency, he called for work on "smoking as a psycho-physiological phenomenon with not just difficult biological consequences but also biological causes." Mikhailov proposed that taking this refined stand could lead to true progress, because "only 'Sunday sermons,' only 'frightening propaganda,' only appeals to rationality are not enough."[78] He praised the lowering of tar and nicotine content, more filters, and even "nicotine-free" cigarettes, but he observed that while filters decreased nicotine, they caused deeper inhalations, and "ersatz" cigarettes held little promise. For successful cessation he recommended recognizing smoking as a social, economic, biological, and medical problem and acknowledging that smokers needed "not propaganda and not persuasion but serious medical help."[79] Rather than just an attack on the established system, Mikhailov's essay also suggested alternatives. He said there needed to be a new category for smokers akin to drug addict.

He detailed the work of F. Birch of England into the possible genetic makeup of smokers. He recounted an experiment conducted at the Max Planck Institute where different cessation methods were weighed: smokers forced to indulge until they blacked out or compelled to join inhalations with electric shocks and verbal warnings of impending death. He claimed that the most successful method was from the Americans and based on "self-control and social control" with individualized supervision, but he dismissed this treatment as unrealistic for mass application. Instead he lauded the success of certain chemical methods, including cytisine, an alkaloid that binds with nicotine receptors in the brain, stopping the release of dopamine, which had been marketed since 1964 in Bulgaria and across Eastern Europe.[80] Mikhailov reported a 90 percent success rate with these drugs.[81]

Mikhailov's approach to addiction resonated with the readership of *Literaturnaia gazeta*. In June the gazette responded to the letters of readers with another nearly full page on tobacco with one sample "angry letter," a question-and-answer session with a doctor, a recommended method of quitting smoking from the west, and a request for more responses.[82] Mikhailov's sophistication regarding dependency was missing. The "Angry Letter" from a teacher began with a lamentation that nearly all the boys smoked and ended disparagingly that it was the "teachers and the school" that were to blame by being hypocritical, bad examples.[83] The question-and-answer portion with a doctor focused on tobacco and children, blaming adult examples. He proposed more propaganda and giving preference to hiring nonsmokers.[84] The thirteen-point questionnaire for readers started with six questions about smoking's dangers presented in push-poll style. These were followed by queries about quitting with prewritten responses that followed Mikhailov's derided psychological reasoning. The final section asked, without any follow-up, whether smoking was a "social evil akin to alcoholism" and whether current cessation work was sufficient. Here the preselected answers were more propaganda, pack warnings, sales prohibitions, advertising, and media representation, stopping production of lower-grade tobacco products, public smoking prohibitions, and organizing an institute to study the problem.[85] These suggestions reflected the British and US anti-tobacco campaigns.[86] Finally, an American five-day smoking cure from the foreign press recommended cravings be "doused" with two to three glasses of water along with breathing exercises; a strict dietary regimen; the elimination of soft furniture, television, and alcohol; and thoughts to "strengthen the will."[87]

In 1976 *Literaturnaia gazeta* published a rough statistical outline of the nearly eleven thousand answers they received to the questionnaire. Of these, 66.9 percent thought tobacco sales to minors should be forbidden. The next most popular idea was banning public smoking, winning the votes of 62.4 percent (82.5 percent of nonsmokers and 50.3 percent of smokers). Limiting media images of smoking concerned 45.2 percent. Contrasts appeared between users and non-smokers. The 58.9 percent of respondents who were smokers were more wary of antismoking efforts than were nonsmokers. For instance, prohibitions on color advertisements appealed to 37.4 percent of nonsmokers and 25.6 percent of smokers; pack warnings were deemed warranted by 37.8 percent of nonsmokers and 24.5 percent of smokers. Like Mikhailov, the readers demanded more than propaganda. They asked for a sympathetic portrait of smokers and remained skeptical of packaging, warnings, and sales restrictions.[88] Just over half (50.4 percent) believed that it was time to diminish the productions of low-quality goods. Such a move would not be easy, according to the science editors of *Literaturnaia gazeta*, responsible for putting together the results. Their correspondent to Glavtabak, A. Vokov, argued that low-nicotine tobacco (0.8–0.9 percent) would be difficult to produce, because eastern tobacco types had nicotine content of up to 1.8 percent and "demand among smokers is usually for the strongest cigarettes." Tobacco producers blamed smokers for wanting a product they had to produce. Even smokers agreed that it was not the availability of cigarettes that drove demand; rather, demand drove availability. Similarly, smokers said that advertisements and pack design did not compel purchases and that warnings would not stop the "dedicated smoker—without these he well knows the dangers of tobacco." The coverage of the questionnaire results ended in a call to workers of the ministries of health, food, and manufacture to stop making a deadly product.[89]

Despite the anger expressed in the journal, there was a large dose of defeatism in coverage. For instance, in a 1976 piece the author asked why cessation languished in the Soviet Union: "We have experience in quickly solving difficult problems. We clearly identified the necessity of a solution with a concrete goal and found an effective target. We focused intense strength and materials on it and achieved success. This, for instance, was the way we conquered the core of atomic energy and how we stepped into the cosmos. But with smoking it is a different thing. Here . . . the need for some kind of radical decision has not been fully realized, and the concrete goal is very difficult to see. What, in the end, do we want? That there are no smokers? That's utopia. At least it looks like a utopia today."[90] Outside the Soviet Union, the increasing animosity to tobacco from *Literaturnaia gazeta* merited notice. An essay in 1977 in *La Suisse* singled out the journal for generating pack warnings, reduction in nicotine content, and sales restrictions. They pointed out that industrial and trade groups continued to invest time and energy in tobacco production and the state plans for increased production ensured that popular cessation concerns, as voiced in *Literaturnaia gazeta* and elsewhere, would take a back seat to production.[91]

In 1978, on the ten-year anniversary of "Save the Men!," *Literaturnaia gazeta* returned to the question. Urlanis now emphasized there was a ten-year gap between male and female average age of death. Drinking was increasing. He condemned Minzdrav for inaction and asked for more active antismoking work, because "the more we try to save the men, the more they'll endanger themselves again."[92]

Social Pressure and Government Action

By the mid-1970s Soviet citizens and journalists shared a strong interest in smoking cessation, but their concepts of how to fight tobacco diverged. Central to this difference of opinion was understanding cigarette dependency.[93] Rather than seeing smoking as a biological, social, and psychological problem, as Mikhailov argued, different groups interpreted smoking in distinct ways. Many officials and doctors did consider smoking dangerous, but not dangerous enough to merit quitting themselves or increasing regulations. Lectures and posters on tobacco abuse appeared throughout the era, but without a strong supporting example from medical professionals many found the warnings less than meaningful. Critics lamented a system where "these same doctors, who as a duty of service explained to patients the dangers of smoking, did not themselves stop smoking even in the presence of patients."[94] The Soviet medical community resisted, but mounting evidence of the general wasting of the population was becoming hard to ignore.[95] As late as 1983, medical students complained that it was hard to quit when most of their teachers continued to smoke.[96] Even as medical professionals resisted, the statistics for Soviet morbidity and mortality grew ever more grim. Probably embarrassed by the implications and fearful of what the west or their own citizens would do with such knowledge of Soviet weakness, the government hid the extent of the problem while it searched for a solution.[97]

A 1971 report from Dr. L. V. Orlovskii, of Minzdrav's Central Scientific Research Institute for Sanitary Enlightenment, described at length the dangers of tobacco and called for "clarification" of this to the public. He maintained that "if the population were well aware of what a great threat tobacco carries not just to the user but also the health of those around them, then the number of tobacco slaves . . . would be incomparably fewer." He urged better therapies, noting that three-quarters of smokers who wanted to quit could not. He called for propaganda aimed at young boys that emphasized a smoker could not be a "cosmonaut, pilot, submariner, or sportsmen-champion."[98] For girls, he argued, the focus should be on yellow teeth, wrinkles, bad breath, and pregnancy complications, since girls smoked for fashion and weight loss. Like his ideas for why people smoked, Orlovskii's advice for quitting echoed calls of the 1920s about strength of will, communal responsibility, and aversion therapies. He mentioned the new tablet options of *Tabeks* and *Lobesil* but did not give success rates for these or any of the other therapies.[99] Produced in Poland, the cytisine-based *Tabeks* went through clinical trials in the 1960s and was introduced over the counter in the 1970s.[100]

In 1975—hounded by the popular press, pressured by sanitary enlightenment advocates, and inspired by international example—Deputy Minister of Health A. G. Safonov sent out a directive for the "Strengthening of Propaganda on the Danger of Smoking." The short document argued for the need to build on previous work while acknowledging it as "insufficient."[101] This time, the focus was on medical workers. The directive condemned the large number of doctors and nurses who smoked. To fight this, it suggested prohibiting medical personnel from smoking in the presence of patients and increasing propaganda.[102] Records from within Minzdrav suggested a flurry of paper and concrete action such as phasing in a prohibition on smoking by personnel at hospitals, polyclinics, and dispensaries and eventually restricting smoking by visitors, in cafeterias, and in leisure areas.[103] More than just restrictions, the ministry included special attention to medical, psychotherapeutic, and even acupuncture therapies.[104] Reports from sanitary enlightenment workers across the Soviet Union flowed in, documenting initiatives begun in response to the directive.[105] For instance, Andijan oblast in Uzbekistan promised more sanitary enlightenment work in schools, a ban on smoking by teachers in front of students, and the organization of cessation exhibitions. In addition, recommendations came in to get teachers to police common areas, report smoking students to parents, and shame smokers "at meetings, in wall newspapers and on school radio programs."[106]

Measures for the general public moved forward in 1977, when the Central Committee of the Communist Party and the Council of Ministers of the USSR proposed new and extensive intrusions into smoking behavior as part of their general program no. 870, "Measures for the Further Betterment of Health." The proposal did not focus entirely on smoking but emphasized attacking "bad habits," among which they included a call "to clarify to the wider population the dangerous effects of smoking for the purpose of the gradual elimination of the habit."[107] In 1978 this directive was followed up by a decree with more specifics, signed by Chairman of the Council of Ministers of the USSR A. N. Kosygin, "On Measures for the Fight with Smoking." The Council of Minsters called for no smoking in spaces of cultural, trade, and social interaction; no sales by schools or to those under sixteen; more cessation posters; articles and information on radio, movie, and television programs; and wider anti-tobacco actions to prevent uptake and help current smokers quit. The plan included providing more antismoking drugs, decreasing nicotine content, and adding warning labels by July 1, 1979, to all tobacco products, including matches. In a repeat of Semashko's disastrous 1920 meeting, Kosygin asked Gosplan—along with the Ministries of Finance, Trade, and Food Industry—to "investigate the question of the gradual reduction of the sale and production of tobacco products."[108]

Many took their recommendations to increase propaganda or distribute cessation messages in radio or television in stride, but the Ministry of Trade countered that diminishing the number of places to buy tobacco did "not help decrease the number of smokers and users" but instead lead to consumer anger and shortages. Gosplan warned it would just increase imports and advised waiting for propaganda to work and demand to decrease before curtailing production. The Ministry of Finance only asked that a plan be put in place for other goods to be produced to replace the income from tobacco sales. Just as in 1920, the discussion of the proposed decree at the Council of Ministers meeting on December 21, 1978, was split. The propaganda resolution sailed through, but the drive for a gradual reduction in production was turned into a call for decreasing supply only after demand decreased.[109] There was no debate about the danger of smoking. The contention was over how best to pursue a cessation agenda.

The final decree appeared in December 1978. The plan tasked authorities in health, education, film, and physical culture to join representatives in trade, production, and agriculture to work together to fight tobacco. Smoking was forbidden on transport vehicles and smoking areas established. Antismoking propaganda expanded. New points of sale could not be opened or operated near schools. Children under sixteen could not purchase tobacco products. Filter cigarette production would be expanded and better filters developed. Pack warnings would be prepared by July 1, 1980, and tobacco would be engineered to contain fewer toxic elements. A full group of planners and the Ministries of Finance, Trade, and Food Industry were told to "investigate measures for the gradual decrease of sales and production of tobacco products for the population with consideration for change in demand for these products." Additionally, Minzdrav would research newer, more effective mean of cessation.[110]

The national program drew heavily on reports from initiatives undertaken in Krasnodarskii Krai, a region on the Black Sea Coast famous for its health resorts. In 1976 officials there decided on local "measures for the strengthening of the fight with smoking." They instituted innovative antismoking initiatives, especially in the city of Sochi, where a special commission addressed creating "an 'antinicotine' psychological climate" using propaganda and therapeutic methods and prohibiting smoking in social spaces, on beaches, and in all therapeutic institutions. In 1979 alone, thirteen thousand antismoking lectures were read in the region. The report elaborated: "On average every resident of the krai participates in various forms of smoking control at least five times a year." As a result, after four years of work, Sochi claimed that over seventy thousand people had quit smoking.[111]

Two years later, to enhance "popular opinion against smoking," Minzdrav increased national propaganda and research. The Ministry of Education should intensify the fight against smoking in schools. The Ministry of Trade was instructed to stop the placement of kiosks near schools and sales of tobacco to children under sixteen, the Ministry of Culture to work with movies and publishing, and the Ministry of Food Industry to curtail production of unfiltered cigarettes, finalize warnings on packs, remove advertisements from packs, and engineer tobacco to include fewer harmful elements (a charge also given to the Ministry of Agriculture). Tobacco industry researchers had been pursuing this course since Schmuk, but now it was official.[112] As an alternative to smoking, Gosplan was to increase the assortment of chewing gums and decrease production of unfiltered cigarettes.[113]

Industry was ahead of the government. Engineering of low-nicotine leaf had been attempted for decades, and the Iava Factory began production of cigarettes with a lower nicotine content in 1975 because of directives from Glavtabak.[114] Sinel'nikov remembered them—*Vechernie* (Evenings)—as "cigarettes for gourmets." The name implied a milder effect on the smoker, something calming for the end of the day. Low-nicotine and low-tar Russian cigarettes took their naming from the western marketing innovation of "light" cigarettes. Ironically in Russian, the words "light" and "lung" are the same—*legkii*.[115] The 1978 Iava Factory history declared that the factory produced tobacco not only to satisfy demand but because they "cared for the health of smokers," contrasting themselves with capitalist manufacturers who tried to increase use. They instead stressed that they tried to limit nicotine and use special filters.[116] *Iava,* one of the most popular cigarettes among youth, produced the first packs with warning labels in 1978, well before the 1980 deadline.[117] Under orders from the Central Committee of the Communist Party, which according to Iava's director Sinel'nikov felt pressured because "the entire civilized world had a warning about smoking," the factory made a small run of *Iava miagkaia* with a label reading, "The Ministry of Health warns that smoking is hazardous to your health." The government was worried of a backlash from smokers and preferred testing with the "highest-deficit cigarette."[118]

The management of Iava, along with representatives of the party and the Russian food ministry closely monitored the first sales of the newly labeled packs when they were launched on the outskirts of Moscow. A long line formed for the cigarettes. As each customer was shown the new warnings, responses ranged from "this is nonsense" to the pragmatic worry that the label would raise the price. According to Sinel'nikov, it had no effect on sales. Everyone bought the one-carton limit.[119] The labeling message became a feature of propaganda, as seen in the 1988 poster "Minzdrav Warned . . ." (Figure 9.11). The striking visual

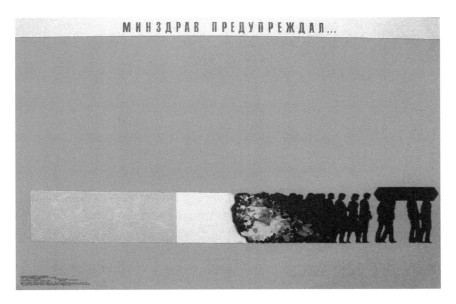

FIGURE 9.11. Poster. "Minzdrav Warned . . ." 1988. Courtesy Russian State Library.

shows a filtered cigarette lying on its side against a bright red background. Instead of smoke issuing from the ashy butt, a line of men and women, with a group of pallbearers supporting a coffin, solemnly trudge forward. The past tense of the pack warning along with the funeral procession make clear that the wages of smoking are death.

Regulation of spaces for smoking also progressed quickly. The ban against smoking on flights created in 1973 was expanded in 1977 to include longer flights. In the same year smoking in sports facilities, schools, dormitories, libraries, and medical facilities was restricted. Tobacco was banned in many social spaces as smokers were segregated into special areas. Enforcement of these bans, however, was not spelled out and adherence uneven. Reports circulated of individuals pushing for enforcement rather than authorities[120] With time, imposition of smoking spaces changed the scentscapes of urban life. Smokers moved to stairwells and clogged corridors or bathrooms and indulged in mass at the exits of subway stations and public buildings. The relative absence of smoking in classrooms changed the experience of tobacco in the city and the smell of buildings.[121] For smokers, it stretched the span between nicotine doses and perhaps encouraged cutting down or even quitting. For nonsmokers, the deodorization of some spaces likely made the odor of tobacco unexpected, more unpleasant, and therefore more confrontational when they encountered it.[122]

Internal documents of Minzdrav from 1978 implied that interest was building for more attacks on smoking. The unsigned report "Information on the Standing of the Fight with Smoking in the USSR" outlined the problems of smoking and the number of smokers in Moscow—60 percent of men and 10 percent of women in 1978. The document noted that World Health Organization (WHO) figures placed most smokers in the sixteen- to eighteen-year-old age group. In addition, the number of cigarettes consumed per person had increased.[123] Since the decree, the ministry had engaged in propaganda against smoking among medical workers and the general population. It had organized lectures, seminars, advertisements, posters, brochures, and even films regarding the dangers of cigarettes, but it now requested more direct intervention from the government. Specifically, it wanted a "special directive document on the fight with smoking."[124]

On June 4, 1980, the Presidium of the Council of Ministers of the USSR discussed how to promote work against smoking. On June 12, 1980, a decree from the Central Committee of the CPSU along with the Council of Ministers of the USSR outlined "Measures for Strengthening the Fight against Smoking."[125] The new decree praised Sochi as a nonsmoking city while recognizing that efforts fell woefully short "especially among the young." The same advice echoed throughout: produce propaganda to "clarify" the danger of tobacco, increase information at medical establishments, and involve all means of general communication (radio, television, print, etc.). Pack warnings were to become standard, as were "diminishing the production of unfiltered cigarettes . . . increasing the production of higher sorts of tobacco. . . [and] chewing gum."[126] Therapeutics, however, remained relatively unexplored even as psychotherapy gained ground as a specialty.[127]

In 1981 the republics and autonomous regions reported back on their progress. The medical workers' union in Armenia declared little: meetings at all institutions regarding the decree, a few dozen stories in central and regional newspapers, four radio programs, three for television, and two posters and one brochure with print runs of ten thousand copies.[128] Some areas attempted more. Voroshilovgrad promised future smoke-free zones. Tashkent oblast forbade sales of tobacco at buffets. Gorkii oblast prohibited smoking by doctors, medical students, and patients during consultations and promised special therapeutics for quitting, including drugs, psychotherapeutics, and acupuncture.[129] In Leningrad medical workers created a new form of televised collective therapy, with nine programs directed by a doctor.[130]

Gorbachev returned to the problem of smoking in 1987–1989. Minzdrav detailed that tobacco agriculture and tobacco imports had decreased, and the sales of tobacco had stayed largely stable. Still, there were "serious shortcomings." Filters had not improved. Propaganda was not effective. Academics and the public critiqued health work, and the number of smokers was not decreasing.

Minzdrav proposed strictures on where to smoke and sell tobacco (no schools, medical, sport, cultural, or leisure spaces, excluding restaurants), bans on aromatic tobaccos and sales to those under eighteen, institution of plain packaging, and new labels declaring "Smoking is a danger to your health and the health of those around you and does not make you an attractive person."[131] They asked for a continued campaign against unfiltered smokes, more chewing gum, and more stringent demands for industry and agriculture, including the planned reduction of tobacco crops, the decrease in the dangerous components within smoke, the gradual reduction of production of unfiltered and lower-sort tobacco, higher-quality anti-tobacco propaganda, and greater research into "effective methods" of treatment. Perhaps most importantly, they begged "for research on effective, new methods for forming a negative social opinion toward smoking and smokers."[132] The party and ministers proposed "further measures in the fight with smoking," following the recommendations of Minzdrav regarding diminishing production, restricting sales points, disincentivizing trade, establishing smoke-free spaces, increasing effective propaganda, instituting plain packaging, and bettering therapy.[133] The majority offered no critique. Agricultural representatives agreed to the move on reducing land sown and moving to healthier leaf. The Ministry of Finance requested different ways to allow stores to fulfill plans outside of tobacco.[134] In 1988, the Soviets participated in the first "day without tobacco" as part of global antismoking initiatives.[135] In 1990 a new journal against bad habits (alcohol, tobacco, and narcotics) started up to preach abstention.[136] And in 1991 Minzdrav put out revised norms for tar and nicotine content.[137] Educational groups clarified in 1991 how to move forward with better propaganda, but the collapse of the system forestalled any legislative moves.[138]

Professor A. K. Demin, in his massive excavation of the tobacco epidemic in the Russian 1990s, dismissed the Soviet anti-tobacco policies of the 1970s as "declarative in nature" and toothless, since "there was no real control of their implementation." Although Demin contended that oncologists and sanitary enlightenment activists actively championed a cessation agenda, he dismissed the pack warnings as mild and remembered that doctors continued to smoke in front of patients. Further, psychiatric-narcology specialists, charged with fighting tobacco, lacked the will to do much as "there was a widespread opinion that smoking was 'better' than alcohol abuse and alcohol abuse was 'better' than the use of narcotics." Progress on the question he credited to increased interest engendered by the European Regional branch of the World Health Organization's conference on "Smoking and Health" that took place in 1983 in Suzdal, the subsequent pressure by the government on Minzdrav to take action, and the uptick in research in the period after 1985.[139] This was well after major decrees had already been hammered out.

From Demin's viewpoint in 2000 it may have seemed like little to nothing was working on the cessation front, and his condemnation of the 1970s legislation as largely impotent and the medical professionals as recalcitrant is fair. Looking through the press and archives reveals anti-tobacco work and discontent were far more active earlier, and more broadly based, than his narrative indicates. The 1960s propaganda campaigns and popular press articles broke through into more regular features in the 1970s, and reception of these pieces indicated increasing discontent with medical and governmental inaction. These popular groups, aided by editors who asked for answers, pushed a cessation campaign in the 1970s that was accelerated by foreign inspiration and intervention in the 1980s. This mirrored the success of antismoking campaigns in the same period in the US, where grassroots activism and local legislation advanced cessation and smoke-free spaces against entrenched lobbying groups and a stubborn political system.[140] In the USSR it would be a similar swelling of popular anger, as channeled through the press and into public, that would propel tobacco cessation measures.

The Soviets entered the 1960s crowing of their immense strides in public health. By the end of the decade these boasts were brought into question. Urlanis and his call to "Save the Men!" revealed a state in decline and a public willing to hear and act. In letters and laments it became clear that many were ready for a renewed attack on tobacco culture in the Soviet Union. Particularly important were articles in the press asking government ministers for answers and action. In *Literaturnaia gazeta*, and other journals and newspaper pieces, appeals for better therapies, restriction of public smoking, and manipulation of tobacco products broke into the scene—echoing many of the same ideas that had floated around Semashko's proposed ban in 1920. The Soviets had come full circle, but this time instead of calls for a top-down change, it was the public demanding action.

Spurred by public interest, international example, and the increasingly dire demographic news, first Minzdrav and then the party and government finally moved against tobacco and for public health. Their proposals included increased propaganda and attention to construction of tobacco products, the marketing of them, and ways to decrease their manufacture. They attended to therapies and social messaging. It was a massive set of plans that were circulated, discussed, and finally implemented, but even as increased attention was given to cessation, so did the government give heightened attention to production, allowing PM in and increasing quotas. The Tenth Five-Year Plan (1976–1980) included plans for more cigarettes, especially blended products. Output surged from 1960 to 1982 by 69 percent. Consumption per person also nearly doubled from an estimate of 1,059 cigarettes in 1962 to 1,786 by 1980.[141] Increasing numbers of men and women smoked with every year.[142] The time to save the men was running out.

Epilogue

THE POST-SOVIET SMOKER

By 1982, when Sinel'nikov stepped in as director of Iava Soviet tobacco was in crisis. Sinel'nikov remembered: "The market for tobacco products was constantly balanced on the edge of uncontrollable deficit." From 1970 to 1980 the use of tobacco products rose in the USSR by 50 billion items, from 375 to 425 billion, but industry equipment was aging and not being replaced. Agriculture output continued to decline, and cigarette shortages intensified. The tobacco industry experimented with new tobaccos and utilizing waste products (dust and veins), and as a result, quality suffered. Complaints rose. For workers times were tough. Raw materials and transport were a problem, and work discipline fell off. What money there was had little buying power. The Iava Factory put together a special service on site to help employees manage the worst deficits of soap and other necessities.[1]

Neither Iurii Andropov nor Konstantin Chernenko managed to revive the industry as they stepped in—and were carried out—of power. Gorbachev rose with great hopes for reviving the economic system and creating a market, but he was no friend to tobacco. Gorbachev's economic policy of perestroika, coupled with his campaigns for sobriety, put immense pressures on alcohol and tobacco. Wine production was severely curtailed by a quarter or even half, depending on the type of wine, and vodka output dramatically reduced.[2] Production of cigarettes and farming of tobacco in the Soviet Union declined from 1986 to 1991 by 38 percent. In the same years, the economic dislocation of Gorbachev's programs entailed a decrease in imported tobacco by 46 percent.[3] To have any tobacco had become a luxury. As the founder of the mega-band Kino, Viktor Tsoi sang in his 1988 "Pachka sigaret," "But if you have in your pocket a pack of cigarettes/ that means it's really not so bad today." In the summer of 1989, in connection with protests in Bulgaria, tobacco went unharvested, and deliveries to the Soviet Union collapsed.[4]

By the summer of 1990 things were looking dire for cigarette smokers. Eleven of the fifty Soviet tobacco factories were shut down because of broken machinery, lack of spare parts, and deficits of tobacco, filters, paper, and inks. Farm workers in Tomsk struck over tobacco deficits, and other workers threatened work stoppages. Black-market prices for tobacco rose over ten to twenty times normal pack prices as rationing began in some areas.[5] Old women trolling the subway could reportedly sell a jar of collected tobacco butts for two rubles to a desperate smoker. Protests and riots erupted over the lack of tobacco.[6] Western manufacturers watched as two hundred people in Leningrad, three hundred in Gorkii, and some three thousand in Iaroslavl gathered to protest the shortages.[7] In Moscow disgruntled smokers rioted, blocked Gorbachev's path to Red Square, and demanded more smokes. Sinel'nikov, as director of Iava, remembered having a tense time escorting the representatives of an irate crowd around the floor of the factory to prove that they were producing, not hoarding, cigarettes.[8] Sinel'nikov's efforts might have calmed the group, but they could not conjure up tobacco. Instead, western manufacturers swooped in with cigarettes to save the state.[9] Between 1990 and 1991 RJR (makers of *Camel* and *Winston*) and PM, who had seeded the ground with *Marlboro*, sent in thirty-four billion cigarettes.[10] The influx of American cigarettes stabilized the tobacco situation, even as the government deteriorated. In August 1991 an unsuccessful coup revealed the growing power vacuum at the center, and on December 31, 1991, the Soviet Union dissolved.

Postcollapse Marketing and Skyrocketing Use

The collapse of the Soviet Union dramatically changed the previous relationship of the tobacco business and the state, with consequences for production, marketing, and consumption. Western firms came in eagerly, trying to scoop up shares of the established smokers, and with aggressive marketing attempted to hook new smokers—the younger the better. Even as smoking rates skyrocketed, the collapse of the state and economy led to a complete deterioration of the public health system.

Boris Yeltsin became president of Russia in 1990 and oversaw the transition for Russia after the fall of the USSR. The collapse left each republic's tobacco agriculture and production independent of the center and prepared the way for some 40 percent of the world's smokers to be offered up to international tobacco

in a largely unregulated and exceedingly rapid transition. Some domestic factories produced illicit runs of cigarettes at night while counterfeit international
brand cigarettes were snuck over borders.[11] In the chaos, international tobacco
companies imported legally, and smuggled surreptitiously, large amounts of
cigarettes, which were sold at extremely low prices, as they worked to secure
control of a newly independent tobacco industry and create new brand-loyal
smokers.[12] In Ukraine alone, in just 1996, 25 billion cigarettes were sold on the
black market.[13]

Several companies started a step ahead because of their early entries into
the Soviet bloc, the personal relationships built over decades, and the already
established brand recognition. Sinel'nikov recalled that the tobacco situation was
very different at the fall of the Soviet Union than that of other food industries.
"Among our industry there were already close ties with the west," Sinel'nikov
commented.[14] Not only had he established relationships with PM during the
production of *Soiuz-Apollon* and *Marlboro*, in 1989 he was brought to the US
and toured RJR factories. These early relationships helped foreign tobacco
assess the situation and profit quickly. Internal documents of BAT from October 1992 recount the potential they saw in partnering with the Iava Factory and
Sinel'nikov, who was "shrewd, capable and has good contacts both in the Moscow
Government and in the tobacco/cigarette industry."[15] The plan called for taking
the current 13.2 billion cigarettes produced per year to twenty billion by 1998.
Sinel'nikov was not the only Soviet tobacco man courted by foreign interests.
While Iava-Tabak was privatized and brought together with BAT, the Uritskii
Factory of St. Petersburg ended up with RJR and Krasnodar with PM.[16] As the
industry privatized, it was made more efficient and productive, nearly tripling
output, but worker protections and perks fell by the wayside.[17]

Ownership was not the only changeover as the tobacco industry transitioned
from communism to capitalism and from a command to a create-demand economy. As Sinel'nikov recalled, it was an entirely new way of working. No longer
did they just follow the state plan, now they "worked on how to interest users,
increase the market share of our product, and increase the effectiveness of production." Focus groups, testing, and new specialists in marketing, construction,
and sales meant "a different level of approaching the problem."[18] By the mid-
1990s a Muscovite could expect foreign tobacco to be advertised on radio and
television and on half of city billboards. Beautiful full-screen cinematic love letters to *Marlboro* with cowboys and desert sunsets ran before movies in theaters.
At sporting events or concerts, roving brand representatives gave away tobacco
swag to promote different brands. In some areas of the Former Soviet Union
(FSU) like Uzbekistan, Kyrgyzstan, Kazakhstan, Tajikistan, and the Caucasus,
bans on advertising and no-smoking zones were reversed.[19] Marketing to youth

became particularly blatant in the next several years with websites, comics, and other campaigns targeting school-age children.[20]

In 1993 an attempt was made to curtail at least advertising of tobacco products (along with alcohol). The tobacco industry responded quickly with the formation of the Coalition for Objective Information and proposed a compromise by which advertisements for tobacco and alcohol products would be relegated to the evening hours. While Russian Health Ministry officials resisted, the power of money was strong, and advertisements continued to be sold despite the ban.[21] A second round in 1995 did succeed in getting advertisements off televisions; however, the ban did not carry the hoped-for stringency.[22] Even as prohibitions went into effect, foreign companies shifted tactics.[23] In 2001 another round of legislation emerged significantly watered down because of industry influence.[24]

By 2001 PM had 19.5 percent of market share in Russia, BAT 13.3 percent, Liggett Ducat 12.3 percent, and Japan Tobacco International 20 percent.[25] Cheap papirosy continued to find a market among the poorest smokers, those down on their luck, or even many who preferred the taste.[26] Nostalgia brands made a resurgence with collector tins and appeals to "old-style" smoking.[27] The rampant marketing of cheap, easily accessible cigarettes led to massive increases in smoking across Russia and the FSU. From 1992 to 2003 smoking prevalence skyrocketed as the number of female smokers more than doubled, from 7 to 15 percent, and the number of male smokers rose from 57 to 63 percent or even higher. In some countries of the FSU per capita consumption increased by 56 percent.[28] By 2003 Russia was consuming about 240–250 packs per capita per year.[29] Fascination with foreign, especially western, lifestyles fueled demand for imported cigarettes while the quality of domestic tobacco products dropped.[30]

Iava had its own revival as it bet on consumer preferences for new tobacco in old packs by launching *Iava zolotaia* (Iava Gold). The slogan for the brand, "The Empire Fights Back," offered smokers, according to one analyst, "a new cigarette which, although of the same quality as the international brands, does not require them to abandon their national identity in favour of a global culture. Yava Gold foreshadowed Vladimir Putin."[31]

Public Health and Post-Soviet Cessation

The increase in smoking occurred even as public health provision collapsed. The fall of the Soviet Union brought with it an accompanying starvation of the health system. Although health standards had been falling for some time, steadily decreasing funding and personnel problems after 1991 showed a new level of danger.[32] Demographic trends visible before the fall of the Soviet Union intensified throughout the 1990s as funding, accessibility, and quality of medical care deteriorated. These problems with health care combined with dire financial conditions for those already food-insecure and living at a subsistence level. Many men, in particular, sought solace in alcohol and tobacco with tragic results.[33] Male life expectancy dropped to 57.5 years in 1994.[34]

A disturbing change was the numbers of young people taking up tobacco even as their elders died from its use. In Russia in 1996 some 65 percent of eighteen- to twenty-four-year-old and 73 percent of twenty-five- to thirty-four-year-old males smoked. Among women 27 percent of eighteen- to twenty-four-year-olds and 28 percent of twenty-five- to thirty-four-year-olds smoked.[35] The rise in young women's smoking was particularly striking. By 1990 more than twice as many women smoked in the thirty-to fifty-year-old age group compared to 1990 and of women over age fifty 40 percent more smoked.[36] These increased smoking rates were found to be similarly marked in Ukraine and the Baltic states, whereas Armenia, Georgia, Kyrgyzstan and Moldova had lower rates of female smoking.[37]

Public health efforts to fight tobacco continued, if weakened. Since 1992 Russia has participated in the annual "Worldwide Day without Tobacco." Radio, television, and school participation assured a much greater visibility for anti-tobacco propaganda than in Soviet years.[38] Russia became involved in the WHO campaign and in more conferences regarding antismoking work. Still, legislation that was passed by the state, such as a 2001 effort, remained largely ignored; even when enforced, the penalties were largely benign.[39] FSU countries had greater success in combatting tobacco, joining WHO's Framework Convention on Tobacco Control (FCTC) in batches starting with Lithuania and Armenia in 2004 followed by Belarus and the other Baltic nations in 2005 and Ukraine and others in 2006. Russia lagged.

In 2007 *Literaturnaia gazeta* republished Urlanis's "Save the Men!" and gave an assessment of the current situation. Far from getting better in Russia, the distance between male and female average life spans had increased to fourteen years, and men's average life span was fifty-nine years. Whereas in 1968 Soviet life spans had been close to those of the west, now the average Russian woman lived ten fewer years than her West European counterpart.[40] Tobacco was a deadly contributor to these poor health outcomes—responsible for 220,000 to 300,000 premature deaths per year.[41]

Opposed Again

Russian President Vladimir Putin shifted the focus to health as a leading problem of the Russian state when he returned to office in 2008. Putin's frequent public portrayals of his own strength have served as a symbolic assertion of Russia's strength as a nation even as public health messaging and regulation have been beefed up.[42] In 2008 Russia joined the FCTC and with that moved toward bans on advertising, promotion, and event sponsorship by tobacco companies along with stronger health warnings on packs.[43] Putin's government took aim at alcohol with regulations on prices, sales, and advertising. Alcohol was blamed for 43 percent of premature deaths and implicated in suicides, accidental deaths, and homicides. In the next five years alcohol consumption fell by almost 20 percent.[44] In 2013 Putin signed broad legislation including forbidding smoking in public, banning sales of tobacco in kiosks, instituting graphic warning labels, and raising taxes. In 2014 smoking was banned in restaurants and bars, and the prohibition was strictly enforced. In 2017 Putin increased tobacco taxes again (including for e-cigarettes) and made smoking workers responsible for making up their work hours lost on "smoking breaks." Overall, Putin's measures seem to have been very effective.[45] If in 2009 more than 60 percent of Russian males smoked, as of 2016 that number was about 50 percent, according to data from WHO's Global Adult Tobacco Survey.[46]

The spaces and scentscapes of today's Russia have been transformed with these restrictions and impositions of no-smoking spaces. Stairwells and entryways no longer reek of tobacco. Tobacco butts have diminished. The smell of tobacco on people's clothing in buildings is not nearly as sensible. It is a new world. The halls of the Russian State Library in Moscow give evidence of these changes. The smoking room in the basement and near the toilets, which through the 1990s overflowed with young students chattering and puffing away has been repurposed even as the ironically cheeky antismoking posters of the 1930s that decorated the lounge hang around. The censorious eyes of the pioneers now fall on just a few stragglers who wait for friends to exit the bathroom. The rank tobacco smell no longer belches into the corridor to permeate the landing nor does the haze climb up the stairs. Time and schedules are disturbed. Smokers must now exit the building to rush out and get their nicotine fix, then risk the inconvenience of a long security line to reenter. The outside is also changed. The courtyard of the library has been transformed. Smokers, forced to indulge meters away from entrances, are rarely visible. On rainy days one might catch a furtive puff of smoke and whiff of tobacco from a contraband cigarette sucked down under the wide portico, but for the most part, tobacco is no longer embedded in the texture of the city. Tobacco, the odor of an era, is sensible no more. While the durability of these changes is still to be seen, perhaps, finally, Semashko's "comic" story will find its happy ending.

Notes

INTRODUCTION

1. Michael Pearson, *The Sealed Train* (New York: G. P. Putnam's Sons, 1975), 85; Faith Hillis, *Utopia's Discontents: Russian Émigrés and the Quest for Freedom, 1830s–1930s* (New York: Oxford University Press, 2021), 211.

2. Karl Radek, *Through Germany in the Sealed Coach*, trans. Ian Birchall (2005) https://www.marxists.org/archive/radek/1924/xx/train.htm; Pearson, *Sealed Train*, 85.

3. Vladimir Bonch-Bruevich, "Lenin o durmanakh," *Trezvost' i kul'tura*, no. 7–8 (1931): 14.

4. N. Semashko, *Nezabyvaemyi obraz* (Moscow: Gosizdat, 1959), 11.

5. D. N. Loranskii and E. B. Popova, "Kurenie i ego vliianie na zdorov'e cheloveka," *Sovetskoe zdravookhranenie*, no. 11 (1980): 49. The article cited the following sources for these numbers: D. N Loransky, "Smoking Control Programs in the U.S.S.R.: Proceedings of the Third World Conference 'Smoking and Health'" (1977), 2:791–93; and L. V. Orlovskii, "Mesto sanitarnogo prosveshcheniia v bor'be s kureniem," in *Materialy vyezdnogo zasedaniia problemnoi komissii "Sanitarnoe prosveshenie" pri Prezidiume AMN SSSR* (Arkhangel'sk, June 29–July 1, 1977), 122–30.

6. Dean R. Lillard and Zlata Dorofeeva, "Smoking in Russia and Ukraine before, during, and after the Soviet Union," in *Life Course Smoking Behavior: Patterns and National Context in Ten Countries*, ed. Dean Lillard and Rebekka Christopoulou (Oxford: Oxford University Press, 2015), 117–40, here 124.

7. American Lung Association, "Overall Tobacco Trends," https://www.lung.org/research/trends-in-lung-disease/tobacco-trends-brief/overall-tobacco-trends.

8. World Health Organization, "Tobacco," May 27, 2020, https://www.who.int/newsroom/fact-sheets/detail/tobacco; "The Toll of Tobacco in the Russian Federation," https://www.tobaccofreekids.org/problem/toll-global/eurasia/russian-federation; "Current Cigarette Smoking among Adults in the United States," https://www.cdc.gov/tobacco/data_statistics/fact_sheets/adult_data/cig_smoking/index.htm.

9. Leon Trotsky, "Attention to Trifles!," in *Problems of Everyday Life: And Other Writings on Culture and Science* (New York: Monad, 1973), 74–75, repr. in *The Military Writings of Leon Trotsky* (New York: New Park Publications, 1979), 4.

10. Works on Russian and Soviet tobacco are limited in number and scope—the charming, popular history by Igor' Bogdanov, *Dym otechestva, ili kratkaia istoriia tabakokureniia* (Moscow: Novoe literaturnoe obozrenie, 2007); the memoirs of Leonid Sinel'nikov as director of Iava, in English as *Smoke and Mirrors: From the Soviet Union to Russia, the Pipedream Meets Reality* (London: Unicorn Publishing, 2020) and in Russian in expanded form in *Delo—Tabak: Polveka fabriki "Iava" glazami ee rukovoditelia* (Moscow: Delo, 2017); and two works both published by the industry funding press—A. V. Malinin's *Tabak: O chem umolchal MINZDRAV* (Moscow: Russkii tabak, 2003) and *Tabachnaia istoriia Rossii* (Moscow: Russkii tabak, 2006). For tobacco and public health there is a short historical introduction in L. N. Federenko, *Kurenie v Rossii* (Slavianskii filial Armavirskogo gosudarstvennogo pedagogicheskogo instituta, 2002) and two edited volumes by A. K. Demin, *Kurenie ili zdorov'e v Rossii* (Moscow: Fond "Zdorov'e i okruzhaiushchaia sreda,"

1996), and *Rossiia: Delo tabak. Rassledovanie massovogo ubiistva* (Moscow: Rossiiskaia assotsiatsiia obshchestvennogo zdorov'ia, 2012).

11. Matthew P. Romaniello, "Muscovy's Extraordinary Ban on Tobacco," in *Tobacco in Russian History and Culture: From the Seventeenth Century to the Present*, ed. Matthew P. Romaniello and Tricia Starks (New York: Routledge, 2009), 9–25.

12. A. I. Il'inskii, *Tri iada: Tabak, alkogol' (vodka) i sifilis*, 2nd ed. (Moscow: Kh. Barkhudarian, 1898), 24.

13. Lev Borisovich Kafengauz, *Evoliutsiia promyshlennogo proizvodstva Rossii (posledniaia tret' XIX v.–30-e gody XX v.)* (Moscow: Epifaniia, 1994), 166, 198, 265.

14. Joel R. Bius, *Smoke 'em if You Got 'em: The Rise and Fall of the Military Cigarette Ration* (Annapolis, MD: Naval Institute Press, 2018), 8.

15. Anon., "Tabachnaia promyshlennost' za 40 let sovetskoi vlasti," *Tabak*, no. 3 (1957): 6.

16. Ivan Ivanovich Priklonskii, *Upotrebelenie tabaka i ego vrednoe na organizm cheloveka vliianie* (Moscow: K. Tikhomivor, 1909), 5; I. Tregubov, *Normal'nyi sposob brosit' kurit'* (Batum: D. L. Kapelia, 1912), 3; "Russian Paper Trade: The Manufacture of Paper Cigarette Tubes," *The World's Paper Trade Review*, 29 March 1907, 8; Bogdanov, *Dym otechestva*, 78; F. V. Greene, *Sketches of Army Life in Russia* (New York: Charles Scribner's Sons, 1880), 14.

17. Anon., "Tabachnaia promyshlennost' za 40 let," 11.

18. Tricia Starks, "'Constant Companions': Fabergé Tobacco Cases and Sensory Prompts to Addiction in Late Imperial Russia," in *The Life Cycle of Russian Things: From Fish Guts to Fabergé, 1600–Present*, ed. Matthew P. Romaniello, Alison K. Smith, and Tricia Starks (London: Bloomsbury, 2021), 135–52.

19. Jordan Goodman, *Tobacco in History: The Cultures of Dependence* (London: Routledge, 1993), 94. China was close behind Russia in the turn to cigarettes, but there advertising and mechanization remained important: see Carol Benedict, *Golden-Silk Smoke: A History of Tobacco in China, 1550–2010* (Berkeley: University of California Press, 2011), 133–39; and Matthew Kohrman, "Introduction," in *Poisonous Pandas: Chinese Cigarette Manufacturing in Critical Historical Perspectives*, ed. Matthew Kohrman, Gan Quan, Liu Wennan, and Robert N. Proctor (Stanford, CA: Stanford University Press, 2018), 8.

20. V. A. Kholostov and G. L. Dikker, "Tabachnaia promyshlennost' za 50 let sovetskoi vlasti," *Tabak*, no. 4 (1967): 8; Jack E. Henningfield, Emma Calvento, and Sakire Pogun, *Nicotine Psychopharmacology* (Bethesda, MD: Springer, 2009), 62–63; 468–69.

21. Nicotine concentrations changed with time and technology, but a 1959 article gave makhorka's content as 4.57 percent of dried weight versus broadleaf at 0.98 and Maryland at 0.79 (M. F. Mashkovtsev, "O snizhenii norm soderzhaniia nikotina v kuritel'nykh izdeliiakh," *Tabak*, no. 2 [1959]: 15–17).

22. Kathleen Sebelius, *How Tobacco Smoke Causes Disease: The Biology and Behavioral Basis for Smoking-Attributable Disease. A Report of the Surgeon General* (Rockville, MD: US Department of Health and Human Services, 2010), 111; Goodman, *Tobacco in History*, 5–6; Gary S. Cross and Robert N. Proctor, *Packaged Pleasures: How Technology and Marketing Revolutionized Desire* (Chicago: University of Chicago Press, 2014), 61–87; Robert N. Proctor, *Golden Holocaust: Origins of the Cigarette Catastrophe and the Case for Abolition* (Berkeley: University of California Press, 2011), 33–34; David T. Courtwright, *Forces of Habit: Drugs and the Making of the Modern World* (Cambridge, MA: Harvard University Press, 2002), 97–98.

23. Karl Schlögel, *The Scent of Empires: Chanel No. 5 and Red Moscow*, trans. Jessica Spengler (Cambridge: Polity, 2020), 21–30; Alexander Martin, "Sewage and the City: Filth, Smell, and Representations of Urban Life in Moscow, 1770–1880," *Russian Review* 67, no. 2 (2008): 243–74.

24. Jan Plamper, "Sounds of February, Smells of October: The Russian Revolution as Sensory Experience," *American Historical Review* 126, no. 1 (2021): 146–47, 149, 153, butts 151–52; Sheila Fitzpatrick and Yuri Slezkine, eds., *In the Shadow of Revolution: Life Stories of Russian Women from 1917 to the Second World War* (Princeton, NJ: Princeton University Press, 2000), 35, 64, 91, 136, 145, 154.

25. John Reed, *Ten Days That Shook the World* (New York: Vintage, 1960), 123.

26. Robert N. Proctor, *The Nazi War on Cancer* (Princeton, NJ: Princeton University Press, 1999); Frances L. Bernstein, Christopher Burton, and Dan Healey, "Introduction—Experts, Expertise, and New Histories of Soviet Medicine," in *Soviet Medicine: Culture, Practice, and Science,* ed. Frances L. Bernstein, Christopher Burton, and Dan Healey (DeKalb: Northern Illinois University Press, 2010), 3–26.

27. Plamper, "Sounds of February," 151.

28. Jane Bennett, *Vibrant Matter: A Political Ecology of Things* (Durham, NC: Duke University Press, 2010), vii–ix, 1–19, 39–51.

29. Emilia Koustova, "Equalizing Misery, Differentiating Objects: The Material World of the Stalinist Exile," in *Material Culture in Russia and the USSR: Things, Values, Identities,* ed. Graham H. Roberts (London: Bloomsbury, 2017), 29–53.

30. Jennifer J. Carroll, *Narkomania: Drugs, HIV, and Citizenship in Ukraine* (Ithaca, NY: Cornell University Press, 2019), 5–10.

31. Alexey Golubev, *The Things of Life: Materiality in Late Soviet Russia* (Ithaca, NY: Cornell University Press, 2020), 4–8; Christina Kiaer, *Imagine No Possessions: The Socialist Objects of Russian Constructivism* (Cambridge, MA: MIT Press, 2005), 53–64; Svetlana Boym, *Common Places: Mythologies of Everyday Life in Russia* (Cambridge, MA: Harvard University Press, 1994), 73–102; Igor Kopytoff, "The Cultural Biography of Things: Commoditization as Process," in *The Social Life of Things,* ed. Arjun Appadurai (Cambridge: Cambridge University Press, 1986), 64–91; Daniel Miller, *Stuff* (Cambridge: Polity, 2010), 23–31.

32. Emma Widdis, *Socialist Senses: Film, Feeling, and the Soviet Subject, 1917–1940* (Bloomington: Indiana University Press, 2017), 3–6; Tricia Starks, *The Body Soviet: Propaganda, Hygiene, and the Revolutionary State* (Madison: University of Wisconsin Press, 2008), 12–36.

33. Nikolai Krementsov, "Introduction: On Words and Meanings" and "New Sciences, New Worlds, and 'New Men,'" in *The Art and Science of Making the New Man in Early-Twentieth-Century Russia,* ed. Nikolai Krementsov and Yvonne Howell (London: Bloomsbury, 2021), 1–23, 85–104; Andy Willimott, *Living the Revolution: Urban Communes and Soviet Socialism, 1917–1932* (Oxford: Oxford University Press, 2017).

34. Igal Halfin, *Terror in My Soul: Communist Autobiographies on Trial* (Cambridge, MA: Harvard University Press, 2003), 1–6; Jochen Hellbeck, *Revolution on My Mind: Writing a Diary under Stalin* (Cambridge, MA: Harvard University Press, 2009), 1–15.

35. Tim Vihavainen, "The Spirit of Consumerism in Russia and the West," in *Communism and Consumerism: The Soviet Alternative to the Affluent Society,* ed. Timo Vihavainen and Elena Bogdanova (Leiden: Brill, 2015), 1–6.

36. Demin, *Rossiia,* 61.

37. Richard Kluger, *Ashes to Ashes: America's Hundred-Year Cigarette War, the Public Health, and the Unabashed Triumph of Philip Morris* (New York: Knopf, 1996); Sarah Milov, *The Cigarette: A Political History* (Cambridge, MA: Harvard University Press, 2019); Pamela E. Pennock, *Advertising Sin and Sickness: The Politics of Alcohol and Tobacco Marketing, 1950–1990* (DeKalb: Northern Illinois University Press, 2007); Benedict, *Golden-Silk Smoke;* Allan M. Brandt, *The Cigarette Century: The Rise, Fall, and Deadly Persistence of the Product That Defined America* (New York: Basic Books, 2007); Iain Gately, *Tobacco: The Story of How Tobacco Seduced the World* (New York: Grove, 2001); Barbara Hahn, *Making*

Tobacco Bright: Creating an American Commodity, 1617–1937 (Baltimore: Johns Hopkins University Press, 2011); Mary C. Neuburger, *Balkan Smoke: Tobacco and the Making of Modern Bulgaria* (Ithaca, NY: Cornell University Press, 2013); Proctor, *Golden Holocaust*; Stephen Lock, Lois Reynolds, and E. M. Tanesey, *Ashes to Ashes: The History of Smoking and Health* (Amsterdam: Rodopi, 1988); Cross and Proctor, *Packaged Pleasures*, 61–87.

38. John C. Burnham, *Bad Habits: Drinking, Smoking, Taking Drugs, Gambling, Sexual Misbehavior, and Swearing in American History* (New York: New York University Press, 1993), 234; David T. Courtwright, *The Age of Addiction: How Bad Habits Became Big Business* (Cambridge, MA: Belknap, 2019), 1–10; quotations 6, 9.

39. Cross and Proctor, *Packaged Pleasures*, 10–13.

40. Stephen V. Bittner, "A Problem of Taste: An American Connoisseur's Travels through the Soviet Union's Black Sea Vineyards and Wineries," *Kritika: Explorations in Russian and Eurasian History* 19, no. 2 (2018): 305–25; Stephen V. Bittner, *Whites and Reds: A History of Wine in the Lands of Tsar and Commissar* (Oxford: Oxford University Press, 2021), 170–99.

1. ATTACKED

1. Semashko, *Nezabyvaemyi obraz*, 11–12.

2. Sheila Fitzpatrick, *The Russian Revolution* (Oxford: Oxford University Press, 2001); Alexander Rabinowitch, *Prelude to Revolution: The Petrograd Bolsheviks and the July 1917 Uprising* (Bloomington: Indiana University Press, 1991), and *The Bolsheviks Come to Power: The Revolution of 1917 in Petrograd* (New York: W. W. Norton, 1978).

3. Michael Zdenek David, "The White Plague in the Red Capital: The Control of Tuberculosis in Russia, 1900–1941" (PhD diss., University of Chicago, 2007); Bertrand M. Patenaude, *The Big Show in Bololand: The American Relief Expedition to Soviet Russia in the Famine of 1921* (Stanford, CA: Stanford University Press, 2002); K. David Patterson, "Typhus and Its Control in Russia, 1870–1940," *Medical History* 37, no. 4 (1993): 361–81.

4. N. A. Semashko, ed. *Desiat' let oktiabria i sovetskaia meditsina* (Moscow: NKZ RSFSR, 1927), and *Health Protection in the USSR* (London: Victor Gollancz, 1934); Starks, *Body Soviet*, 12–36; Tricia Starks, "Propagandizing the Healthy, Communist Life," *American Journal of Public Health* 107, no. 11 (2017): 1718–24.

5. Susan Gross Solomon, "Social Hygiene in Soviet Medical Education, 1922–1930," *Journal of the History of Medicine and Allied Sciences* 45, no. 4 (1990): 607–43, and "David and Goliath in Soviet Public Health: The Rivalry of Social Hygienists and Psychiatrists for Authority over the Bytovoi Alcoholic," *Soviet Studies* 41, no. 2 (1989): 254–75.

6. Henry Sigerist, *Medicine and Health in the Soviet Union* (New York: Citadel Press, 1947), 29; E. D. Ashurkov et al., eds., *N. A. Semashko: Izbrannye zdravookhranenie* (Moscow: Meditsinskaia literatura, 1954), 5–49.

7. T. H. Rigby, *Lenin's Government: Sovnarkom, 1917–1922* (Cambridge: Cambridge University Press, 1979), 76, 80.

8. Rossiiskii gosudarstvennyi arkhiv sotsial'no-politicheskoi istorii (RGASPI) f. 19, op. 1, d. 405, l. 4; Gosudarstvennyi arkhiv Rossiiskoi Federatsii (GARF) f. A-482, op. 1, d. 155, l. 445.

9. GARF f. A-482, op. 1, d. 155, l. 444.

10. Leon Trotsky, *My Life* (New York: Pathfinder Press [1930], 1970), 342; V. I. Lenin, "Communism and the New Economic Policy" (speech at the Eleventh Party Congress, March–April 1922), in *The Lenin Anthology*, ed. Robert C. Tucker (New York: W. W. Norton, 1975), 530; as quoted in Elizabeth Wood, *The Baba and the Comrade: Gender and Politics in Revolutionary Russia* (Bloomington: Indiana University Press, 1997), 49.

11. Protocol no. 2, December 28, 1920, GARF f. A-482, op. 1, d. 288, l. 120; Protocol no. 3 January 5, 1921, GARF f. A-482, op. 1, d. 288, l. 122. Protocol no. 1 was not in the file.

12. GARF f. A-482, op. 1, d. 288, l. 109; GARF f. A-482, op. 1, d 288, l. 120.

13. GARF f. A-482, op. 1, d. 288, l. 112.

14. The protocol of the second meeting set the next meeting for December 31, but no protocol was in the file. Protocol no. 3 instead came from the meeting of January 5, 1921, in GARF f. A-482, op. 1, d. 288, l. 112.

15. GARF f. A-482, op. 1, d. 155, l. 453.

16. GARF f. A-482, op. 1, d. 288, l. 107.

17. GARF f. A-482, op. 1, d. 155, ll. 446–46 ob.

18. Tricia Starks, *Smoking under the Tsars: A History of Tobacco in Imperial Russia* (Ithaca, NY: Cornell University Press, 2018), 162–200; A. P. Nechaev, *Tabak i ego vliianie na umstvennuiu deiatel'nost' vzroslykh i detei* (Moscow: Zhizn' i znanie, 1925), 4; Ia. E. Shostak, *Kurevo* (Ul'ianovsk: Izdatel'stvo Ul'ianovskogo gubzdravotdela, 1925); V. N. Zolotnitskii, *O vrede kureniia tabaka* (Moscow: G. F. Mirimanov, 1925), 5; A. M. Rapoport, *Tabak i ego vliianie na organizm* (Moscow: Gosmedizdat, 1929), 32–36.

19. "Issledovaniia i otkrytiia: Bor'ba s tabakom v Germanii," *Gigiena i zdorov'e rabochei sem'i* (hereafter *GiZRS*), no. 6 (1924): 16.

20. S. Nezlin, *O vrede kureniia tabaka* (Moscow: Doloi negramotnost', 1926), 21–22; D. M. Rossiiskii, *O tabake i vrede ego kureniia* (Moscow: G. F. Mirimanov, 1925), 22; Zolotnitskii, *O vrede*, 15.

21. GARF f. A-482, op. 1, d. 155, l. 505.

22. RGASPI f. 19, op. 2, d. 627, ll. 1–3; GARF f. A-482, op. 1, d. 155, l. 546.

23. GARF f. A-482, op. 1, d. 155, l. 711.

24. V. V. Belousov, *Izuchenie truda v tabachnom proizvodstve* (Petersburg: Gosizdat, 1921), 177–79.

25. I. M. Varushkin, *Pochemu vreden tabak* (Moscow: Gosizdat, 1926), 19.

26. I. A. Pridonov, ed., *Bros'te kurit'! Populiarnoe izlozhenie o vrede tabaka* (Kostroma: Gosudarstvennaia Tipo-litografiia, 1922), 3, 12.

27. D. N. Lukashevich, *"Nevinnaia privychka" (tabakokurenie)* (Leningrad: Priboi, 1925).

28. Laura L. Phillips, *Bolsheviks and the Bottle: Drink and Worker Culture in St. Petersburg, 1900–1929* (DeKalb: Northern Illinois University Press, 2000), 17.

29. Bittner, *Whites and Reds*, 20; Kathy S. Transchel, *Under the Influence: Working-Class Drinking, Temperance, and Cultural Revolution in Russia, 1895–1932* (Pittsburgh: University of Pittsburgh Press, 2006), 69–75; Phillips, *Bolsheviks and the Bottle*, 19–20.

30. Starks, *Smoking under the Tsars*, 226.

31. Romaniello, "Muscovy's Extraordinary Ban," 9–25.

32. I. V. Sazhin, *Pravda o kurenii* (Leningrad: Leningradskaia pravda, [1926] 1930), 28.

33. Nezlin, *O vrede*, 49.

34. Nezlin, *O vrede*, 49–50.

35. S. N. Boginskii, *Tabak i ego kurenie* (Nizhnii Novgorod: Nizhpoligraf, 1925), 9.

36. Nezlin, *O vrede*, 50.

37. "Revoliutsionnyi voennyi sovet respubliki," GARF f. A-482, op. 1 d. 162, l. 22. See also Ia. A. Violin, *Tabak i ego vred dlia zdorov'ia* (Kazan: Shtaba zapasnoi armii, 1920), 17.

38. A similar banner adorned the podium at the September 1917 Democratic State Conference in Pushkin. See Rabinowitch, *Bolsheviks Come to Power*, 177; and Karen F. A. Fox, "'Tobacco Is Poison!': Soviet-Era Anti-Smoking Posters," in *Tobacco in Russian History and Culture*, 183.

39. Bednota, "Doloi kurenie!" *Izvestiia Narodnogo komissariata zdravookhraneniia*, no. 1–4 (1921): 42.

40. Popov, *Vred tabakokureniia: Sotsial'no-gigienicheskii ocherk* (Perm: Sanprosveta Permskogo okradrava, 1926), 22; Vl. Al'tman, "Pokolenie oktiabria v bor'be za novyi byt (Dostizheniia i zadachi komsomola)," in *Za novyi byt: Posobie dlia gorodskikh klubov*, ed. M Epshtein (Moscow: Doloi negramotnost', 1925), 22–43; L. M. Vasilevskii, *Gigiena pionera* (Moscow: Novaia Moskva, 1925), 29–30.

41. "Pro zdrav"izcheiku: Chastushki," *ZNB*, no. 1 (1925): 5; Zina Antonova, "Kurit' vredno," *ZNB*, no. 8–9 (1925): 15–16; I. G., "Novyi byt idet," *ZNB*, no. 4–5 (1926): 8–9; "V obednyi pereryv," *ZNB*, no. 22 (1926): 7.

42. "Po Moskve," *Izvestiia*, September 5, 1924, 4; "Khronika: Bor'ba s kureniem," *GiZRS*, no. 21 (1924): 16.

43. "Druzhno rabotaem," *Za novyi byt* (hereafter *ZNB*), no. 17–18 (1925): 20; Nezlin, *O vrede*, 55; on the discussion, see Gromakova, "Pora pereiti ot slova k delu," *ZNB*, no. 10–11 (1926): 23.

44. Diane Koenker, *Moscow Workers and the 1917 Revolution* (Princeton, NJ: Princeton University Press, 1981), 158.

45. "Po Moskve," *Izvestiia*, June 1, 1924, 5.

46. "Obiazatel'noe postanovlenie," *Izvestiia*, July 2, 1926, 6.

47. "Sud: O protivopozharnykh merakh na postroikakh," *Izvestiia*, July 31, 1926, 6; B. S. Sigal, *Vrednaia privychka (Kuren'e tabaka)* (Moscow: Gosmedizdat, 1929), 12.

48. Starks, *Body Soviet*, 14–16.

49. Neil B. Weissman, "Origins of Soviet Health Administration: Narkomzdrav, 1918–1928," in *Health and Society in Revolutionary Russia,* ed. Susan Gross Solomon and John F. Hutchinson (Bloomington: Indiana University Press, 1990), 97–120; I. P. Avdeichik and G. K. Iukhnovich, eds., *Plakaty pervykh let sovetskoi vlasti i sotsialisticheskogo stroitel'stva (1918–1941)* (Minsk: Plymia, 1985).

50. Theodore Dreiser, *Dreiser Looks at Russia* (New York: Horace Liveright, 1928), 91–92. See E. V. Barkhatova, *Iz istorii russkogo plakata:"Okna" ROSTA i Glavpolitprosveta 1919–1922* (St. Petersburg: Rossiskaia natsional'naia biblioteka, 2000).

51. Alexander Wicksteed, *Life under the Soviets* (London: John Lane the Bodley Head, 1928), 119; Susan Gross Solomon, "Thinking Internationally, Acting Locally: Soviet Public Health as Cultural Diplomacy in the 1920s," in *Russian and Soviet Health Care from an International Perspective: Comparing Professions, Practice and Gender, 1880–1960*, ed. Susan Grant (Basingstoke: Palgrave Macmillan, 2017), 193–216; Michael David-Fox, *Showcasing the Great Experiment: Cultural Diplomacy and Western Visitors to the Soviet Union, 1921–1941* (Oxford: Oxford University Press, 2012), 29.

52. K. Gorokhov, *Zlaia travka (tabachnoe zasil'e)* (Odessa: Avtora, 1929), 31.

53. T. F. Markarova, "Meditsinskaia pechat'," in *Okhrana narodnogo zdorov'ia v SSSR*, ed. M. D. Kovrigin (Moscow: Meditsinskaia literatura, 1957), 481–82; Jeffrey Brooks, "The Breakdown in Production and Distribution of Printed Material, 1917–1927, in *Bolshevik Culture: Experiment and Order in the Russian Revolution*, ed. Abbott Gleason, Peter Kenez, and Richard Stites (Bloomington: Indiana University Press, 1985), 151–73, as referenced in Nikolai Krementsov, *Revolutionary Experiments: The Quest for Immortality in Bolshevik Science and Fiction* (Oxford: Oxford University Press, 2014).

54. Wood, *Baba and the Comrade*, 194–98.

55. Ralph Talcott Fisher, Jr., *Pattern for Soviet Youth: A Study of the Congresses of the Komsomol, 1918–1954* (New York: Columbia University Press, 1959), 82.

56. Lukashevich, *Nevinnaia privychka*, 40.

57. Solomon, "David and Goliath," 254–75; Patricia Herlihy, *The Alcoholic Empire: Vodka and Politics in Late Imperial Russia* (Oxford: Oxford University Press, 2002); Phillips, *Bolsheviks and the Bottle*; Transchel, *Under the Influence*; Stephen White, *Russia Goes Dry: Alcohol, State, and Society* (Cambridge: Cambridge University Press, 1996); Mark

Lawrence Schrad, *Vodka Politics: Alcohol, Autocracy, and the Secret History of the Russian State* (New York: Oxford University Press, 2014); Daniel Beer, "The Medicalization of Religious Deviance in the Russian Orthodox Church, 1880–1905," *Kritika: Explorations in Russian and Eurasian History* 5, no. 3 (2004): 451–82, and *Renovating Russia: The Human Sciences and the Fate of Liberal Modernity, 1880–1930* (Ithaca, NY: Cornell University Press, 2008); Golfo Alexopoulos, *Stalin's Outcasts: Aliens, Citizens, and the Soviet State, 1926–1936* (Ithaca, NY: Cornell University Press, 2003); Julie A. Cassiday, "Flash Floods, Bedbugs, and Saunas: Social Hygiene in Maiakovskii's Theatrical Satires of the 1920s," *Slavic and East European Review* 76, no. 4 (1998): 643–57, and *The Enemy on Trial: Early Soviet Courts on Stage and Screen* (DeKalb: Northern Illinois University Press, 2000); Igal Halfin, *Intimate Enemies: Demonizing the Bolshevik Opposition, 1918–1928* (Pittsburgh: University of Pittsburgh Press, 2007).

58. Susan Gross Solomon, "Social Hygiene and Soviet Public Health," in *Health and Society in Revolutionary Russia*, 175–99. See Pavel Vasil'ev, "Evoliutsiia predstavlenii o narkotikakh v rossiiskikh meditsinskikh tekstakh (1890–1930-e gody): Ot 'iadov tsivilizatsii' k 'perezhitkam kaptializma,'" in *Biulleten' Germanskogo istoricheskogo institute v Moskve*, ed. Katja Bruisch (Moscow: Germanskii istoricheskii institut v Moskve, 2012), 52–65.

59. For the intersection of gender, ethnicity, politics, and medicine, see Frances Lee Bernstein, *The Dictatorship of Sex: Lifestyle Advice for the Soviet Masses* (DeKalb: Northern Illinois University Press, 2007); Dan Healey, *Homosexual Desire in Revolutionary Russia: The Regulation of Sexual and Gender Dissent* (Chicago: University of Chicago Press, 2002); Paula Michaels, *Curative Powers: Medicine and Empire in Stalin's Central Asia* (Pittsburgh: University of Pittsburgh Press, 2003), and *Lamaze: An International History* (Oxford: Oxford University Press, 2014); Eric Naiman, *Sex in Public: The Incarnation of Early Soviet Ideology* (Princeton, NJ: Princeton University Press, 1997); Starks, *Body Soviet*, 31–34, 81, 176–77; and Cassandra Cavanaugh, "Backwardness and Biology: Medicine and Power in Russian and Soviet Central Asia, 1868–1934" (PhD diss., Columbia University, 2001).

60. D. Rossiiskii, "O nikotinizme," *Meditsina: Ezhemesiachnyi zhurnal dlia usovershchenstvovaniia*, no. 7 (1926): 89–10.

61. Nezlin, *O vrede*, 51–53.

62. Transchel, *Under the Influence*, 75.

63. Sazhin, *Pravda*, 25–27.

64. Ia. I. Lifshits, *Doloi kurenie i p'ianstvo!* (Kharkov: Nauchnaia mysl', 1928), 24.

65. K. Shapshev, "Predislovie," to Popov, *Vred tabakokureniia*, 5.

66. Lukashevich, *Nevinnaia privychka*, 7–8 (story), 14–19 (individual and social effects), quotations 19.

67. S. Kal'manson and D. Bekariukov, *Beregi svoe zdorov'e! Sanitarnaia pamiatka dlia rabochikh podrostkov* (Leningrad: Molodaia gvardiia, 1925), 18.

68. E. I. Berman, *O stol' tsenimom tabake i trudovom molodniake: S pit'iu diagrammami v tekste* (Moscow: Zhizn' i znanie, 1926), 6.

69. E. B. Bliumenau, *Okhmeliaiushchie durmany: Tabak, opii i morfii, kokain, efir i gashish, ikh vred i posledstviia* (Leningrad: Seiatel', 1925).

70. A. S. Sholomovich, *Detskii pokhod na vzroslykh* (Moscow: Mozdravotdel, 1926), 10–11.

71. Sazhin, *Pravda o kurenii*, 17.

72. Boginskii, *Tabak i ego kurenie*, 10.

73. A. Press, "Otravlenie vsego naseleniia tabachnym dymom (chast 1)," *GiZRS*, no. 18 (1924): 2–3.

74. Zolotnitskii, *O vrede*, 10.

75. Popov, *Vred tabakokureniia*, 14.

76. Varushkin, *Pochemu vreden tabak*, 7.

77. Nezlin, *O vrede*, 22.

78. Sholomovich, *Detskii pokhod na vzroslykh*, 30, 37; Il'ianskii and Lapin, "Beregi zdorov'e i nikakikh gvozdei!," *ZNB*, no. 4–5 (1925): 10.

79. I. G. Uporov, *Tabak, ego kurenie i vliianie na organizm* (Sverdlovsk: Izdatel'stvo Sanepida Sverdlovskogo okzdravotdela, 1925), 10.

80. "Issledovaniia i otkrytiia: O kurki papiros, kak rasprostraniteli tuberkuleza," *GiZRS*, no. 4 (1923): 15.

81. Popov, *Vred tabakokureniia*, 19–20.

82. I. Sazhin, "O kurenii," *Gigiena i zdorov'e rabochei i krest'ianskoi sem'i* (hereafter *GiZRiKS*), no. 13 (1926): 8.

83. Nechaev, *Tabak i ego vliianie*, 31–32.

84. Nechaev, *Tabak i ego vliianie*, 32.

85. A. Press, "Bor'ba s tabachnoiu raspushchennost'iu," *GiZRS*, no. 3 (1925): 2–4.

86. I. V. Sazhin, "Pochemu nado brosit' kurit'?" *GiZRiKS*, no. 1 (1928): 5.

87. Violin, *Tabak i ego vred*, 5–6.

88. Sholomovich, *Detskii pokhod na vzroslykh*, 10.

89. Boginskii, *Tabak i ego kurenie*, 8.

90. Lukashevich, *Nevinnaia privychka*, 20–26; Sazhin, "Pochemu nado brosit' kurit'?," 5.

91. N. A. Semashko, "Rabochaia zhizn'," *Pravda*, May 26, 1921, 2.

92. Lukashevich, *Nevinnaia privychka*, 27–29; Berman, *O stol' tsenimom tabake*, 4–5; Nezlin, *O vrede*, 41–42; Sazhin, *Pravda o kurenii*, 21–23; Rossiiskii, "O nikotinizme," 10.

93. Starks, *Body Soviet*, 183–87; Zolotnitskii, *O vrede*, 14–15.

94. Nezlin, *O vrede*, 26.

95. Popov, *Vred tabakokureniie*, 16.

96. Nechaev, *Tabak i ego vliianie*, 4–8, 20–21.

97. Varushkin, *Pochemu vreden tabak*, 11–12.

98. Varushkin, *Pochemu vreden tabak*, 22; Nezlin, *O vrede*, 49; "Pervaia obraztsovaia tipografiia," *Izvestiia*, September 24, 1924, 5; "Rol' Komsomola v podniatii proizvoditel'nosti truda," *Izvestiia*, October 15, 1924, 5.

99. Iu. Ostrovskii, "Kak mozhno dostignut' ekonomii," *Pravda*, July 2, 1926, 5; V. Zhuravlev, "Bol'she vnimaniia bor'be s progulami!," *Pravda*, April 7, 1927, 5.

100. "Iz zhizni izcheiki N.O.T.," *V akademii i shkole* 2, no. 17 (1923), quoted in A. Gastev, *Iunost' idi!* (Moscow: VTsSPS, 1923), 61.

101. Nezlin, *O vrede*, 1–4, 7, 54.

102. Starks, *Smoking under the Tsars*, 164, 192, 221–22.

103. Lukashevich, *Nevinnaia privychka*, 29; Varushkin, *Pochemu vreden tabak*, 18.

104. Nezlin, *O vrede*, 4–5.

105. Berman, *O stol' tsenimom tabake*, 14.

106. "Pozharnaia okhrana vystavki," *Izvestiia*, August 11, 1923, 3; "Pozhar na putinskikh neftepromyslakh," *Pravda*, June 10, 1927, 4; "Pozharnaia okhrana fabrik i zavodov," *Izvestiia*, July 15, 1927, 3; "Finansovoe izdatel'stvo NKF SSSR," *Izvestiia*, June 28, 1928, 4; D. Shvartsman, "Snizhenie sebestoimosti i voprosy trudovoi distsipliny," *Izvestiia*, February 19, 1929, 2.

107. L. M. Vasilevskii, *Gigiena propagandista (agitatora, lektora, prepodavatelia)* (Moscow: Molodaia gvardiia, 1924), 21–22.

108. Nezlin, *O vrede*, 20.

109. Sazhin, *Pravda o kurenii*, 11.

110. Trotsky, "Attention to Trifles!," 74–75.

111. *Krasnaia gazeta*, December 17, 1920, 3, as referenced in Julie Hessler, *A Social History of Soviet Trade: Trade Policy, Retail Practices, and Consumption, 1917–1953* (Princeton, NJ: Princeton University Press, 2004), 64.

112. *Trud* (1928), as referenced in William J. Chase, *Workers, Society, and the Soviet State: Labor and Life in Moscow, 1918–1929* (Urbana: University of Illinois Press, 1987), 191.

113. Viaznikov, "Vygovor nekul'turnomy," *Krokodil*, no. 30 (1929): 4.

114. Tsentral'nyi arkhiv obshchestvennykh dvizhenii Moskvy (TsAODM) f. 634, op. 1, d. 15 l, 142.

115. Lukashevich, *Nevinnaia privychka*, 34–35.

116. Nezlin, *O vrede*, 48.

117. Popov, *Vred tabakokureniia*, 21; Nezlin, *O vrede*, 25; "Issledovaniia i otkrytiia: Preduprezhdenie raka iazyka," *GiZRiKS*, no. 24 (1928): 16; Rossiiskii, *O tabake*, 13–14.

118. GARF f. A-482, op. 1, d. 562, ll. 299–302.

119. The listing of titles from the press would put this in the late 1920s (N. N. Petrov, *Chto nado znat' o rake* [Leningrad: Leningradskaia pravda, n.d.], 15).

120. Nezlin, *O vrede*, 8–15.

121. Violin, *Tabak i ego vred*, 9.

122. A. Polianskii, ed., *Deistvie tabachnago dyma na zhivotnykh i cheloveka (Stoit'-li kurit? Kak rekomenduetsia kurit'?)* (Novo-Nikolaevsk: Soiuz-Bank, 1919), 1, 3–12; Rossiiskii, "O nikotinizme," 8; Sazhin, *Pravda o kurenii*, 5–10.

123. Nezlin, *O vrede*, 24; Sazhin, *Pravda o kurenii*, 13–14; Rossiiskii, "O nikotinizme," 9.

124. Krementsov, *Revolutionary Experiments*, 130, 157.

125. A. G. Kagan, *Rabochaia molodezh' na otdykhe* (Leningrad: Priboi, n.d), 8.

126. N. A. Semashko, *Sotsial'nye bolezni i bor'ba s nimi* (Moscow: Voprosy truda, 1925), 13.

127. N. Semashko, "Molodezh' i zdorovyi byt," *Pravda*, September 8, 1927, 5.

128. Boginskii, *Tabak i ego kurenie*, 8.

129. Sigal, *Vrednaia privychka*, 9.

130. Rossiiskii, "O nikotinizme," 9.

131. Sazhin, *Pravda o kurenii*, 12.

132. Polianskii, *Deistvie tabachnago dyma*, 10.

133. Nezlin, *O vrede*, 23–24.

134. Sazhin, *Pravda o kurenii*, 12.

135. V. Belousov, "Okhrana truda: Kurenie tabaka v svete okhrany truda," *GiZRS*, no. 4 (1923): 7.

136. Nechaev, *Tabak i ego vliianie*, 5.

137. Zolotnitskii, *O vrede*, 9.

138. Bernstein, *Dictatorship of Sex*, 62, 84. Healey, *Homosexual Desire*, 70, 84, 86, 90, 104–7; Olga Matich, *Erotic Utopia: The Decadent Imagination in Russia's Fin de Siècle* (Madison: University of Wisconsin Press, 2005), 83, 232, 246–55; Zolotnitskii, *O vrede*, 13.

139. Zolotnitskii, *O vrede*, 13; Nezlin, *O vrede*, 25.

140. Violin, *Tabak i ego vred*, 16.

141. Rossiiskii, "O nikotinizme," 9. Violin presented the same anecdote from a Professor Sherbak (*Tabak i ego vred*, 15).

142. Shostak, *Kurevo*, 11.

143. L. Tagir, "Otravlenie zritel'nykh nervov alkogolem i tabakom," *GiZRiKS*, no. 14 (1927): 5.

144. Nezlin, *O vrede*, 18–20; See also Sazhin, *Pravda o kurenii*, 10–11; and Popov, *Vred tabakokureniia*, 14.

145. Varushkin, *Pochemu vreden tabak*, 8.

146. Laura Goering, "'Russian Nervousness': Neurasthenia and National Identity in Nineteenth-Century Russia," *Medical History* 47, no. 1 (2003): 24–25.

147. Susan K. Morrissey, "The Economy of Nerves: Health, Commercial Culture, and the Self in Late Imperial Russia," *Slavic Review* 69, no. 3 (2010): 645–49.

148. Nikolai Krementsov, *A Martian Stranded on Earth: Alexander Bogdanov, Blood Transfusions, and Proletarian Science* (Chicago: University of Chicago Press, 2011), 61–68.

149. Irina Sirotkina, *Diagnosing Literary Genius: A Cultural History of Psychiatry in Russia, 1880–1930* (Baltimore: Johns Hopkins University Press, 2002), 97.

150. Goering, "Russian Nervousness," 26.

151. Morrissey, "Economy of Nerves," 649.

152. Uporov, *Tabak*, 12.

153. As referenced in Shostak, *Kurevo*, 6.

154. Sazhin, *Pravda o kurenii*, 16.

155. Violin, *Tabak i ego vred*, 12.

156. Bliumenau, *Okhmeliaiushchie durmany*, 9.

157. Zolotnitskii, *O vrede*, 19.

158. Goering, "Russian Nervousness," 30; Eliot Borenstein, *Men without Women: Masculinity and Revolution in Russian Fiction, 1917–1929* (Durham, NC: Duke University Press, 2000), 4.

159. "Eshche o vrede tabaka," *GiZRiKS*, no. 9 (1927): 5.

160. Sazhin, *Pravda o kurenii*, 8.

161. "Issledovaniia i otkrytiia: Nikotin i polovye zhelezy," *GiZRiKS*, no. 17 (1927): 15–16.

162. Berman, *O stol' tsenimom tabake*, 11–12; Nezlin, *O vrede*, 34–35; Violin, *Tabak i ego vred*, 12.

163. "Prichiny prezhdevremennoi starosti zhenshchiny," *GiZRS*, no. 22 (1927): 2–4.

164. Popov, *Vred tabakokureniia*, 17; Nezlin, *O vrede*, 34–36.

165. Popov, *Vred tabakokureniia*, 17; Sazhin, *Pravda o kurenii*, 19–20.

166. L. M. Vasilevskii, *Gigiena molodoi devushki* (Moscow: Novaia Moskva, 1926), 31–32.

167. Goering, "Russian Nervousness," 30.

168. Shostak, *Kurevo*, 6; Popov, *Vred tabakokureniia*, 16.

169. Zolotnitskii, *O vrede*, 16–17.

170. "Izuchenie byta detskoi prostitutsii," *ZNB*, no. 8–9 (1925): 13–14; "Vopiiushchie bezobraziia v institute sotsial'no-individual'nogo vospitaniia," *Izvestiia*, June 30, 1928, 4; Catriona Kelly, *Children's World: Growing up in Russia, 1890–1991* (New Haven: Yale University Press, 2007), 434–35.

171. Mikhail Kol'tsov, "Deti smeiutsia," *Pravda*, May 1, 1927, 3.

172. "Krasnyi Petrograd: Bor'ba s kureniem," *Izvestiia*, June 19, 1920, 2.

173. Nezlin, *O vrede*, 37.

174. Sazhin, *Pravda o kurenii*, 20; Violin quoted from prerevolutionary studies by Mendel'son (*Tabak i ego vred*, 11); Starks, *Smoking under the Tsars*, 162–200.

175. Sazhin, *Pravda o kurenii*, 20–21.

176. L. M. Basserman, ed., *Trud, zdorov'e, byt Leningradskoi rabochei molodezhi*, vol. 1: *Rabochie podrostki i shkoly fabzavucha (po dannym obsledovanii 1923–24 gg.)* (Leningrad: Izdatel'stvo Sanprosveta Leningradskogo gubzdravotdela, 1925), 20.

177. Varushkin, *Pochumu vreden tabak*, 20.

2. RESURRECTED

1. V. I. Lenin, "Razvitie kapitalizma v Rossii," in *Polnoe sobranie sochinenii* (Moscow: Gosizdat, 1958), 3:543.

2. I. Stal'skii, ed., *Donskaia gosudarstvennaia tabachnaia fabrika: Ocherk po materialam starykh kadrovikov DGTF A. K. Vasil'eva, E. I. Riabininoi, O. P. Ogarenko, i V. I. Shcherbakava* (Rostov-on-Don: Gosizdat, 1938), 3–4; Worker memoir from Dobrynin

in GARF f. R-5667, op. 10, d. 83, l. 2; K. Markovich, *Otchet: Po sboru papiros, tabaku i kuritel'nykh prinadlezhnostei, proizvedennomu v g. Rostove n/D. i po nekotorym stantsiiam Vladinavnazskoi zheleznoi dorog* (Rostov-on-Don: S. P. Iakovlev, 1904), 6.

3. V. G. Novikova and N. N. Shchemelev, *Nasha marka: Ocherki istorii Donskoi gosudarstvennoi tabachnoi fabriki* (Rostov-on-Don: Rostovskoi knizhnoe izdatel'stvo, 1968), 89–90.

4. Diane Koenker, William G. Rosenberg, and Ronald Grigor Suny, eds., *Party, State, and Society in the Russian Civil War: Explorations in Social History* (Bloomington: Indiana University Press, 1989); Timothy J. Colton, *Moscow: Governing the Socialist Metropolis* (Cambridge, MA: Harvard University Press, 1996), 71–151; Mauricio Borrero, *Hungry Moscow: Scarcity and Urban Society in the Russian Civil War, 1917–1921* (New York: Peter Lang, 2003); Starks, *Body Soviet*, 14–16.

5. William G. Rosenberg, "Introduction: NEP Russia as a 'Transitional' Society," in *Russia in the Era of NEP: Explorations in Soviet Society and Culture*, ed. Sheila Fitzpatrick, Alexander Rabinowitch, and Richard Stites (Bloomington: Indiana University Press, 1991), 1.

6. Lewis H. Siegelbaum, *Soviet State and Society between Revolutions, 1918–1929* (New York: Cambridge University Press, 1992).

7. Novikova and Shchemelev, *Nasha marka*, 90–95, 101–3, 107–8, 109–11; Stal'skii, *Donskaia gosudarstvennaia tabachnaia fabrika*, 20.

8. Novikova and Shchemelev, *Nasha marka*, 90–95, 106, 109–16.

9. Lifshits, *Doloi kurenie i p'ianstvo*, 39.

10. Romaniello, "Muscovy's Extraordinary Ban," 9–25.

11. *Kratkii ocherk tabakokureniia v Rossii, v minuvshev 19-m stoletii: Za period vremeni s 1810 po 1906 god* (Kiev: Petr Varskii, 1906); "Tabak," in *Entsiklopedicheskii slovar'*, ed. F. A. Brokgauz and I. A. Efron (St. Petersburg: I. A. Efron, 1901), 32:431–33.

12. M. V. Dzhervis, *Russkaia tabachnaia fabrika v XVIII i XIX vekakh* (Leningrad: Akademiia nauk SSSR, 1933), 16.

13. A. A. Arakelov, "Monopolizatsiia tabachnoi promyshlennosti Rossii," *Voprosy istorii*, no. 9 (1981): 18.

14. William Augustine Brennan, *Tobacco Leaves: Being a Book of Facts for Smokers* (Menasha, WI: Index Office, 1915), 32–33.

15. V. I. Korno and M. I. Kitainer, *Balkanskaia zvezda: Stranitsy istorii* (Iaroslavl: Niuans, 2000), 3; N. I. Umnova, "Tabachnaia promyshlennost' za 15 let (s. 1890–1904)," in *Sbornik statei i materialov po tabachnomu delu*, ed. S. A. Egiz (Peterburg: V. F. Kirshbaum, 1913), 140.

16. Bogdanov, *Dym otechestva*, 80.

17. Boginskii, *Tabak i ego kurenie*, 3.

18. Isaac Babel, "Tobacco," in *The Complete Works of Isaac Babel*, ed. Nathalie Babel (New York: W. W. Norton, 2002), 263–66.

19. Anatolii Kaplan, "Kak spast' tabachnuiu promyshlennost'," *Pravda*, July 18, 1918, 4; "Sostoianie tabachnoi promyshlennosti," *Pravda*, August 14, 1918, 4; "Tabak," *Pravda*, August 28, 1918, 3.

20. "Tabachnaia monopoliia," *Pravda*, November 24, 1918, 3; N. Sharov, "Nasha tabachnaia promyshlennost'," *Rabotnitsa*, no. 10 (1923): 15–16.

21. "K vosstanovleniiu promyshlennosti: Tabachnaia promyshlennost'," *Pravda*, May 19, 1921, 2.

22. Sharov, "Nasha tabachnaia promyshlennost'," 15–16.

23. S. Narkir'er, "Tabachnaia promyshlennost' i snabzhenie naseleniia tabachnymi izdeliami v gody revoliutsii," *Vestnik tabachnoi promyshlennosti*, no. 1 (1922): 19–30.

24. Sharov, "Nasha tabachnaia promyshlennost'," 15–16.

25. Iu. P. Bokarev, "Tobacco Production in Russia: The Transition to Communism," in *Tobacco in Russian History and Culture from the Seventeenth Century to the Present*, 151.

26. "Tabachnaia promyshlennost," *Izvestiia*, March 20, 1918, 1.

27. V. Boiadzhi, "Eksport tabaka i sostoianie tabachnoi promyshlennosti," *Pamiatka tabakovoda*, no. 3 (1923): n.p.

28. Bogdanov, *Dym otechestva*, 196–97.

29. "Zakrytie tabachnykh fabrik," *Pravda*, November 5, 1918, 4.

30. "Ostanovka tabachnykh fabrik," *Pravda*, April 14, 1918, 2.

31. Bokarev, "Tobacco Production in Russia," 151.

32. Kafengauz, *Evoliutsiia promyshlennogo proizvodstva Rossii*, 156, 198, 265.

33. GARF f. R-5558, op. 4, d. 44, ll. 1–13, quotation l. 13.

34. Bokarev, "Tobacco Production in Russia," 151.

35. S. Narkir'er, *Proizvodstvo tabachnykh fabrik RSFSR v 1919 godu (v tsifrakh): Po materialam Statisticheskogo otdela Glavnogo upravleniia gosudarstvennoi tabachnoi promyshlennosti* (Moscow: Vysshii sovet narodnogo khoziastva, 1921), 12.

36. Korno and Kitainer, *Balkanskaia zvezda*, 134.

37. Korno and Kitainer, *Balkanskaia zvezda*, 114–16.

38. "Chislo kuriashchikh v Moskve," *Pravda*, November 12, 1918, 4. Colton gives the Moscow population as 1,716,000 in April 1918 and 1,316,000 in September 1919 (*Moscow*, 124).

39. S. Egiz, "Polozhenie tabakovodstva v Sovetskoi Rossii," *Vestnik tabachnoi promyshlennosti*, no. 1 (1922): 4.

40. Egiz, "Polozhenie," 9.

41. Dr. Rokau, *Interesnaia i liubopytnaia istoriia kurivshikh, niuchavshikh i zhevashikh tabak: S legendarnym pravdivym skazaniem o ego pagubnom vliianii na zdorovy cheloveka* (Moscow: Tipografiia byvshei A. V. Kudriavtsevoi, 1885–1886), 3; Goodman, *Tobacco in History*, 4.

42. Benedict, *Golden-Silk Smoke*, 11.

43. Narkir'er, "Tabachnaia promyshlennost," 21.

44. Narkir'er, "Tabachnaia promyshlennost," 24.

45. Courtwright, *Forces of Habit*, 141.

46. Aaron Retish, *Russia's Peasants in Revolution and Civil War: Citizenship, Identity, and the Creation of the Soviet State, 1914–1922* (Cambridge: Cambridge University Press, 2008), 27.

47. Retish, *Russia's Peasants*, 118.

48. Zosa Szajkowski Collection, Box 1, Folder "Fliers and Open Letters," Bakhmeteff Archive of Russian and East European Culture, Rare Book and Manuscript Library, Columbia University Libraries. Thank you to Faith Hillis for bringing these materials to my attention and to Vladimir Davidenko for obtaining images of them. See Brendan McGeever, *Antisemitism and the Russian Revolution* (Cambridge: Cambridge University Press, 2019), 19–37, 140–82.

49. Herlihy, *Alcoholic Empire*, 146–51; Transchel, *Under the Influence*, 69–75; Narkir'er, "Tabachnaia promyshlennost," 19–30.

50. Narkir'er, "Tabachnaia promyshlennost," 19–30.

51. Narkir'er, "Tabachnaia promyshlennost," 19–30.

52. Boginskii, *Tabak i ego kurenie*, 4.

53. "Tabachnye kartochki," *Pravda*, November 22, 1918, 3; "Tabachnye kartochki," January 16, 1919, 3; "Makhorka," *Pravda*, June 11, 1919, 2; "K prodazhe tabaku i papiros," *Pravda*, August 5, 1919, 2; Reed, *Ten Days*, 12.

54. "Prodovol'stvennoe delo: Poluchenie tabaku i spichek," *Izvestiia*, November 19, 1918, 4.

55. Iu. Larin, "Snabzhenie Rossii v 1919-m godu," *Pravda*, February 1, 1919, 1.

56. "Voprosy prodovol'stviia," *Pravda*, July 15, 1920, 2; "Voprosy prodovol'stviia," *Pravda*, July 21, 1920, 2; "Voprosy prodovol'stviia," *Pravda*, July 30, 1920, 2.

57. *Krasnaia Moskva* (Moscow: Izd. Moskovskogo soveta RKiKrD, n.d.), 320–23.

58. "Na makhorke," *Pravda*, August 6, 1924, 3; S. Narkir'er, "Ocherki po ekonomike tabachnogo proizvodstva," *Vestnik tabachnoi promyshlennosti*, no. 3 (1923): 26–33; "Na papirosy," *Pravda*, August 22, 1924.

59. Alan Ball, "Private Trade and Traders during NEP," in *Russia in the Era of NEP*, 94–95.

60. "Zaderzhanie spekuliantor," *Izvestiia*, August 9, 1918.

61. Hessler, *Social History*, 26–37.

62. See, for example, "Melochi zhizni," *Pravda*, November 30, 1918, 3.

63. Hessler, *Social History*, 10, 68.

64. Bogdanov, *Dym otechestva*, 197–98.

65. Hessler, *Social History*, 40.

66. Sergei V. Iarov, "Workers," in *Critical Companion to the Russian Revolution, 1914–1921*, ed. Edward Acton, Vladimir Iu. Cherniaev, and William G. Rosenberg (Bloomington: Indiana University Press, 1997), 604–17.

67. Mat', "Posobie dlia kuriashchikh mladentsev," *Krokodil*, no. 14 (1924): 14.

68. Rosenberg, "Introduction," 5–6.

69. Rosenberg, "Introduction," 5.

70. Pav. Abaimov, "Kak prigotovit' khoroshii kuritel'nyi tabak," *Kooperativnoe delo*, no. 6 (1922): 17–18.

71. S. V. Kifuriak, *Tabachnaia fabrika "Iava"* (Moscow: Pishchevaia promyshlennost', 1978), 33.

72. Korno and Kitainer, *Balkanskaia zvezda*, 119.

73. "Organizatsiia tabachnoi promyshlennosti v SSSR," in *Tabachnaia promyshlennost'*, ed. S. A. Gol'dshtein (Moscow: RIO TsK VSRPVP, 1929), 6:71.

74. Narkir'er, *Proizvodstvo tabachnykh fabrik RSFSR*, 5, 8; Demin gives the Sovnarkom decree as June 28, 1918 (*Rossiia*, 46).

75. N. Sharov, "K voprosu o chastnykh predpriiatiiakh tabachnoi promyshlennosti v SSSR," *Vestnik tabachnoi promyshlennosti*, no. 9–10 (1923): 2–5.

76. Bokarev, "Tobacco Production," 152.

77. Korno and Kitainer, *Balkanskaia zvezda*, 126–30.

78. Sharov, "Nasha tabachnaia promyshlennost'," 15–16.

79. Kifuriak, *Tabachnaia fabrika "Iava,"* 16; A. A., "Po fabrikam i zavodam," *Izvestiia*, December 17, 1921, 4.

80. Kifuriak, *Tabachnaia fabrika "Iava,"* 33.

81. Rosenberg, "Introduction," 6.

82. Sharov. "Nasha tabachnaia promyshlennost'," 15–16.

83. GARF f. R-6889, op. 1, d. 434, ll. 1–9.

84. Sharov, "Nasha tabachnaia promyshlennost'," 15–16.

85. Kifuriak, *Tabachnaia fabrika "Iava,"* 25.

86. "Ispytaniia pervoi sovetskoi papirosno-nabivnoi mashiny," *Pravda*, June 10, 1927, 4.

87. "Khronika," *Pravda*, March 6, 1926, 5; Malinin, *Tabachnaia istoriia Rossii*, 155.

88. Bokarev, "Tobacco Production in Russia," 152.

89. D. Sokolovskii, "K voprosu o emkosti vsesoiuznogo i ukrainskogo tabachnykh rynkov v sviazi s piatiletnim planom razvertyvaniia promyshlennosti," in *Tabachnaia promyshlennost' i tabakovodstvo*, ed. Ia. M. Gol'bert (Moscow: Mospoligraf, 1926), 2–10.

90. Hessler, *Social History*, 81, 104.

91. "Tabak v Rossii," subsection of "Tabak" in *Entsiklopedicheskii slovar'*, 32:428–36.

92. Dzhervis, *Russkaia tabachnaia fabrika*, 12.

93. Osipov, "Tabak v Rossii," 429.

94. E. S. Krymskii, *Vred dlia zdorov'ia ot kureniia i niukhaniia tabaku i sredstva peres-tat' kurit'* (Evenigorodka: E. S. Krymskii, 1889), 4; N. P. Pomerantsev, *O tabake i vrede ego kureniia* (Moscow: M. M. Tarchigin, 1908), 2.

95. Gregory Y. Sokolnikov, *Soviet Policy in Public Finance, 1917–1928* (Stanford, CA: Stanford University Press, 1931), 50.

96. Transchel, *Under the Influence*, 32.

97. Sokolnikov, *Soviet Policy in Public Finance*, 23.

98. See, for example, the Sovnarkom decree of 1921 taxing cartridges and tobacco: "Dekret: Soveta narodnykh komissarov ob aktsize s tabachnykh i gil'zovykh izdelii," *Sbornik dekretov, postanovlenii, instruktsii, Sovnarkoma, VTsIKa i dr. organov pravitel'stvennoi vlasti, noiabr'–dekabr', 1921* (Novo-Nikolaevsk: Sibirskii otdeleniia Tsentrosoiuza, 1921), 27–28.

99. "Tabachnaia promyshlennost'," *Izvestiia*, March 20, 1918, 1.

100. Demin, *Rossiia*, 46.

101. Neil Weissman, "Prohibition and Alcohol Control in the USSR: The 1920s Campaign against Illegal Spirits," *Soviet Studies* 38, no. 3 (1986): 354–55.

102. Weissman, "Prohibition and Alcohol Control," 355–58.

103. GARF f. R-5446, op. 7, d. 1069, ll. 1–8.

104. Sokolovskii, "K voprosu," 2–10.

105. Evsei Kogan, "Sovetskii eksport listovogo tabaka," in *Sbornik materialov po tabachnoi promyshlennosti*, ed. A. A. Rozhnov (Moscow: Gosudarstvennoe tekhnicheskoe izdatel'stvo, 1930), 300.

106. "K voprosu o vyvoze tabachnogo syr'ia za granitsu," *Vestnik tabachnoi promyshlen-nosti*, no. 4 (1923): 1.

107. Boiadzhi, "Eksport tabaka," n.p.

108. Malinin, *Tabachnaia istoriia Rossii*, 134.

109. "Dukat," *Izvestiia*, February 14, 1923, 2; M. D. Stepanov, "O gosudarstvennoi i chastnoi tabachnoi promyshlennosti," in *Vestnik tabachnoi promyshlennosti*, no. 5–6 (1923): 2–8; "Sovetskii sud," *Izvestiia*, March 16, 1925, 4.

110. Lukashevich, *Nevinnaia privychka*, 5.

111. Wicksteed, *Life under the Soviets*, 15.

112. Malinin, *Tabachnaia istoriia Rossii*, 132.

113. Malinin, *Tabachnaia istoriia Rossii*, 132.

114. Wicksteed, *Life under the Soviets*, 16.

115. Régine Robin, "Popular Literature in the 1920s: Peasants as Readers," in *Russia in the Era of NEP*, 256.

116. Orlando Figes, "The Peasantry," in *Critical Companion to the Russian Revolution*, 549; V. I. Lenin, "The Work of the People's Commissariat for Education," *Pravda*, February 9, 1921, 1, repr. in his *Collected Works* (Moscow: Progress Publishers, 1960–1970), 29:436–53.

117. K. Romov, "Poleznoe primenenie knigi," *Krokodil*, no. 12 (1924): 16.

118. "Chetyre vida smychki s derevnei," *Krokodil*, no. 10 (1924): 16.

119. The paper attacked was *Krasnyi luch*. "O pol'ze kureniia tabaka," *Krokodil*, no. 31 (1926): 10.

120. D. Dolev, "Lit-kuril'shchik," *Krokodil*, no. 17 (1924): 10.

121. Bogdanov, *Dym otechestva*, 201.

122. Malinin, *Tabachnaia istoriia Rossii*, 135.

123. Kafengauz, *Evoliutsiia promyshlennogo proizvodstva Rossii*, 265.

124. P. Nikitin, "Shto pokazano obsledovanie Lentabaktresta," *Pravda*, August 4, 1926, 6.

125. "Delo tabak," *Krokodil*, no. 10 (1924): 14.

126. Al. Alevich., "Delo—tabak!," *Izvestiia*, January 30, 1926, 3.

127. "Bor'ba za kachestva papiros," *Izvestiia*, February 13, 1926, 4.

128. D. Chk-ai, "Vot vam i etiketki," *Pravda*, September 7, 1926, 6; "Papirosnoe klad-bishche," *Pravda*, September 25, 1926, 5; G—, "Za poriadok i ekonomiiu: Vnimanie melo-cham," *Pravda*, April 18, 1926, 6.

129. Malinin, *Tabachnaia istoriia Rossii*, 141–43; "Ratsionalizatsiia proizvodstva," *Pravda*, May 31, 1927, 5.

130. Stal'skii, *Donskaia gosudarstvennaia tabachnaia fabrika*, 24.

131. Korno and Kitainer, *Balkanskaia zvezda*, 134.

132. Kifuriak, *Tabachnaia fabrika "Iava,"* 16, 33.

133. Brokgauz and Efron, *Entsiklopedicheskii slovar'*, 32:422; Umnova, "Tabachnaia promyshlennost'," 129–31; Dzhervis, *Russkaia tabachnaia fabrika*, 100.

134. Starks, *Smoking under the Tsars*, 55–101.

135. "Chislennost' i sostav rabochei sily, zaniatoi v tabachnom proizvodstve," in *Tabachnaia promyshlennost'*, 6:69.

136. Victoria Bonnell, "Introduction," in *The Russian Worker: Life and Labor under the Tsarist Regime*, ed. Victoria Bonnell (Berkeley: University of California Press, 1983); Wood, *Baba and the Comrade*, 44.

137. Narkir'er, *Proizvodstvo tabachnykh fabrik RSFSR*, 9, 12; N. D. Rozenbaum, *Tabach-noe proizvodstvo: Sanitarno-gigienicheskie ocherki* (Moscow: Voprosy truda, 1924), 11.

138. "V soiuze rabochikh tabachnogo, gil'zovogo i makhorochnogo proizvodstva," *Pravda*, July 23, 1919, 2.

139. GARF f. R-6889, op. 1, d. 434, l. 1.

140. Emma Goldman, *My Disillusionment in Russia* (Mineola, NY: Dover Publications, 1923), 56–57.

141. Belousov, *Izuchenie truda*, 5, 12, 55.

142. "Professional'nye vrednosti tabachnogo proizvodstva," in *Tabachnaia promyshlen-nost'*, 6:64; Shostak, *Kurevo*, 7–9; Violin, *Tabak i ego vred*, 10; Belousov, *Izuchenie truda*, 61–66; Dr. N. Rozenbaum, "Otravliaiutsia li rabochie tabachnykh fabrik nikotinom?," *Vestnik tabachnoi promyshlennosti*, no. 4 (1923): 50–55.

143. "Khronika," *Voprosy narkologii*, no. 1 (1926): 87–94; Rozenbaum, *Tabachnoe proiz-vodstvo*, 34–35, 49–60, 67.

144. "Issledovaniia i otkrytiia: Deistvie tabachnoi pyli," *GiZRS*, no. 2 (1924): 15; "Issle-dovaniia i otkrytiia: Deistvie tabachnoi pyli na desna," *GiZRS*, no. 10 (1924): 15; Starks, *Smoking under the Tsars*, 73–74; Starks, *Body Soviet*, 105–6.

145. Berman, *O stol' tsenimom tabake*, 4–5.

146. "Telegramma komanduiushchego voiskami Petrogradskogo voennogo okruga Avrora predsedateliu revvoensoveta Trotskomu," in *Kronshtadt 1921*, ed. V. P. Naumov and A. A. Kosakovskii (Moscow: Fond "Demokratiia," 1997), no. 6: 49, 194–201. See also Vladimir N. Brovkin, *Behind the Front Lines of the Civil War: Political Parties and Social Movements in Russia, 1918–1922* (Princeton, NJ: Princeton Legacy Library, 1994), 392.

147. Vladimir N. Brovkin, *The Mensheviks after October: Socialist Opposition and the Rise of the Bolshevik Dictatorship* (Ithaca, NY: Cornell University Press, 1991), 243; Ronald I. Kowalski, *The Russian Revolution, 1917–1921* (London: Routledge, 1997), 219.

148. "Iz operativno-shifroval'noi svodki sekretno-operativnogo upravleniia VChK Leninu i Stalinu," in *Kronshtadt 1921*, no. 24: 91.

149. John B. Hatch, "Labor Conflict in Moscow, 1921–1925," in *Russia in the Era of NEP*, 64–67.

150. Wood, *Baba and the Comrade*, 153.

151. Narkir'er, *Proizvodstvo tabachnykh fabrik RSFSR*, 9; Rozenbaum, *Tabachnaia proizvodstvo*, 11; "Chislennost' i sostav rabochei sily," 69–70.

152. "Chislennost' i sostav rabochei sily," 69–70.

153. "Zarobotnaia plata v tabachoi promyshlennosti," in *Tabachnaia promyshlennost'*, 6:70.

154. "Zarobotnaia plata," 70–71.

155. Wendy Z. Goldman, *Women at the Gates: Gender and Industry in Stalin's Russia* (Cambridge: Cambridge University Press, 2002), 17.

156. Wood, *Baba and the Comrade*, 123–26.

157. A. A. Nosova, "38 let raboty na fabrike," *Tabak*, no. 1 (1953): 17.

158. "Rabotnitsa u stanka," *Pravda*, March 6, 1926, 5.

159. Kal't, "Nasha fabrika—nasha gordost'" *Pravda*, November 29, 1924, 3.

160. A. Shumskii, "U tabachnits," *Rabotnitsa*, no. 1 (1927): 16.

161. Kifuriak, *Tabachnaia fabrika "Iava,"* 33.

162. Stal'skii, *Donskaia gosudarstvennaia tabachnaia fabrika*, 23.

163. A. I. Levin, "Obespylivanie vrednykh tsekhov tabachnoi fabriki," in *Tabachnaia promyshlennost' i tabakovodstvo*, 46.

164. Levin, "Obespylivanie vrednykh tsekhov," 46, 46–52.

165. Starks, *Smoking under the Tsars*, 55–101.

166. Kifuriak, *Tabachnaia fabrika "Iava,"* 33–35.

167. Shumskii, "U tabachnits," 16.

168. Sokolovskii, "K voprosu," 2–10.

3. SOLD

1. Richard Stites, *Revolutionary Dreams: Utopian Visions and Experimental Life in the Russian Revolution* (New York: Oxford University Press, 1988), 85.

2. Karen Petrone, *The Great War in Russian Memory* (Bloomington: Indiana University Press, 2011), 5.

3. Randi Cox, "'NEP without Nepmen!': Soviet Advertising the Transition to Socialism," in *Everyday Life in Early Soviet Russia: Taking the Revolution Inside*, ed. Christina Kiaer and Eric Naiman (Bloomington: Indiana University Press, 2006), 119–22.

4. Randi Barnes Cox, "The Creation of the Socialist Consumer: Advertising, Citizenship, and NEP" (PhD diss., Indiana University, 1999), 274.

5. Cox, "Creation of the Socialist Consumer," 10–11, 16–17, 19–25; Cox, "'NEP without Nepmen!,'" 122–24.

6. Aleksandr Snopkov, Pavel Snopkov, and Aleksandr Shkliaruk, eds., *Reklama v plakate: Russkii torgovo-promyshlennyi plakat za 100 let (Advertising Art in Russia)* (Moscow: Kontakt-kul'tura, 2007), 93.

7. Cox, "Creation of the Socialist Consumer," 10–11, 16–17, 19–25, 40.

8. Cox, "Creation of the Socialist Consumer," 10–11, 16–17, 19–22, 135–36.

9. Amy E. Randall, *The Soviet Dream World of Retail Trade and Consumption in the 1930s* (New York: Palgrave, 2008), 2–8; Cox, "'NEP without Nepmen!,'" 128–29.

10. Naiman, *Sex in Public*, 5–24; David L. Hoffmann, *Cultivating the Masses: Modern State Practices and Soviet Socialism, 1914–1939* (Ithaca, NY: Cornell University Press, 2011), 200–202.

11. Bernstein, *Dictatorship of Sex*; Naiman, *Sex in Public*, 181–207; Wood, *Baba and the Comrade*, 201–7; Starks, *Body Soviet*, 12–36.

12. Cox, "Creation of the Socialist Consumer," 33–36. See, for example, "Vnimanie," *Izvestiia* July 15, 1922, 4; and "Krytorgsiab," *Izvestiia*, July 15, 1922, 4.

13. "Krymtabaktrest," *Izvestiia*, November 27, 1923, 9.

14. Relli Shechter, "Reading Advertisements in a Colonial/Development Context: Cigarette Advertising and Identity Politics in Egypt, c. 1919–1939," *Journal of Social History* 39, no. 2 (2005): 483–503.

15. Snopkov, Snopkov, and Shkliaruk, *Reklama v plakate*, 93.

16. Cox, "Creation of the Socialist Consumer," 242–50; Cox, "'NEP without Nep-men!,'" 131–51; O. I. Budanova, "Problema tabakokureniia v otechestvennom plakate: Ot reklamy tabaka do antitabachnoi propagandy," in *Rumiantsevskie chteniia—2015*, ed. E. A. Ivanova (Moscow: Pashkov dom, 2015), 35–38.

17. Cox, "Creation of the Socialist Consumer," 5.

18. S. Vysheslavtseva, "Reklama i lozung-plakat Maiakovskogo," *Literaturnaia gazeta*, no. 15 (1937): 3.

19. Snopkov, Snopkov, and Shkliaruk, *Reklama v plakate*, 93.

20. Mollie Arbuthnot, "The People and the Poster: Theorizing the Soviet Viewer, 1920–1931," *Slavic Review* 78, no. 3 (2019): 728.

21. Cox, "Creation of the Socialist Consumer," 40–42.

22. Wicksteed, *Life under the Soviets*, 15.

23. David Howes, "HYPERESTHESIA, or, The Sensual Logic of Late Capitalism," in *Empire of the Senses: The Sensual Culture Reader*, ed. David Howes (London: Bloomsbury Academic, 2005), 284–92.

24. Miller, *Stuff*, 23–31.

25. Sebelius, *How Tobacco Smoke Causes Disease*, 181; J. E. Rose, "Multiple Brain Pathways and Receptors underlying Tobacco Addiction," *Biochemical Pharmacology* 74, no. 8 (2007): 1263–70; K. Fagerstrom, "Determinants of Tobacco Use and Renaming the FTND to the Fagerstrom Test for Cigarette Dependence," *Nicotine Tobacco Research* 14, no. 1 (2012): 75–78.

26. Michael Brake, *The Sociology of Youth Culture and Youth Subcultures* (New York: Routledge, 2013), 13–19.

27. B. S. Trazhevskii, "Emkost' rynka i zadachi tabachnoi promyshlennosti," *Vestnik tabachnoi promyshlennosti*, no. 1–2 (1925): 10–16.

28. Sholomovich, *Detskii pokhod na vzroslykh*, 10.

29. Wood, *Baba and the Comrade*, 150.

30. B. B. Kogan and M. S. Lebedinskii, *Byt rabochei molodezhi* (Moscow: Moszdravot-del, 1929), 72–73.

31. Dated and reproduced in Snopkov, Snopkov, and Shkliaruk, *Reklama v plakate*, 104.

32. Dated and reproduced in Snopkov, Snopkov, and Shkliaruk, *Reklama v plakate*, 106.

33. Colton, *Moscow*, 119–28.

34. Dated, attributed, and reproduced in Snopkov, Snopkov, and Shkliaruk, *Reklama v plakate*, 106.

35. Dated, attributed, and reproduced in Snopkov, Snopkov, and Shkliaruk, *Reklama v plakate*, 117.

36. Klaus Vashik and Nina Baburina, *Real'nost' utopii: Iskusstvo russkogo plakata XX veka* (Moscow: Progress-Traditsiia, 2003), 79.

37. Tricia Starks, "A Community in the Clouds: Advertising Tobacco, Gender, and Liberation in Pre-Revolutionary Russia," *Journal of Women's History* 25, no. 1 (2013): 62–84.

38. Benedict, *Golden-Silk Smoke*, 199–236; Carol Benedict, "Bourgeois Decadence or Proletarian Pleasure? The Visual Culture of Male Smoking in China across the 1949 Divide," in *Poisonous Pandas*, 95–132.

39. Matthew Hilton, *Smoking in British Popular Culture, 1800–2000* (Manchester: Manchester University Press, 2000), 145–47; Jarret Rudy, *The Freedom to Smoke: Tobacco Consumption and Identity* (Montreal: McGill-Queen's University Press, 2005), 148–50; Penny Tinkler and Cheryl Krasnick Warsh, "Feminine Modernity in Interwar Britain and North America: Corsets, Cars, and Cigarettes," *Journal of Women's History* 20, no. 3 (2008): 113–43; Neuburger, *Balkan Smoke*, 91–95.

40. Helena Goscilo and Andrea Lanoux, "Introduction: Lost in the Myths," in *Gender and National Identity in Twentieth-Century Russian Culture*, ed. Helen Goscilo and Andrea Lanoux (DeKalb: Northern Illinois University Press, 2006), 6–7.

41. Goscilo and Lanoux, "Introduction," 11–12.

42. N. A. Semashko, "Nuzhna li zhenstvennost'?," *Molodaia gvardiia*, no. 6 (1924): 205–6, as referenced in Bernstein, *Dictatorship of Sex*, 71.

43. Burnham, *Bad Habits*, 95–96; Hilton, *Smoking in British Popular Culture*, 145–51; Rudy, *Freedom to Smoke*, 160–64.

44. Bogdanov, *Dym otechestva*, 192–94; Galina Petrovna Sidorova, "Semiotika povsednevnosti: Zhenskoe kurenie kak tekst v kontekste sovetskoi kul'tury (na material-akh khudozhestvennoi literatury i kino)," *Voprosy kul'turologii*, no. 8 (2009): 86–90.

45. Wood, *Baba and the Comrade*, 2–3.

46. Wood, *Baba and the Comrade*, 49–56, 106–11.

47. Cox, "Creation of the Socialist Consumer," 278–82.

48. V. N. Liakov attributes the poster to Rodchenko in his *Sovetskii reklamnyi plakat i reklamnaia grafika, 1933–1973* (Moscow: Sovetskii khudozhnik, 1977), plate 22.

49. Brandt, *Cigarette Century*, 31.

50. Marjorie L. Hilton, "Retailing the Revolution: The State Department Store (GUM) and Soviet Society in the 1920s," *Journal of Social History* 37, no. 4 (2004): 954.

51. Starks, *Smoking under the Tsars*, 194.

52. Dated and reproduced in Snopkov, Snopkov, and Shkliaruk, *Reklama v plakate*, 105.

53. Aleksandr Snopkov, Pavel Snopkov, and Aleksandr Shkliaruk, eds., *Sovetskii reklamnyi plakat, 1923–1941/Soviet Advertising Posters* (Moscow: Kontakt, 2013), 68, plate 54.

54. Cox, "Creation of the Socialist Consumer," 289–91.

55. Cox, "'NEP without Nepmen!,'" 130.

56. "Nash panoptikum," *Krokodil*, no. 28–29 (1924): 7.

57. Phillips, *Bolsheviks and the Bottle*, 36–38.

58. Jessica Smith, *Women in Soviet Russia* (New York: Vanguard, 1928), 126.

59. Plamper, "Sounds of February," 151.

60. V. I. Lenin, "All Out for the Fights against Denikin!" *Collected Works*, 29:436–53.

61. Henri Beraud, *The Truth about Moscow: As Seen by a French Visitor,* trans. John Peile (London: Faber and Gwyer, 1925), 157.

62. Richard Stites, "The Role of Ritual and Symbols," in *Critical Companion to the Russian Revolution*, 568.

63. N. N. Sukhanov, *The Russian Revolution, 1917*, ed. and trans. Joel Carmichael (Princeton, NJ: Princeton University Press, 1984), 193, 579, quotation 595.

64. David G. Horn, *The Criminal Body: Lombroso and the Anatomy of Deviance* (New York: Routledge, 2003), 93–94; Bittner, *Whites and Reds*, 220.

65. Yulia Karpova, *Comradely Objects: Design and Material Culture in Soviet Russia, 1960s–1980s* (Manchester: Manchester University Press, 2020), 3, 48.

66. D. Sokolovskii, "K voprosu o emkosti Vsesoiuznogo Ukrainskogo tabachnykh rynkov v sviazi s piatiletnim planom razvertyvaniia promyshlennosti," in *Tabachnaia promyshlennost' i tabakovodstvo*, 6. Malinin found similar commentaries (*Tabachnaia istoriia Rossii*, 144–46).

67. "Novye tseny na papirosy," *Izvestiia*, April 18, 1926, 6.

68. "O vrede kureniia," *Krokodil*, no. 6 (1925): 10.

69. Mikhail Bulgakov, *Notes on the Cuff and Other Stories*, trans. Alison Rice (Ann Arbor, MI: Ardis, 1991), 132–35.

70. Weissman, "Prohibition and Alcohol Control."

71. Nezlin, *O vrede*, 1.

72. Dated, attributed, and reproduced in Snopkov, Snopkov, and Shkliaruk, *Reklama v plakate*, 107.

73. Dated, attributed, and reproduced in Snopkov, Snopkov, and Shkliaruk, *Reklama v plakate*, 139.

74. Dated and reproduced in Snopkov, Snopkov, and Shkliaruk, *Reklama v plakate*, 109.

75. N. Kopovalova, *Konstantin Stepanovich Mel'nikov (1890–1974)* (Moscow: Komsomol'skaia pravda, 2016), 4–7; Anna Petrova, ed., *Arkhitektor Konstantin Mel'nikov: Pavil'ony, garazhi, kluby i zhil'e sovetskoi epokhi* (Moscow: Gosudarstvennyi muzei arkhitektury im. A. V. Shchuseva, 2015), 30–33; A. A. Strigaleva and I. V. Kokkinaki, eds., *Konstantin Stepanovich Mel'nikov* (Moscow: Iskusstvo, 1985), 156–57.

76. Snopkov, Snopkov, and Shkliaruk, *Reklama v plakate*, 106.

77. For a different interpretation, see Cox, "'NEP without Nepmen!,'" 139.

78. Vasilevskii, *Gigiena propagandista*, 20.

79. Cox considered this woman to be the wife of the bureaucrat, but no signs of intimacy, such as those between the NEP-man and NEP-woman, betray this. The clerk instead is looking back at the NEP-man or perhaps the peasant, not down and back to the woman ("Creation of the Socialist Consumer," 276–78).

80. Stephen Kotkin, *Magnetic Mountain: Stalinism as a Civilization* (Berkeley: University of California Press, 1995), 198–236.

81. Starks, *Body Soviet,* 16. Naiman, *Sex in Public,* 208–49.

4. TREATED

1. Sholomovich, *Detskii pokhod na vzroslykh*, 21; A. S. Sholomovich, "Bor'ba s kureniem i lechenie kuril'shchikov," *Voprosy narkologii* 2 (1928): 81.

2. The specialized dispensaries were called narkodispensaries. Here they are grouped into the general system of dispensarization (Solomon, "David and Goliath," 263; Transchel, *Under the Influence,* 83–89; Mary Schaeffer Conroy, "Abuse of Drugs other than Alcohol and Tobacco in the Soviet Union," *Soviet Studies* 42, no. 3 [1990]: 447–80).

3. Starks, *Body Soviet*, 50–53.

4. Zolotnitskii, *O vrede*, 5. See also B. Sigal, *Trud i zdorov'e rabochei molodezhi* (Leningrad: Molodaia gvardiia, 1925), 43.

5. A. S. Sholomovich, "Kratkii ocherk chetyrekh let raboty," *Voprosy narkologii* 2 (1928): 104–8.

6. Zababurina, "Boremsia s narkotizmom," *ZNB*, no. 8–9 (1925): 17.

7. "Bor'ba s narkotikami," *Izvestiia*, April 7, 1926, 5.

8. Sholomovich, "Kratkii ocherk," 105–6.

9. "Khronika: K bor'be s kureniem," *GiZRiKS*, no. 14 (1928): 14.

10. Sholomovich, "Bor'ba s kureniem," 82.

11. "Bor'ba s narkotikami."

12. A. S. Sholomovich, "Otchet dispensernoi bor'by s narkotizmom v Moskve," *Voprosy narkologii* 1 (1926): 71–86.

13. Sebelius, *How Tobacco Smoke Causes Disease*, 105–6.

14. Sholomovich, "Bor'ba s kureniem," 82–83.

15. On other addictive substances, see Pavel Vasilyev, "War, Revolution, and Drugs: The 'Democratization' of Drug Abuse and the Evolution of Drug Policy in Russia, 1914–24," in *Russia's Home Front in War and Revolution, 1914–22, 2: The Experience of War and Revolution*, ed. Adele Lindenmeyr, Christopher Read, and Peter Waldron (Bloomington, IN: Slavica Publishers, 2016), 411–30.

16. V. A. Trofimov, *Tabak—vrag zdorov'ia* (Leningrad: Meditsinskaia literatura, 1959), 14. The story actually appeared in 1939. See Mikhail Mikhailovich Zoshchenko, "O tom, kak Lenin brosil kurit'," *Shestaia povest' Belkina*, vol. 6 (Moscow: Vremia, 2008), https://ruslit.

traumlibrary.net/book/zoschenko-ss07-06/zoschenko-ss07-06.html#work002013004; Catriona Kelly, *Refining Russia: Advice Literature, Polite Culture, and Gender from Catherine to Yeltsin* (Oxford: Oxford University Press, 2001), 258.

17. L. N. Tolstoy, "Dlia chego liudi obdurmanivaiutsia," *Polnoe sobranie sochinenii* (Moscow: Gosizdat, 1937), 25:269–85. See Starks, *Smoking under the Tsars*, 162–16; Lukashevich, *Nevinnaia privychka*, 3, 36; Gorokhov, *Zlaia travka*, 22–23.

18. P. Polunim, "Rabochie o ploshchadke: Mnogoe dala ploshchadka," *ZNB*, no. 4–5 (1925): 15.

19. Lukashevich, *Nevinnaia privychka*, 36.

20. Sholomovich, *Detskii pokhod na vzroslykh*, 20.

21. A. L. Mendel'son, *Vospitanie voli* (Leningrad: Leningradskaia pravda, 1928), 21–22, 28.

22. Violin, *Tabak i ego vred*, 16; I. Sazhin, "Kak deistvuet kurenie na zdorov'e i trudosposobnost' (chast' 2)," *GiZRS*, no. 14 (1924): 8.

23. Nezlin, *O vrede*, 27–28.

24. "Pis'mo v redaktsiiu," *Izvestiia*, January 17, 1924, 6.

25. K. Kaplan, *Ne kuri* (Kharkov: Nauchnaia mysl', 1930), 3–4.

26. Ia. I. Lifshits, *Doloi kurenie i p'ianstvo!*, 31.

27. Pridonov, *Bros'te kurit'!*, 11.

28. Berman, *O stol' tsenimom tabake*, 14.

29. Basserman, *Trud, zdorov'e, byt*, 21.

30. Lifshits, *Doloi kurenie i p'ianstvo!*, 6–7.

31. Sazhin, *Pravda o kurenii*, 25–26.

32. Nezlin, *O vrede*, 51.

33. Sigal, *Vrednaia privychka*, 13.

34. Violin, *Tabak i ego vred*, 16.

35. Conroy, "Abuse of Drugs," 455–56.

36. Rossiiskii, *O tabake*, 9.

37. Zolotnitskii, *O vrede*, 17–19.

38. Boginskii, *Tabak i ego kurenie*, 7–8.

39. Berman, *O stol' tsenimom tabake*, 15–16.

40. Popov, *Vred tabakokureniia*, 13.

41. Bliumenau, *Okhmeliaiushchie durmany*, 10, 16.

42. Conroy, "Abuse of Drugs," 462.

43. Sazhin, *Pravda o kurenii*, 16.

44. Morrissey, "Economy of Nerves," 649.

45. Sirotkina, *Diagnosing Literary Genius*, 126; Simon Pawley, "Revolution in Health: Nervous Weakness and Visions of Health in Revolutionary Russia, c. 1900–31," *Historical Research*, no. 90 (2017): 191–209.

46. M. G. Trakhman, *Materialy po zdravookhraneniiu na transporte za 1924 god* (Moscow: Mediko-sanitarnyi otdel putei soobshcheniia Narodnogo komissariata zdravookhraneniia RSFSR, 1926), 23–25, 27.

47. Nezlin, *O vrede*, 30–33.

48. Krementsov, *Revolutionary Experiments*, 27–28.

49. Rosenberg, "Introduction," 4–5.

50. Popov, *Vred tabakokureniia*, 18–19.

51. Violin, *Tabak i ego vred*, 13–15.

52. Tsentral'nyi munitsipal'nyi arkhiv Moskvy (TsMAM) f. 634, op. 1, d. 39, l. 201.

53. Vasilevskii, *Gigiena pionera*, 29.

54. Sholomovich, *Detskii pokhod na vzroslykh*, 23.

55. As quoted in Berman, *O stol' tsenimom tabake*, 18–19.

56. Sigal, *Vrednaia privychka*, 11.

57. Basserman, *Trud, zdorov'e, byt*, 18–19.

58. Basserman, *Trud, zdorov'e, byt*, 22.

59. "Otvety na voprosy chitatelei," *GZRS*, no. 11 (1927): 17; Tikhon Kholodnyi, "Komsomol v pokhode," *Pravda*, August 9, 1927, 3.

60. Elizabeth Wood, *Performing Justice: Agitation Trials in Early Soviet Russia* (Ithaca, NY: Cornell University Press, 2005); Lynn Mally, *Revolutionary Acts: Amateur Theater and the Soviet State, 1917–1938* (Ithaca, NY: Cornell University Press, 2000).

61. B. Sigal, *I. Sud nad pionerom kuril'shchikom i II. Sud nad neriashlivym pionerom: Dve intsenorovki* (Moscow: Zhizn' i znanie, 1927), quotation 11.

62. Violin, *Tabak i ego vred*, 16.

63. Popov, *Vred tabakokureniia*, 22.

64. Popov, *Vred tabakokureniia*, 23. On drunkenness, see N. B. Lebina, *Rabochaia molodezh' Leningrada: Trud i sotsial'nyi oblik, 1921–1925 gody* (Leningrad: Nauka, 1982), 146.

65. Nezlin, *O vrede*, 54.

66. Varushkin, *Pochemu vreden tabak*, 26.

67. Sazhin, *Pravda o kurenii*, 16.

68. Starks, *Body Soviet*, 118–20.

69. I. G., "Novyi byt idet," *ZNB*, no. 4–5 (1926): 8–9.

70. Zdraviachek 12-i sov. Shkoly Zamraiona, "Nasha rabota," *ZNB*, no. 10–11 (1926): 24.

71. Sholomovich, "Kratkii ocherk," 106–7; Sholomovich, "Bor'ba s kureniem," 82.

72. Sholomovich, *Detskii pokhod na vzroslykh*, 22.

73. Sholomovich, "Kratkii ocherk," 81.

74. Nezlin, *O vrede*, 56.

75. Sholomovich, "Otchet," 83.

76. Zina Antonova, "Kurit' vredno," *ZNB*, no. 8–9 (1925): 15–16.

77. I. Mil'man, "Bortsy za zdorovyi byt," *ZNB*, no. 13–14 (1927): 16.

78. P. Dem'ianov, "Kak okhraniat' detei ot tabachnogo dyma," *GiZRiKS*, no. 13 (1926): 9.

79. N. Rablova, "Vred kureniia," *Krokodil*, no. 9 (1924): 10.

80. Sholomovich, "Otchet," 71–86.

81. Budnitskii, "Skopom na bor'bu s kureniem," *GZRS*, no. 17 (1924): 13.

82. Zolotnitskii, *O vrede*, 15.

83. Transchel, *Under the Influence*, 89, 96.

84. I. D. Strashun, "Desiat' let bor'by proletariata za zdorov'e," in *Desiat' let oktiabria*, 59; *Vsia Moskva* (Moscow: Moskovskii rabochii, 1928), 39.

85. "Polgoda ne kuriat," *ZNB*, no. 14–15 (1926): 24.

86. "Khronika: Bor'ba s kureniem," *GiZRiKS*, no. 7 (1928): 14.

87. Zh., "Predlagaem sledovat' nashemu primery," *ZNB*, no. 3 (1927): 16, referencing a challenge from the journal's issue no. 2 (1927), "Durnoi primer."

88. Lukashevich, *Nevinnaia privychka*, 38–39.

89. Lukashevich, *Nevinnaia privychka*, 38–39.

90. Sholomovich, "Bor'ba s kureniem," 82.

91. B. S. Kovgankin, *Komsomol na bor'bu s narkotizmom: Kak molodezhi pobedit' bolezni byta. P'ianstvo i kurenie tabaka* (Moscow: Molodaia gvardiia, 1929), 37–38.

92. Gorokhov, *Zlaia travka*, 26.

93. A. G. Stoiko, "O lechenii tabakokureniia i kollektivnoi psikhoterapii ego, kak osobom metode," *Voprosy narkologii*, 2:84.

94. Stoiko, "O lechenii tabakokureniia," 84.

95. Sirotkina, *Diagnosing Literary Genius*, 150–59.

96. V. M. Bekhterev, *Gipnoz, vnushenie, telepatiia* (repr. Moscow: Mysl', 1994).

97. Stoiko, "O lechenii tabakokureniia," 84–85.

98. Stoiko, "O lechenii tabakokureniia," 84–85.

99. Widdis, *Socialist Senses*, 11–14.

100. Daniel P. Todes, *Ivan Pavlov: A Russian Life in Science* (Oxford: Oxford University Press, 2014), 464–81.

101. Carroll, *Narkomaniia*, 11.

102. Widdis, *Socialist Senses*, 15–17.

103. Stoiko, "O lechenii tabakokureniia," 86.

104. Stoiko, "O lechenii tabakokureniia," 86.

105. David Joravsky, *Russian Psychology: A Critical History* (Oxford: Basil Blackwell, 1989), 235–36; Sarah Marks, "Suggestion, Persuasion, and Work: Psychotherapy in Communist Europe," *European Journal of Psychotherapy and Counselling* 20, no. 1 (2018): 3–16; Martin Allan Miller, *Freud and the Bolsheviks: Psychoanalysis in Imperial Russia and the Soviet Union* (New Haven: Yale University Press, 1998).

106. Stoiko, "O lechenii tabakokureniia," 86.

107. Stoiko, "O lechenii tabakokureniia," 87. A similar argument dominated discussion of birth pain as a learned response. See Michaels, *Lamaze*, 33–44.

108. Stoiko, "O lechenii tabakokureniia," 87–88.

109. Polianskii, *Deistvie tabachnago dyma*, 15.

110. Bliumenau, *Okhmeliaiushchie durmany*, 38.

111. "Otvety na voprosy chitatelei," *GiZRiKS*, no. 10 (1928): 16.

112. Zolotnitskii, *O vrede*, 20.

113. Violin, *Tabak i ego vred*, 16.

114. Zolotnitskii, *O vrede*, 29; Boginskii, *Tabak i ego kurenie*, 9; Popov, *Vred tabakokureniia*, 21.

115. *Give the Boy a Square Deal! Annual Report* (Chicago: Anti-Cigarette International League, 1921), 7.

116. Zolotnitskii, *O vrede*, 20.

117. "Vy kurite?," *Pravda*, November 26, 1927, 8; "Vred ot kureniia," *Pravda*, December 21, 1927, 6; "Novosti gigienicheskogo mundshtuka," *Pravda*, December 7, 1927, 6; "Antinikotin: Gigienicheskii mundshtuk," *GiZRiKS*, no. 5 (1928): inside front cover.

118. Sazhin, *Pravda o kurenii*, 27–28.

119. Lukashevich, *Nevinnaia privychka*, 36.

120. Berman, *O stol' tsenimom tabake*, 8.

121. Nezlin, *O vrede*, 46–47.

122. Nezlin, *O vrede*, 46–47.

123. B. Samsonov, with drawings by K. Eliseev, "V Narkodispansere," *Krokodil*, no. 11 (1928): 5.

124. Gol'dshtein, *Tabachnaia promyshlennost'*, 54.

125. Sholomovich, *Detskii pokhod na vzroslykh*, 45.

126. "V tabachnom dymu," *ZNB*, no. 3–4 (1929): 13–14.

127. Bulgakov, *Notes on the Cuff*, 135–36.

128. S. Gershtein, "Pomnite, rebiata," *Krokodil*, no. 43 (1928): 3.

129. David L. Hoffmann, *Stalinist Values: The Cultural Norms of Soviet Modernity, 1917–1941* (Ithaca, NY: Cornell University Press, 2003), 81.

130. S. Egiz, "Polozhenie tabakovodstva v Sovetskoi Rossii," *Vestnik tabachnoi promyshlennosti*, no. 1 (1922): 7.

131. Varushkin, *Pochemu vreden tabak*, 15–17.

132. A. Press, "Otravlenie vsego naseleniia tabachnym dymom (chast 2)," *GZRS*, no. 20 (1924): 4–5.

133. Zolotnitskii, *O vrede*, 21–23.

134. "Issledovaniia i otkrytiia: O kurenii," *GiZRiKS*, no. 14 (1928): 15.

135. Popov, *Vred tabakokureniia*, 21; "Issledovaniia i otkrytiia: Opyty s kureniem tabaku," *GiZRS*, no. 5 (1924): 15; Nezlin, *O vrede*, 43–45.

136. Zolotnitskii, *O vrede*, 29.

137. Sazhin, *Pravda o kurenii*, 24; Polianskii, *Deistvie tabachnago dyma*, 13–14.

138. Nezlin, *O vrede*, 16.

139. Polianskii, *Deistvie tabachnago dyma*, 1.

140. Popov, *Vred tabakokureniia*, 10–13; K. N. Shapshev, "O soderzhanii nikotina v makhorkakh i papirosakh," *Gigiena i epidemiologiia*, no. 1 (1925).

141. Sazhin, *Pravda o kurenii*, 5.

142. Lifshits, *Doloi kurenie i p'ianstvo!*, 28.

143. I. Sarygin, "Vred i pol'za upotrebleniia tabaka," *Vestnik tabachnoi promyshlennosti*, no. 11 (1923): 50.

144. Sarygin, "Vred i pol'za upotrebleniia tabaka," 51.

145. Sarygin, "Vred i pol'za upotrebleniia tabaka," 51. Zolotnitskii opposed this (*O vrede*, 10). See also Starks, *Smoking under the Tsars*, 81–82, 204.

146. Sarygin, "Vred i pol'za upotrebleniia tabaka," 52–53.

147. Egiz, "Polozhenie tabakovodstva," 8.

148. *Give the Boy*, 4–5.

149. "Na transporte: Bor'ba za zdorovyi byt," *Biulleten' NKZ*, no. 9 (1926): 34–38.

150. *Putevoditel' po Muzeiu zdravookhraneniia Leningradskogo obzdravotdela* (Leningrad: Leningradskii meditsinskii zhurnal, 1928).

151. D. Zabolotnyi, "Vrednye privychki," *GiZRiKS*, no. 24 (1926): 1–2; Mendel'son, *Vospitanie voli*, 29.

152. M. Kovarskii, "Kak dolzhen byt' ustroen klub," *ZNB*, no. 7 (1925): 12.

153. V. V. Maiakovskii, *Polnoe sobranie sochinenii* (Moscow: Khudozhestvennaia literatura, 1958), 10:116–18.

154. A. S. Utekhin, *Doloi kurevo, s 8 risunkami* (Leningrad: Fizkul'tura i sport, 1930); Tiapugin, *Pochemu i kak dolzhna molodezh' borot'sia s tabakom* (Moscow: Gosmedizdat, 1930); Sazhin, *Pravda o kurenii*; Kaplan, *Ne kuri*.

155. The subject of the review was the Utekhin volume. See A. Grigor'ev, "Chitatelei: Protiv p'ianstva i kureniia," *Trezvost' i kul'tura*, no. 17 (1930): 19.

5. UNFULFILLED

1. Edward Geist, "Cooking Bolshevik: Anastas Mikoian and the Making of the 'Book about Delicious and Healthy Food,'" *Russian Review* 71, no. 2 (2012): 297–98.

2. A. Mikoian, "Zadachi tabachnoi promyshlennosti," *Tabachnaia promyshlennost'*, no. 8 (1931): 4–7. See short discussions in Malinin, *Tabachnaia istoriia Rossii*, 155–56; Bogdanov, *Dym otechestva*, 194–95; and Malinin, *Tabak*, 109.

3. Mikoian, "Zadachi tabachnoi promyshlennosti," 5.

4. Mikoian, "Zadachi tabachnoi promyshlennosti," 5.

5. Mikoian, "Zadachi tabachnoi promyshlennosti," 7.

6. I. V. Stalin, "The Tasks of Business Executives," *Collected Works*, vol. 13 (Moscow: Foreign Languages Publishing House, 1954). https://www.marxists.org/reference/archive/stalin/works/1931/02/04.htm.

7. Karl Radek, "Revoliutsiia i kontrrevoliutsiia na novom etape i podgotovka interventsii," *Izvestiia*, January 1, 1931, 2.

8. Mikoian, "Zadachi tabachnoi promyshlennosti," 5.

9. Mikoian, "Zadachi tabachnoi promyshlennosti," 5, 7.

10. David L. Hoffmann, *Peasant Metropolis: Social Identities in Moscow, 1929–1941* (Ithaca, NY: Cornell University Press, 1994), 1, 33–42.

11. Alec Nove, "Victims of Stalinism: How Many?," posits ten to eleven million. S. G. Wheatcroft gives four to five million in "More Light on the Scale of Repression and Excess Mortality in the Soviet Union in the 1930," both in *Stalinist Terror: New Perspectives*, ed. J. Arch Getty and Roberta T. Manning (Cambridge: Cambridge University Press, 1993), 261–74 and 275–90, respectively.

12. Malinin, *Tabachnaia istoriia Rossii*, 155–56.

13. Transchel, *Under the Influence*, 149.

14. See similarly China's 1950s policies, as detailed in Huangfu Qiushi and Matthew Kohrman, "The Chinese Cigarette during the 'Great Leap Forward,'" in *Poisonous Pandas*, 73–92.

15. "Nashi zadachi," *Tabachnaia promyshlennost'*, no. 1–2 (1930): 1–2.

16. N. Mirkin, "Zadachi tabachno-makhorochnoi promyshlennosti vo vtoroi piatiletke," *Tabachnaia promyshlennost'*, no. 10 (1931): 3.

17. V. Grigor'ian, *Tabak: Pavil'ion gruzinskoi SSR* (Tbilisi: Zaria vostoka, 1935), 2.

18. Ruth Mandel, "Cigarettes in Soviet and Post-Soviet Central Asia," in *Smoke: A Global History of Smoking*, ed. Sander L. Gilman and Zhou Xun (London: Reaktion Books, 2004), 182; Sarah Cameron, *The Hungry Steppe: Famine, Violence, and the Making of Soviet Kazakhstan* (Ithaca, NY: Cornell University Press, 2020); Robert Kindler, *Stalin's Nomads: Power and Famine in Kazakhstan* (Pittsburgh: University of Pittsburgh Press, 2018).

19. Harvard Project on the Soviet Social System. Schedule A, Vol. 7, Case 94 (interviewer A.P., type A4). Female, 40, Ukrainian, Various occupations: since 1937, kolkhoznik. Widener Library, Harvard University, 5.

20. Robert Conquest, *Harvest of Sorrow: Soviet Collectivization and the Terror-Famine* (New York: Oxford University Press, 1986); Lynne Viola, *Peasant Rebels under Stalin: Collectivization and the Culture of Peasant Resistance* (New York: Oxford University Press, 1996).

21. Novikova and Shchemelev, *Nasha marka*, 118, 128–31; Lynne Viola, *The Best Sons of the Fatherland: Workers in the Vanguard of Soviet Collectivization* (Oxford: Oxford University Press, 1987), 121–51.

22. Mikoian, "Zadachi tabachnoi promyshlennosti," 4–7.

23. A. O. Matsiuk, "Syr'evuiu bazu na revoliutsionnye tempy," *Tabachnaia promyshlennost'*, no. 1–3 (1931): 1–4.

24. R. W. Davies, *The Soviet Economy in Turmoil, 1929–1930* (Cambridge, MA: Harvard University Press, 1989), 58.

25. Malinin, *Tabachnaia istoriia Rossii*, 155–56.

26. A. Levin, "Ispol'zovanie starogo oborudovaniia na tabachnykh fabrikakh," *Tabachnaia promyshlennost'*, no. 1–2 (1930): 7–11; "Novaia tabachnaia fabrika," *Pravda*, May 14, 1934, 6; "Tsennoe izobretenie," *Pravda*, November 3, 1934, 5; G. P. Emets, "K rekonstruktsii makhorochnykh fabrik," *Tabak*, no. 1 (1939): 8–9; S. N. Gabaev, "Rekonstruktsiia i stroitel'stvo novykh tabachnykh fabrik," *Tabak*, no. 1 (1939): 11–12.

27. Korno and Kitainer, *Balkanskaia zvezda*, 139–40.

28. Norton T. Dodge, *Women in the Soviet Economy: Their Role in Economic, Scientific, and Technical Development* (Baltimore: Johns Hopkins University Press, 1966), 181.

29. Linov, "Sigaretnaia mashina," *Tabak*, no. 4 (1938): 19–26; D. Skovrtsov, "Kapital'nyi remont fabriki 'Dukat,'" *Tabak*, no. 5 (1938): 27–28.

30. GARF f. R-5446, op. 23a, d. 870, ll. 1–7.

31. Davies, *Soviet Economy*, 58–60.

32. "6 milliardov papiros," *Izvestiia*, December 26, 1934, 4.

33. A. Naugol'nov, "Korotkie signaly: V Baku spekuliruiut papirosami," *Pravda*, July 14, 1934, 4; "V Baku spekuliruiut papirosami," *Pravda*, August 8, 1934, 2; Ia. Iashin, "Tabachnaia spekuliatsiia," *Pravda*, August 6, 1934, 4; I. Maliugin, "Irkutskoe papirosniki," *Pravda*, January 10, 1935," 3.

34. S. Orman, "Aromatnye papirosy," *Pravda*, December 30, 1939, 4.

35. Proctor, *Golden Holocaust*, 67.

36. A. A. Schmuk, "The Problem of the Artificial Improvement of Quality in Low Grade Tobaccos," repr. 1931, "The Artificial Improvement of the Quality of Low Grade Tobaccos," repr. 1932, and "Tobacco Substitutes," repr. 1932, all in *The Chemistry and Technology of Tobacco*, vol. 3 (Moscow: Pishchepromizdat, 1953), 465–79, 480–520, 586–611.

37. A. A. Schmuk, "Obtaining Nicotine-Free Cigarettes by the Method of Smoke Filtration," repr. 1932 in *Chemistry and Technology of Tobacco*, 521.

38. A. Koperina and A. Taranova, "O vliianii mundshtuka papiros na sostav tabachnogo dyma," *Tabachnaia promyshlennost'*, no. 1–2 (1930): 59–61.

39. Advertisements for *Astmatol* appear in *GiZRiKS*, no. 7 (1937): 18, and no. 8 (1937): 18.

40. E. E. Kogan, "Metody denikotinizatsii izdelii," *Tabak*, no. 2 (1939): 59–60; "Beznikotinnyi tabak," *Tabak*, no. 6 (1939): 58–60; V. Praiss, "Vliianie fil'truiushchikh vkladyshei iz tselliulozy na soderzhanie nikotina v dyme papirosy," *Tabak*, no. 1 (1939): 62; Bodnar, Nagi, and Veksei (Hungary), "Absorbtsiia nikotina iz tabachnogo dyma razlichnymi poglotiteliami," *Tabak*, no. 1 (1939): 62.

41. A. Kuznetsov, "Perepiska s chitateliami," *GiZRiKS*, no. 1 (1933): 17.

42. A. Koperina and S. Kalibab, "Beznikotinovye papirosy (Khimicheskii sector promfiliala VITIMa," *Tabachnaia promyshlennost'*, no. 3 (1935): 34–35.

43. Stal'skii, *Donskaia gosudarstvennaia tabachnaia fabrika*, 21–27.

44. Novikova and Shchemelev, *Nasha marka*, 116–17, 134.

45. V. Kel'berg, "Shum na tabachnykh fabrikakh i bor'ba s nim," *Tabak*, no. 6 (1937): 11–13; Pukemo, "Ventiliatsiia na tabachnykh fabrikakh," *Tabak*, no. 5 (1938): 21–22.

46. Novikova and Shchemelev, *Nasha marka*, 136.

47. Stal'skii, *Donskaia gosudarstvennaia tabachnaia fabrika*, 30–31.

48. Novikova and Shchemelev, *Nasha marka*, 133, 138, 147–49. On theater cells, see Mally, *Revolutionary Acts*.

49. Grigor'ian, *Tabak*, 8; Stal'skii, *Donskaia gosudarstvennaia tabachnaia fabrika*, 31–32.

50. "Stakhanovskoe dvizhenie v tabachnoi i makhorochnoi promyshlennosti," *Tabachnaia promyshlennost'*, no. 6 (1935): 1–8; Kh. D. Kopa, "Opyt raboty stakhanovskikh brigad, na fabrike 'Dukat' osvoivshikh tekhnicheskie normy," *Tabak*, no. 2 (1937): 4–5; D. Skvortsov, "Stakhanovtsy fabrik 'Dukat' i 'Iava' o svoei rabote," *Tabak*, no. 4–5 (1937): 14–18; "Rech'" tov. Ivanovoi," *Izvestiia*, November 16, 1935, 3. Later memoirs similarly approached the labor heroes: see A. A. Nosova, "38 let raboty na fabrike," *Tabak*, no. 1 (1953): 16–17.

51. M. Ia. Telegina, ed. *Pervyi opyt Stakhanovtsev DGTF* (Rostov-on-Don: Stachin, 1935), 6, 15.

52. Nina Volkova, *Dostignutoe ne predel!* (Moscow: Pishchepromizdat, 1935), 11–15; quotation 14.

53. "Vtoroe rozhdenie," *Izvestiia*, June 12, 1938, 3.

54. Robert Thurston, "The Stakhanovite Movement: The Background to the Great Terror in the Factories, 1935–1938," in *Stalinist Terror*, 142–60; Lewis Siegelbaum, *Stakhanovism and the Politics of Productivity in the USSR, 1935–41* (New York: Cambridge University Press, 1988).

55. A. Mikoian, "V polose velikogo pod"ema," *Pravda*, November 17, 1935, 2.

56. "Okonchanie doklada tov. A. I. Mikoiana," *Izvestiia*, January 25, 1936, 6.

57. "Rech' tov. A. I. Mikoiana na zased. Soveta pri Narkome pishevoi promyshlennosti," *Izvestiia*, July 1, 1936, 2; "Okonchanie doklada tov. A. I. Mikoiana."

58. "Itogi dekabr'skogo plenuma TSK VKP(b)," *Pravda*, January 19, 1936, 2.

59. "Desiatki tysiach ton produktov sverkh plana," *Izvestiia*, April 5, 1938, 2.

60. A. Kh. Buralenko, *Razvitie sovetskoi torgovoi reklamy* (L'vov: n.p., 1959), 19.

61. "Rech' tov. A. I. Mikoiana na zased. Soveta pri Narkome pishevoi promyshlennosti." The effort to acquaint users with products had also been part of 1920s advertising strategies, with soap again used as an example. See Marjorie Hilton, "The Invention of Soviet Advertising," in *Material Culture in Russia and the USSR*, 131.

62. Snopkov, Snopkov, and Shkliaruk, *Sovetskii reklamnyi plakat*, 5–7.

63. "Otovsiudu," *Pravda*, February 17, 1935, 8.

64. "Prazdnichnye podarki," *Pravda*, October 5, 1936, 6.

65. I. M. Gol'dberg, "Obraztsovye tabachnye magaziny v Moskve," *Tabachnaia promyshlennost'*, no. 3 (1936): 29–30.

66. "Gde vy obedaete?," *Izvestiia*, July 23 1937, 3.

67. Proctor, *Golden Holocaust,* 135–36; "Avtomaty dlia prodazhi spichek i papiros," *Pravda*, March 1, 1935, 3.

68. N. A. Kalantarova et al., *Moskva v fotografiiakh, 1920–1930-e gody* (St. Petersburg: Liki Rossii, 2010), 144.

69. "Zapreshchenie prodazhi tabachnykh izdelii detiam," *Pravda*, November 1, 1937, 6.

70. "Etiketka i fabrichnaia marka," *Pravda*, March 15, 1935, 4.

71. Bogdanov, *Dym otechestva*, 208–9.

72. M. M. Gol'dberg, "Papirosnye etikety," *Tabachnaia promyshlennost'*, no. 5 (1935): 5–7.

73. "Vkusy kuril'shchikov," *Izvestiia*, May 5, 1936, 4.

74. Amy E. Randall, "Gender and the Emergence of the Soviet 'Citizen-Consumer' in Comparative Perspective," in *Material Culture in Russia and the USSR*, 142.

75. Randall, "Gender and the Emergence," 143; Karen F. A. Fox, "The History of Marketing in Russia," in *The Routledge Companion to Marketing History*, ed. D. G. Brian Jones and Mark Tadajewski (New York: Routledge, 2016), 438.

76. "Po sovetskoi strane," *Izvestiia*, March 14, 1938, 4.

77. Thurston, "Stakhanovite Movement," 142–60; Siegelbaum, *Stakhanovism and the Politics of Productivity,* 210–46.

78. B. Levin, "O vkusnykh veshchakh," *Pravda*, January 8, 1934, 4.

79. G. Simonenkov, "Skol'ko papiros v pachke," *Pravda*, June 16, 1934, 4; "Barkodely," *Izvestiia*, August 8, 1940, 4; V. V. Sokolov, "Defekty bumagi i kachestvo papiros," *Tabak*, no. 1 (1937): 54–57; L. I. Tifonova, "Defekty gil'zovoi bumagi," *Tabak*, no. 1 (1937): 58–59.

80. Bittner, *Whites and Reds*, 205.

81. S. Grigorenko, "Gde kupit' kuritel'noi bumagi?," *Pravda*, October 7, 1935, 4.

82. "Okonchanie doklada tov. A. I. Mikoiana," *Izvestiia*, January 25, 1936, 6.

83. Sokolov, "Defekty bumagi i kachestvo papiros"; Tifonova, "Defekty gil'zovoi bumagi"; Bogdanov, *Dym otechestva*, 208–9.

84. "Litsom k kachestvu," *Tabak*, no. 6 (1937): 1–2; reprint of "Prikaz po Narodnomu komissariatu pishchevoi promyshlennosti Soiuza SSR," *Tabak*, no. 6 (1937): 3–4; V. S. Kushliu, S. S. Chistov, and E. S. Ermolenko, "O kachestve papiros," *Tabak*, no. 6 (1938): 14–17.

85. Hessler, *Social History*, 5.

86. "Kak spichki stali defitsitnym tovarom," *Izvestiia*, April 8, 1938, 3; "Zasedanie soveta narodnykh komissarov SSSR," *Izvestiia*, August 30, 1938, 2; N. Sidorov, "Nasushchnye voprosy torgovli na sele," *Izvestiia*, February 4, 1939, 3; "Vsemerno uluchshat' torgovliu v derevne," *Izvestiia*, July 8, 1939, 1.

87. "Kak torguiut v Minske," *Izvestiia*, July 17, 1939, 4; P. M., "Na gorodskie temy: V letniuiu noch," *Izvestiia*, July 21, 1939, 4.

88. V. Lavrishchev, "Na bytovye temi: Bobruiskii 'servis,'" *Pravda*, July 4, 1939, 6.

89. "Proisshestviia," *Izvestiia*, March 1, 1935, 4; "Proisshestviia," *Izvestiia*, December 15, 1936, 4. See also "Proisshestviia," *Pravda*, March 7, 1940, 6.

90. "Proisshestviia," *Pravda*, December 27, 1935, 8.

91. "Rezul'taty bespechnosti," *Izvestiia*, April 15, 1937, 4; M. Kuz'min, "Kto vinovat?," *Pravda*, November 2, 1934, 4.

92. F. Barybdin and I. Tikhomirov, "Kuril'shchiki iz Glavtabaka," *Pravda*, May 25, 1940, 4; "Po sledam materialov 'Pravdy,'" *Pravda*, June 8, 1940, 6.

93. Roberta T. Manning, "The Soviet Economic Crisis of 1936–1940 and the Great Purges," in *Stalinist Terror*, 116–41.

94. Mikh. Ido—. "O kachestve papiros," *Pravda*, April 18, 1937, 4.

95. "O vypuske papiros," *Pravda*, January 30, 1938, 6.

96. "Pis'mo shakhterov narkompishchepromu," *Izvestiia*, January 6, 1939, 4.

97. "Kazhdyi poteriannyi chas—prestuplenie," *Izvestiia*, February 17, 1930, 3.

98. "Rabochii klass i tekhnicheskaia intelligentsia v bor'be za piatiletku i novuiu tekhniku," *Pravda*, February 20, 1930, 4; "Prekratit' bezobraziia!," *Pravda*, August 9. 1934, 2. See also "Den' vysokoi proizvoditel'nosti," *Izvestiia*, June 30, 1934, 3; "Polnost'iu zagruzit' rabochii den'," *Izvestiia*, January 3, 1939, 1; and "Prestupnoe popustitel'stvo," *Izvestiia* January 11, 1939, 3.

99. "Shtrafy napravo i nalevo," *Izvestiia*, May 5, 1934, 3; Starks, *Smoking under the Tsars*, 92–93, 138.

100. M. Kaganovich, "Prikaz narodnogo komissara aviatsionnoi promyshlennosti," *Pravda*, January 27, 1939, 3.

101. "Proissshestviia," *Pravda*, April 19, 1935, 6; "Proisshestviia," *Pravda*, July 7, 1935, 6; "Proisshestviia," *Pravda*, April 24, 1936, 6; "Proisshestviia," *Pravda*, August 2, 1939, 6.

102. "Pozhar na mashine," *Izvestiia*, April 16, 1937, 4.

103. "Proisshestviia," *Izvestiia*, September 9, 1937, 4.

104. "Proisshestviia," *Pravda*, February 3, 1937, 6.

105. V. V. Maikovskii, "Pozharnye lozungi," *Polnoe sobranie sochinenii*, 9:418–21. See, for example the poster featured in Trofimov, *Tabak—vrag zdorov'ia*, 12.

106. Kh. Kantor and M. Kureiko, "Sredniaia Volga imeet vse vozmozhnosti zaniat' pochetnoe mesto na vsesoiuznoi krasnoi doske," *Pravda*, July 28, 1933, 3.

107. "K bor'be s kureniem," *GiZRiKS*, no. 13 (1930): 15; Loranskii and Popova, "Kurenie i ego vliianie na zdorov'e cheloveka," 46.

108. "Izzhivem otravlenie tabachnym dymom," "Prizvat' kuril'shchikov k poriadku!" and A. Mendel'son, "Tabak i nervnaia sistema," *GiZRiKS*, no. 11–12 (1931): 6–8; V. S. Fedorov, "Usilim bor'bu s tabachnym durmanom," *GiZRiKS*, no. 33 (1932): 10.

109. "Vspyshka gremuchego gaza v shakhte no. 4," *Izvestiia*, April 22, 1930, 3.

110. A. Topikov, "Soznatel'nyi," *Krokodil*, no. 15 (1930): 8.

111. Utekhin, *Doloi kurevo*, 24–30.

112. Utekhin, *Doloi kurevo*, 31–32.

113. For these posters within the context of anti-tobacco posters of the entire Soviet period, see Fox, "'Tobacco Is Poison!,'" 190–92.

114. D. Midovidov, "Zlo, kotorogo ne zamechaiut," *GiZRiKS*, no. 2 (1929): 7; reader's letter to S. Vorob'ev, *GiZRiKS*, no. 20 (1929): 17; "Perepiska s chitateliami," *GiZRiKS*, no. 1 (1933): 17; Utekhin, *Doloi kurevo*, 5–8; Tiapugin, *Pochemu i kak dolzhna molodezh'*, 5–16; Sazhin, *Pravda o kurenii*, 4–10; Kaplan, *Ne kuri*, 4–10; M. Breitman, "O vrede kureniia dlia zhenskogo organizma," *GiZRiKS*, no. 22 (1929): 6–7; L. Iakobzon, "Tabak i polovaia sposobnost'," *GiZRiKS*, no. 6 (1930): 10.

115. N. Petrov, "Rak iazyka i polosti rta," *GiZRiKS*, no. 7 (1929): 7; reader's letter to Gr—n K—v, *GiZRiKS*, no. 13 (1929), 17; "Otvety na voprosy chitatelei," *GiZRiKS*, no. 23 (1929): 17; N. Petrov, "Voina raku," *GiZRiKS*, no. 6 (1930): 12–13; "Tabak i kurenie ego kak prichina raka," *GiZRiKS*, no. 21 (1930): 17; N. Petrov, "Rakovaia opasnost' i bor'ba s neiu," *GiZRiKS*, no. 7 (1929): 1–2; N. N. Petrov, "Shto nado znat' o rake," *GiZRiKS*, no. 9–10 (1933): 13–14 and *GiZRiKS*, no. 11–12 (1933): 13–16; A. Epshtein, "Kak uberech'sia ot raka," *GiZRiKS*, no. 5 (1937): 2–3; L., "Inostrannaia pechat' o bor'be s rakom," *GiZRiKS*, no. 7 (1929): 11; "Khronika," *GiZRiKS*, no. 21 (1931): 14; Bogorov, "Rak i bor'ba s nim," *GiZRiKS*, no. 15 (1932): 10–11.

116. A. H. Roffo, "Durch Tabak beim Kaninchen entwickeltes Carcinom," *Journal of Cancer Research and Clinical Oncology* 33, no. 1 (1931): 321–32; F. L. Hoffman, "Cancer and Smoking Habits," *Annals of Surgery* 93, no. 1 (1931): 50–67.

117. Only one article on quitting appeared in *GiZRiKS*, coming out in 1936 and focused more on the then popular question of hypnotherapy. See N. K. Bogolepov, *Voprosy nevro-psikhiatricheskoi dispansernoi praktiki* (Moscow: Moskovskii gorodskoi otdel zdravookhraneniia, 1936), 62–63. Readers' letters appeared throughout the period. See "Pisma," *GiZRiKS*, no. 16–17 (1931): 23; "Sovety chitatelei," *GiZRiKS*, no. 25–26 (1931): 23–24; A. Aggev, "Perepiska s chitateliami," *GiZRiKS*, no. 11–12 (1933): 25; Orlov, "Perepiski s chitateliami," *GiZRiKS*, no. 3 (1935): 17; Krainiuk, "Perepiski s chitateliami," *GiZRiKS*, no. 6 (1935): 17; "Perepiska s chitateliami," *GiZRiKS*, no. 6 (1937): 18; "Perepiska s chitateliami—Prof. A. Mendel'son," *GiZRiKS*, no. 3 (1938): 18.

118. Georgii Landau, "Tabak," *Krokodil*, no. 16 (1935): 13; "Nel'zia," *Krokodil*, no. 19 (1935): 14.

119. A. M., "Stranitsa shkol'nika: Shkol'nik, ne kuri!," *GiZRiKS*, no. 11–12 (1931): 18–19; N. D. "Molodezh' v bor'be s kureniem prevratim kurorty v sotsialisticheskie kuznitsy zdorov'ia!," *GiZRiKS*, no. 1–2 (1932): 12–13.

120. "Massovaia rabota Komsomola i partiia," *Izvestiia*, January 21, 1931, 3; Seth Bernstein, *Raised under Stalin: Young Communists and the Defense of Socialism* (Ithaca, NY: Cornell University Press, 2017), 52.

121. N. Sakonskaia, "Ne navisitnyi ugolek," *Krokodil*, no. 15 (1939): 4.

122. Berngard Shul'ts, "A baryshi burzhuaznykh gnev rastut," *Pravda*, March 6, 1930, 2.

123. Cherniak, "Obnishchanie rabochego klassa v Germanii," *Pravda*, April 16, 1933, 4.

124. A—, "Kto grabit i fermera i potrebeitelia," *Pravda*, November 25, 1932, 1.

125. "Uvelichenie nalogov v SShA," *Pravda*, June 24, 1940, 4.

126. Randall, *Soviet Dream World*, 6–10.

127. Sheila Fitzpatrick, *Everyday Stalinism: Ordinary Life in Extraordinary Times. Soviet Russia in the 1930s* (New York: Oxford University Press, 1999), 83.

128. Gol'dshtein, *Tabachnaia promyshlennost'*, 6:54.

129. Randall, "Gender and the Emergence," 147; Bittner, *Whites and Reds*, 115, 137, 141–42; Olga Gurova, "The Ideology of Consumption in the Soviet Union," in *Communism and Consumerism*, 70–75.

130. Sheila Fitzpatrick, *Education and Social Mobility in the Soviet Union, 1921–1934* (Cambridge: Cambridge University Press, 1979), 184–202.

131. "Gazetnye stroki," *Izvestiia*, August 3, 1938, 4; "Tabak novogo urozhaia," *Izvestiia*, October 11, 1939, 4.

132. A. Samoilov, "Dela tabachnye," *Pravda*, February 6, 1938, 6.

133. Victor Gordon Kiernan, *Tobacco: A History* (London: Hutchinson Radius, 1991), 163.

134. Yuri Slezkine, *The House of Government: A Saga of the Russian Revolution* (Princeton, NJ: Princeton University Press, 2017), 533; Sinel'nikov, *Delo—Tabak*, 22.

135. Aleksei Bogomilov, "Voroshilov sovetoval ustroi revoliutsiiu v Irane," *Komsomol'skaia pravda*, December 4–11, 2014, 10.

136. Goscilo and Lanoux, "Introduction," 13.

137. Thomas G. Schrand, "Socialism in One Gender: Masculine Values in the Stalin Revolution," in *Russian Masculinities in History and Culture*, ed. Barbara Evans Clements, Rebecca Friedman, and Dan Healey (London: Palgrave Macmillan, 2002), 194–209.

138. Victoria E. Bonnell, *Iconography of Power: Soviet Political Posters under Lenin and Stalin* (Berkeley: University of California Press, 1997), 161–62.

139. "Papirosy," *Pravda*, June 30, 1940, 3.

6. MOBILIZED

1. GARF f. R-5446, op. 46a, d. 7176, l. 64.

2. GARF f. R-5446, op. 46a, d. 7176, l. 88.

3. Catherine Merridale, *Ivan's War: Life and Death in the Red Army, 1939–1945* (New York: Metropolitan Books, 2006), 266.

4. Merridale, *Ivan's War*, 263–65.

5. Merridale, *Ivan's War*, 266, 274; Brandon Schechter, "The State's Pot and the Soldier's Spoon: Rations (*Paek*) in the Red Army," in *Hunger and War: Food Provisioning in the Soviet Union during World War II*, ed. Donald A. Filtzer and Wendy Z. Goldman (Bloomington: Indiana University Press, 2015), 105.

6. United States President, *Eighteenth Report to Congress on Lend-Lease Operations* (Washington, DC: Government Printing Office, 1944), 15, 52; Bius, *Smoke 'em if You Got 'em*, 68–71.

7. Novikova and Shchemelev, *Nasha marka*, 182.

8. F. S. Saushin, *Khleb i sol'* (Iaroslavl: Verkhne-Volzhskoe, 1983), 87–93, as quoted in Brandon Michael Schechter, *The Stuff of Soldiers: A History of the Red Army in World War II through Objects* (Ithaca, NY: Cornell University Press, 2019), 95.

9. Merridale, *Ivan's War*, 4; Larry E. Holmes, *Stalin's World War II Evacuations: Triumph and Troubles in Kirov* (Lawrence: University Press of Kansas, 2017), 30; Donald Filtzer and Wendy Z. Goldman, "Introduction: The Politics of Food and War," in *Hunger and War*, 11–12.

10. Starks, *Smoking under the Tsars*, 17–54.

11. Proctor, *Golden Holocaust*, 44.

12. Mikoian, "Zadachi tabachnoi promyshlennosti," 7.

13. Bor. Koval', "Tsennaia posylka," *Pravda*, July 7, 1934, 3.

14. "Papirosy vmesto vzryvchatykh veshchestv," *Izvestiia*, April 14, 1937, 2; "Nashimi ispanskim tovarishcham," *Pravda*, April 14, 1937, 5.

15. "Bratskaia pomoshch'," *Izvestiia*, October 4, 1939, 1.

16. "Zhizn' b'et kliuchom," *Izvestiia*, October 4, 1939, 1.

17. "V boiakh o Belofinnami," *Izvestiia*, December 5, 1939, 4.

18. John Barber and Mark Harrison, *The Soviet Home Front, 1941–1945: A Social and Economic History of the USSR in World War II* (London: Longman, 1991), 127; Holmes, *Stalin's World War II Evacuations*, 14–16; Wendy Z. Goldman and Donald Filtzer, *Fortress Dark and Stern: The Soviet Home Front during World War II* (New York: Oxford University Press, 2021), 2–9.

19. Rebecca Manley, *To the Tashkent Station: Evacuation and Survival in the Soviet Union at War* (Ithaca, NY: Cornell University Press, 2009), 1.

20. Holmes, *Stalin's World War II Evacuations*, 14; Lerri E. Kholms, [Larry Holmes] "Posle potopa: Soprotivlenie sovetskoi evakuatsii voennogo vremeni na mestakh

(1941–1945 gg.),'' in *Sovetskii tyl 1941–1945: Povsednevnaia zhizn' v gody voiny*, ed. Beate Fizeler [Fieseler] and Rodzher D. Markvik [Roger D. Markwick] (Moscow: Rosspen, 2019), 236–56; Goldman and Filtzer, *Fortress Dark and Stern*, 11–13.

21. Manley, *To the Tashkent Station*, 30–40.

22. Holmes gives an estimated span of 1,500–2,600 (*Stalin's World War II Evacuations*, 16).

23. Barber and Harrison, *Soviet Home Front*, 128–31; A. V. Khrulev, "Stanovlenie strategicheskogo tyla v Velikoi Otechestvennoi voine," *Voennyi-istoricheskii zhurnal*, no. 6 (1961): 64–80, as translated and excerpted in Seweryn Bialer, ed., *Stalin and His Generals: Soviet Military Memoirs of World War II* (New York: Pegasus, 1969), 369. See also Vasilii Petrovich Kuptsov, "Problemy perestroika narodnogo khoziaistva i evakuatsii mirnogo naseleniia v gody velikoi otechestvennoi voiny" (Doctor of Historical Sciences diss., Rossiiskaia ekonomicheskaia akademiia im. G. V. Plekhanova, Moscow, 2002), 41–43; and Bialer, *Stalin and His Generals*, 372.

24. "Vosstanovlenie tabachnykh plantatsii i fabrik," *Izvestiia*, January 6, 1945, 3; Malinin, *Tabachnaia istoriia Rossii*, 156–57.

25. Kholostov and Dikker, "Tabachnaia promyshlennost' za 50 let," 7; I. V. Moiseev, *Tabak i tabachnaia industriia: Vchera, segodnia, zavtra* (Moscow: Russkii tabak, 2002), 119.

26. Moiseev reported eighteen factories moved. An *Izvestiia* article from 1945 detailed fifteen factories in the outlined regions. Moiseev's connection to industry and later publication probably allowed a fuller accounting ("Vosstanovlenie tabachnykh plantatsii i fabrik," *Izvestiia*, January 6, 1945, 3).

27. Wendy Z. Goldman, "Not by Bread Alone: Food, Workers, and the State," in *Hunger and War*, 44–97; Malinin, *Tabachnaia istoriia Rossii*, 82.

28. Malinin, *Tabachnaia istoriia Rossii*, 237.

29. Kholostov and Dikker, "Tabachnaia promyshlennost' za 50 let," 7–8.

30. Another Leningrad tobacco factory, which was not evacuated, moved to gun, not bullet, production. When there was no metal, they produced wooden wheels for machine gun trolleys. See Bogdanov, *Dym otechestva*, 220. For the rumor, see Mandel, "Cigarettes in Soviet and Post-Soviet Central Asia," 184–85.

31. "Vvedenie," *Sovetskii tyl 1941–1945*, 16.

32. Barber and Harrison, *Soviet Home Front*, 62–63; Holmes, *Stalin's World War II Evacuations*, 30; Manley, *To the Tashkent Station*, 51–53, 104–6; Martin Krag, "Sovetskie zakony o trude v period Vtoroi mirovoi voiny (Na primer predpriiatii voennoi promyshlennosti)," in *Sovetskii tyl 1941–1945*, 69–88.

33. Novikova and Shchemelev, *Nasha marka*, 166–67.

34. Novikova and Shchemelev, *Nasha marka*, 167; Manley, *To the Tashkent Station*, 108–9.

35. Barber and Harrison, *Soviet Home Front*, 64.

36. Novikova and Shchemelev, *Nasha marka*, 188.

37. Novikova and Shchemelev, *Nasha marka*, 169–71; Holmes, *Stalin's World War II Evacuations*, 78.

38. Novikova and Shchemelev, *Nasha marka*, 173–75; Manley, *To the Tashkent Station*, 119–37.

39. Novikova and Shchemelev, *Nasha marka*, 173–75.

40. Holmes, *Stalin's World War II Evacuations*, 31, 33–35.

41. Holmes, *Stalin's World War II Evacuations*, 74–75, 124–46; Novikova and Shchemelev, *Nasha marka*, 173–75.

42. Barber and Harrison, *Soviet Home Front*, 97–98; Goldman and Filtzer, *Fortress Dark and Stern*, 231–62.

43. Holmes, *Stalin's World War II Evacuations*, 31, 33–35.

44. "Sovetskoe informbiuro," *Izvestiia*, July 20, 1941, 1.

45. Novikova and Shchemelev, *Nasha marka*, 155–65.

46. Novikova and Shchemelev, *Nasha marka*, 176–77.

47. Mark Harrison, *Accounting for War: Soviet Production, Employment, and the Defense Burden, 1940–1945* (Cambridge: Cambridge University Press, 1996), 199.

48. Harrison E. Salisbury, *The 900 Days: The Siege of Leningrad* (New York: Harper and Row, 1969), 513–17; Alexis Peri, *The War Within: Diaries from the Siege of Leningrad* (Cambridge, MA: Harvard University Press, 2017), 4; Manley, *To the Tashkent Station*, 55–58.

49. "Simvol trudovoi doblesti—kollektivu 1-i Lenignradskoi tabachnoi fabriki imeni Uritskogo," *Tabak*, no. 4 (1967): 2–3.

50. Barber and Harrison, *Soviet Home Front*, 75.

51. Malinin, *Tabachnaia istoriia Rossii*, 202; Salisbury, *900 Days*, 424.

52. N. Kniazeva, "Etot den' my priblizhali, kak mogli. . .," *Den' Respubliki*, no. 100 (May 24, 2010): 1–3.

53. Peri, *War Within*, 185.

54. Salisbury, *900 Days*, 492, 510.

55. Holmes, *Stalin's World War II Evacuations*, 32.

56. Euridika Charon Kardona, "Dvizhenie ogorodnichstva v sovetskom tylu v 1941–1945 gg.," in *Sovetskii tyl 1941–1945*, 58–59.

57. Barber and Harrison, *Soviet Home Front*, 78–79.

58. For more specific worker experience, see Mikhail Iu. Mukhin, "Sovetskie aviastroiteli v gody Velikoi Otechestvennoi voiny: Povsednevnaia zhizn' na fone voiny," Rodzher D. Markvik and Beate Fizeler, "'Kazhdoe poleno—udar po vragu!': Zhenshchiny v lesnoi promyshlennosti voennogo vremeni," and Dzhuli K. de Graffenrud, [Julie deGraffenried] "Mobilizuia iunost': Trud sovetskikh detei v voennoe vremia," all in *Sovetskii tyl 1941–1945*, 89–102, 103–25, and 126–46, respectively.

59. Donald Filtzer, "Starvation Mortality in Soviet Home-front Industrial Regions during World War II," in *Hunger and War*, 265–66.

60. Merridale, *Ivan's War*, 3, 116–18.

61. Bogdanov, *Dym otechestva*, 216–17.

62. GARF f. R-5446, op. 46a, d. 7176, l. 105.

63. Merridale, *Ivan's War*, 139.

64. William Moskoff, *The Bread of Affliction: The Food Supply in the USSR during World War II* (Cambridge: Cambridge University Press, 1990), 165.

65. Arsenii Formakov, *Gulag Letters*, ed. and trans. Emily D. Johnson (New Haven: Yale University Press, 2017), 65, 76.

66. Steven J. Jug, "Sensing Danger: The Red Army during the Second World War," in *Russian History through the Senses: From 1700 to the Present*, ed. Matthew P. Romaniello and Tricia Starks (London: Bloomsbury, 2016), 222–27.

67. Holmes, *Stalin's World War II Evacuations*, 30. Filtzer and Goldman, "Introduction," 11–12.

68. A. Rozen, "Posylki pribyli na front," *Izvestiia*, September 17, 1941, 3.

69. "Prazdnichnye podarki voinam Krasnoi Armii," *Pravda*, October 23, 1942, 4.

70. E. E. Koloskova, *Moskva v fotografiiakh, 1941–1945* (St. Petersburg: Liki Rossii, 2015), 209.

71. John Armstrong, ed., *The Soviet Partisans in World War II* (Madison: University of Wisconsin Press, 1964); Kenneth Slepyan, *Stalin's Guerrillas: Soviet Partisans in World War II* (Lawrence: University Press of Kansas, 2006), 1–14.

72. Neuburger, *Balkan Smoke*, 154.

73. Earl Ziemke, "Composition and Morale of the Partisan Movement," in *Soviet Partisans in World War II*, 179; and in the same volume, Gerhard L. Weinberg, "Case Studies," 397.

74. GARF f. R-5446, op. 43a, d. 8607, l. 1.

75. GARF f. R-5446, op. 43a, d. 8607, l. 2.

76. GARF f. R-5446, op. 43a, d. 8607, l. 4.

77. Albert L. Weeks, *Russia's Life-Saver: Lend-Lease Aid to the U.S.S.R in World War II* (Lanham, MD: Lexington Books, 2004), 151; George C. Herring, Jr., *Aid to Russia, 1941–1946: Strategy, Diplomacy, the Origins of the Cold War* (New York: Columbia University Press, 1973), 125, 230.

78. Schechter, *Stuff of Soldiers*, 187–88.

79. "Soveshchanie nachal'nikov otdelov agitatsii i propagandy politupravlenii frontov i okrugov," *Agitator i propagandist Krasnoi Armii*, no. 5–6 (1943): 22, as quoted in Schechter, "State's Pot," 129.

80. Schechter, "State's Pot," 111–13.

81. GARF f. R-5446, op. 461, d. 7178, l. 16.

82. GARF f. R-5446, op. 461, d. 7178, l. 14.

83. GARF f. R-5446, op. 461, d. 7178, l. 22; GARF f. R-5446, op. 461, d. 7177, l. 70.

84. GARF f. R-5446 op. 461, d. 7177, ll. 55–56.

85. J. Lucas, *War on the Eastern Front: The German Soldier in Russia, 1941–1945*, 31–33, as referenced in Richard Overy, *Russia's War: A History of the Soviet War Effort, 1941–1945* (New York: Penguin, 1997), 87.

86. Gately, *Tobacco*, 258.

87. Brandon Michael Schechter, "Governmental Issue: The Material Culture of the Red Army, 1941–1945" (PhD diss., University of California, Berkeley, 2015), 114n689.

88. A. P. Chekhov, "O vrede tabaka," *Zagadochnaia natura: Rasskazy* (Moscow: Izdatel'stvo Narodnogo komissariata oborony, 1944), 57–64. For a discussion of the text, see Starks, *Smoking under the Tsars*, 228–29.

89. Anthony Beevor, *The Second World War* (Boston: Little, Brown, 2012), 365.

90. N. A. Panomareva, *O lechenii lits, kuriashchikh tabak (instruktivno-metodicheskoe pis'mo)* (Moscow: Rosglavpoligrafprom, 1965), 14. Later research found that cytisine behaves in a manner like nicotine in the brain and has been found effective in cessation. See Piotr Tutka and Witold Zatoński, "Cytisine for the Treatment of Nicotine Addiction: From a Molecule to Therapeutic Efficacy," *Pharmacological Reports*, no. 58 (2005): 778.

91. GARF f. R-5446, op. 46a, d. 7176, l. 62.

92. GARF f. R-5446, op. 461, d. 7177, l. 62.

93. GARF f. R-5446, op. 461, d. 7177, l. 65.

94. GARF f. R-5446, op. 461, d. 7177, l. 63.

95. GARF f. R-5446, op. 461, d. 7177, ll. 44–43.

96. GARF f. R-5446, op. 461, d. 7178, l. 18; GARF f. R-5446, op. 461, d. 7177, l. 1.

97. GARF f. R-5446, op. 46a, d. 7176, l. 48.

98. Schechter, "Governmental Issue," 112.

99. Sinel'nikov, *Delo—Tabak*, 214.

100. Lev Kopelev, *Khranit' vechno* (Moscow: TERRA, 2004), 1:14, as translated in Schecter, *Stuff of Soldiers*, 140.

101. Gately, *Tobacco*, 258.

102. V. Poltoratskii, "Noch' na perednem krae," *Izvestiia*, September 17, 1941, 3.

103. Schechter, "Governmental Issue," 20.

104. Jug, "Sensing Danger," 231.

105. Schechter, "Governmental Issue," 111.

106. Vasily Grossman, *A Writer at War: A Soviet Journalist with the Red Army, 1941–1945* (New York: Vintage, 2005), 173.

107. P. Rod'kin, "Iz praktiki moei vospitatel'noi raboty," *Agitator i propagandist Krasnoi Armii: Zhurnal glavnogo politicheskogo upravleniia RKKA*, no. 18 (1944): 30. Thanks to Brandon Schechter for this reference.

108. "Davai zakurim," in A. Lukovnikov, *Druz'ia-odnopolchane: Rasskazy pesniakh, rozhdennykh voinoi, melodii i teksty* (Moscow: Muzak, 1985), 32–33, as quoted in Schechter, "State's Pot," 140.

109. Schechter, "Governmental Issue," 133; for full lyrics, see "Davai zakurim," https://победа.екатеринбург.рф/медиа/песни/закурим.

110. K. Listov (music) and M. Ruderman (lyrics), *Makhorochka*, trans. Paula Stone (New York: Russian-American Music Publishers, 1943).

111. Moiseev, *Tabak i tabachnaia industriia*, 119; Novikova and Shchemelev, *Nasha marka*, 196; Malinin, *Tabachnaia istoriia Rossii*, 156.

7. RECOVERED

1. Kholostov and Dikker, "Tabachnaia promyshlennost' za 50 let," 7.

2. Sinel'nikov, *Delo—Tabak*, 21.

3. Sinel'nikov, *Delo—Tabak,* 16; Kifuriak, *Tabachnaia fabrika "Iava,"* 23–24.

4. Sinel'nikov, email correspondence to author, March 10, 2021.

5. Raisa B. Deber, "The Limits of Persuasion: Anti-Smoking Activities in the USSR," *Canadian Journal of Public Health* 72, no. 2 (1981): 119. This article was housed in the industry documents collection for their research wing, https://industrydocuments.library.ucsf.edu/tobacco/docs/jydb0032.

6. Frances Bernstein, "Prosthetic Manhood in the Soviet Union at the End of World War II," *Osiris* 30, no. 1 (2015): 114; Nina Tumarkin, "The Great Patriotic War as Myth and Memory," *European Review* 1, no. 4 (2003): 595–611.

7. Donald Filtzer, "Standard of Living versus Quality of Life: Struggling with the Urban Environment in Russia during the Early Years of Post-war Reconstruction," in *Late Stalinist Russia: Society between Reconstruction and Reinvention*, ed. Juliane Fürst (London: Routledge, 2006), 81–102.

8. Elena Zubkova, *Russia after the War: Hopes, Illusions, and Disappointments, 1945–1957* (Armonk, NY: M. E. Sharpe, 1998), 23–25, 40–47; Kristy Ironside, *A Full-Value Ruble: The Promise of Prosperity in the Postwar Soviet Union* (Cambridge, MA: Harvard University Press, 2021), 1–17.

9. Philip Hanson, *The Rise and Fall of the Soviet Economy* (London: Longman, 2003), 22, 25–28.

10. "Uvelichivaetsia proizvodstvo papiros," *Izvestiia*, June 9, 1945, 1.

11. Malinin, *Tabachnaia istoriia Rossii*, 156–57.

12. "Vosstanovlenie tabachnykh plantatsii i fabrik," *Izvestiia*, January 6, 1945, 3.

13. Novikova and Shchemelev, *Nasha marka*, 179–83; "Vosstanovlenie tabachnykh plantatsii i fabrik"; Malinin, *Tabachnaia istoriia Rossii*, 221.

14. Novikova and Shchemelev, *Nasha marka*, 182.

15. "Vypusk papiros uvelichivaetsia," *Izvestiia*, November 15, 1946, 2; "Ot rabotnits, rabochikh, inzhenerov, tekhnikov i sluzhashchikh tabachnykh fabric ministerstva vkusovoi promyshlennosti Soiuza SSR tovarishchu Stalinu I. V.," *Izvestiia*, April 30, 1947, 2, and May 19, 1947, 1–2; "Vosstanovlenie tabachnykh plantatsii i fabrik."

16. "Vosstanovlenie tabachnykh plantatsii i fabrik."

17. "Milliard papiros."

18. V. Bordonos, *Opyt raboty fabrichnogo komiteta Khar'kovskoi tabachnaia fabrika pro organizatsiia sotsialisicheskogo sorevnovaniia* (Kiev: URSPS, 1954), 3.

19. "Leningradskie papirosy," *Izvestiia*, October 25, 1945, 1.

20. Korno and Kitainer, *Balkanskaia zvezda*, 145.

21. M. Ivanova, "Na 2 milliarda papiros bol'she, chem v proshlom godu," *Pravda*, October 10, 1945, 2.

22. Kholostov and Dikker, "Tabachnaia promyshlennost' za 50 let," 8.

23. S. G. S— (obscured), "Dadim strane bol'she makhorka," *Tabak*, no. 2 (1956): 27–29.

24. Lillard and Dorofeeva, "Smoking in Russia and Ukraine," 124–25.

25. Greta Bucher, *Women, the Bureaucracy, and Daily Life in Postwar Moscow, 1945–1953* (Boulder, CO: East European Monographs, 2006), 27–28, 78–79.

26. Sinel'nikov, *Delo—Tabak,* quotation 14, conditions 42–43.

27. D. Beliaev, "Na torgovye temy: Ost i khvost," *Pravda*, March 20, 1948, 2.

28. M. Gusev, "O tabachnykh izdeliiakh," *Izvestiia*, October 22, 1953, 2.

29. "Soobshchaem adresa," *Krokodil*, no. 13 (1950): 2.

30. V. Klochenko, "Uvazhzevyi krokodil!" *Krokodil*, no. 35 (1950): 15.

31. Bucher, *Women, the Bureaucracy, and Daily Life*, 3–12; Sheila Fitzpatrick, "War and Society in Soviet Context: Soviet Labor before, during, and after World War II," *International Labor and Working-Class History*, no. 35 (1989): 37, 42, 43, 46; Manley, *To the Tashkent Station*, 254, 265; Zubkova, *Russia after the War*, 4–5.

32. Zubkova, *Russia after the War*, 22–25, 36, 401–5.

33. Greta Bucher, "Struggling to Survive: Soviet Women in the Postwar Years," *Journal of Women's History* 12, no. 1 (2000): 139.

34. Zubkova, *Russia after the War*, 20.

35. Mie Nakachi, *Replacing the Dead: The Politics of Reproduction in the Postwar Soviet Union* (New York: Oxford University Press, 2021), 88–152; Claire E. McCallum, *The Fate of the New Man: Representing and Reconstructing Masculinity in Soviet Visual Culture, 1945–1965* (DeKalb: Northern Illinois University Press, 2018), 137.

36. Zubkova, *Russia after the War*, 21.

37. Jennifer Utrata, *Women without Men: Single Mothers and Family Change in the New Russia* (Ithaca, NY: Cornell University Press, 2015), 25–26.

38. Julie Hessler, "A Postwar Perestroika? Toward a History of Private Enterprise in the USSR," *Slavic Review* 57, no. 3 (1998): 516–42.

39. Paulina Bren and Mary Neuburger, "Introduction," in *Communism Unwrapped: Consumption in Cold War Eastern Europe*, ed. Paulina Bren and Mary Neuburger (Oxford: Oxford University Press, 2012), 13; A. V. Mitrofanova, ed., *Rabochii klass SSSR, 1966–1970* (Moscow: Nauka, 1979), 52.

40. Lewis H. Siegelbaum, *Cars for Comrades: The Life of the Soviet Automobile* (Ithaca, NY: Cornell University Press, 2008), 84, 223.

41. Steven Harris, *Communism on Tomorrow Street: Mass Housing and Everyday Life after Stalin* (Baltimore: Johns Hopkins University Press, 2013), 192; Siegelbaum, *Cars for Comrades*, 84; Anna Ivanova, "Socialist Consumption and Brezhnev's Stagnation: A Reappraisal of Late Communist Everyday Life," *Kritika: Explorations in Russian and Eurasian History* 17, no. 3 (2016): 665–78; Christine Varga-Harris, *Stories of House and Home: Soviet Apartment Life during the Khrushchev Years* (Ithaca, NY: Cornell University Press, 2016), 1–10.

42. Susan E. Reid, "Cold War in the Kitchen: Gender and the De-stalinization of Consumer Taste in the Soviet Union under Khrushchev," *Slavic Review* 61, no. 2 (2002): 211–17.

43. Natalya Chernyshova, *Soviet Consumer Culture in the Brezhnev Era* (London: Routledge, 2013), 2–3, 6–7; Ivanova, "Socialist Consumption," 665–78; Lewis H. Siegelbaum, "Cars, Cars, and More Cars: The Faustian Bargain of the Brezhnev Era," in *Borders of Socialism: Private Spheres of Soviet Russia*, ed. Lewis H. Siegelbaum (New York: Palgrave, 2006), 88; James R. Millar, "The Little Deal: Brezhnev's Contribution to Acquisitive Socialism," *Slavic Review* 44, no. 4 (1985): 694–706.

44. Vera Dunham, *In Stalin's Time: Middleclass Values in Soviet Fiction* (New York: Cambridge University Press, 1976); Jukka Gronow, *Caviar with Champagne: Common Luxury and the Ideals of the Good Life in Stalin's Russia* (Oxford: Berg, 2003).

45. David Crowley and Susan E. Reid, "Style and Socialism: Modernity and Material Culture in Post-War Eastern Europe," in *Style and Socialism: Modernity and Material Culture in Post-War Eastern Europe*, ed. Susan E. Reid and David Crowley (Oxford: Berg, 2000), 10–12.

46. Deborah A. Field, *Private Life and Communist Morality in Khrushchev's Russia* (New York: Peter Lang, 2007), 3, 17.

47. Susan E. Reid, "Destalinization and Taste, 1953–1963," *Journal of Design History* 10, no. 2 (1997): 177, 180, 185; Elena Kochetkova, "Milk and Milk Packaging in the Soviet Union: Technologies of Production and Consumption, 1950s–1970s," *Russian History* 46, no. 1 (2019): 30, 46–47.

48. Kurii Gerchuk, "The Aesthetics of Everyday Life in the Khrushchev Thaw in the USSR (1954–64)," in *Style and Socialism*, 81, 89–90.

49. M. V. Kuralev, "Uluchshit' assortiment etiketnoi bumagi dlia tabachnykh izdelii," *Tabak*, no. 5 (1954): 15–17.

50. Anon., "O chem pishut potrebiteli," *Tabak*, no. 5 (1953): 6–8.

51. Sinel'nikov, *Delo—Tabak*, 126.

52. Walter L. Hixson, *Parting the Curtain: Propaganda, Culture, and the Cold War, 1945–1961* (New York: St. Martin's Griffin, 1997), xi–xiv.

53. Milov, *Cigarette*, 88.

54. Sarah Milov, "Smoking as Statecraft: Promoting American Tobacco Production and Global Cigarette Consumption, 1947–1970," *Journal of Policy History* 28, no. 4 (2016): 718–25.

55. Hixson, *Parting the Curtain*, 185–201; Greg Castillo, *Cold War on the Home Front: The Soft Power of Midcentury Design* (Minneapolis: University of Minnesota Press, 2010), xxii–xxiii.

56. Castillo, *Cold War on the Home Front*, xi–xxi, 130–33, and image of smoking in relaxed American home on 31; Elena Kochetkova, "'A Shop Window Where You Can Choose the Goods You Like': Finnish Industrial and Trade Fairs in the USSR, 1950s–1960s," *Scandinavian Journal of History* 43, no. 2 (2018): 1–21.

57. Milov, *Cigarette*, 93.

58. Occasionally prerevolutionary makers stuffed the papirosy tubes with batting. The first manufactured filtered cigarettes in the USSR came out in 1928. From 1947 to 1954 the number of filter cigarettes produced nearly tripled. According to a 1956 article in *Tabak*, the packed tobacco of a cigarette itself worked as a filter, which was why "the taste of the second half of a cigarette always is harsher" (G. L. Dikker, "Sigarety s fil'truiushchimi mundshtukami," *Tabak*, no. 2 [1956]: 27–29). This was an opinion popular in the prerevolutionary period. Smokers were urged to quit a cigarette at halfway.

59. Proctor, *Golden Holocaust*, 343–47, 349, 354–55, 384–88.

60. Sheila Fitzpatrick, "Postwar Soviet Society: 'The Return to Normalcy,' 1945–1953," in *The Impact of World War II on the Soviet Union*, ed. Susan J. Linz (Totowa, NJ: Rowman and Allanheld, 1985), 129–56.

61. "Tabachnaia promyshlennost' za 40 let"; Malinin, *Tabachnaia istoriia Rossii*, 159–60.

62. Kifuriak, *Tabachnaia fabrika "Iava,"* 23–24.

63. Sinel'nikov, *Delo—Tabak*, 28, 51–52.

64. Field, *Private Life and Communist Morality*, 17; Reid, "Destalinization and Taste," 177–201.

65. Sinel'nikov, *Delo—Tabak*, 28, 51–52.

66. Sinel'nikov, *Delo—Tabak*, 40.

67. Sinel'nikov, *Delo—Tabak*, 54–55.

68. Sinel'nikov, *Delo—Tabak*, 54–55.

69. Sinel'nikov, email correspondence to author, March 10, 2021.

70. Elizaveta Gorchakova, "The Iava Tobacco Factory from the 1960s to the Early 1990s: An Interview with the Former Director, Leonid Iakovlevich Sinel'nikov," in *Tobacco in Russian History and Culture*, 213.

71. Francis K. Decker to Frederick P. Haas, VP and General Counsel Liggett and Myers, Inc., "Marketing to Youth," August 1968, https://www.industrydocuments.ucsf.edu/docs/yspj0045.

72. Sinel'nikov, *Delo—Tabak*, 104.

73. Sinel'nikov, *Delo—Tabak*, 54–55.

74. Sinel'nikov, *Delo—Tabak*, 28, 51–52.

75. Gorchakova, "Iava Tobacco Factory," 214.

76. Starks, *Smoking under the Tsars*, 208–11.

77. Kholostov and Dikker, "Tabachnaia promyshlennost' za 50 let," 8. See also "O gosu-darstvennom plane razvitiia narodnogo khoziaistva SSSR na 1971 god," *Izvestiia*, December 8, 1970, 2.

78. Gorchakova, "Iava Tobacco Factory," 217; Neuburger, *Balkan Smoke*, 222.

79. Sinel'nikov, *Delo—Tabak*, 96; Moiseev, *Tabak i tabachnaia industriia*, 121.

80. Sinel'nikov, *Delo—Tabak*, 36–38, 122, 144.

81. Sinel'nikov, *Delo—Tabak*, 31–33.

82. G. L. Dikker, "Patenty: Sposoby snizheniia vrednosti kureniia tabaka," *Tabak*, no. 1 (1974): 57–59; Nina Ivanovna Semenova, "Issledovanie aromaticheskikh veshchestv tabaka i ikh izmenenie v protsessakh tekhnologicheskoi pererabotki" (PhD diss., Krasno-darskii politekhnicheskii institut, 1975).

83. Wjatscheslaw Feonow, "USSR—Tendency to Filter Cigarettes," *Tabak: Journal International* (October 1974), https://www.industrydocuments.ucsf.edu/docs/jppy0124; Demin, *Rossiia*, 49; Neuburger, *Balkan Smoke*, 2, 210–14; Mary Neuburger, "Smokes for Big Brother: Bulgaria, the USSR, and the Politics of Tobacco in the Cold War," in *Tobacco in Russian History and Culture*, 226; Mary Neuberger, "The Taste of Smoke: Bulgartabak and the Manufacturing of Cigarettes and Satisfaction," in *Communism Unwrapped*, 91–115; *Tobacco Reporter*, "Russia's Output for 1974 at 373 Billion Cigarettes," https://www.industry documents.ucsf.edu/docs/htyy0076.

84. James W. Markham, "Is Advertising Important in the Soviet Economy?," *Journal of Marketing* 28, no. 2 (1964): 31.

85. S. V. Serebriakov, *Organizatsiia i tekhnika sovetskoi torgovli* (Moscow: Gostorgizdat, 1956), 76, as quoted in Carter R. Bryan, "Communist Advertising: Its Status and Functions," *Journalism Quarterly* 39, no. 4 (1962): 505–6; Buralenko, *Razvitie sovetskoi torgovoi reklamy*, 21.

86. Markham, "Is Advertising Important," 31–37.

87. "Russian Thinks Again about Advertising," *Times of London*, February 24, 1961, 13.

88. L. V. Orlovskii, "Kurit'—ne tol'ko sebia gubit'," *Gigiena i sanitariia*, no. 9 (1969): 38–39.

89. Zorii Shokin, "Kuril'shik: V sotsiologicheskom i meditsinskom aspektakh," *Literaturnaia gazeta*, August 18, 1971, 13.

90. Sinel'nikov, email correspondence to author, March 10, 2021; Philip Hanson, *Advertising and Socialism: The Nature and Extent of Consumer Advertising in the Soviet Union, Poland, Hungary, and Yugoslavia* (White Plains, NY: International Arts and Sciences Press, 1974), 1–76.

91. Elizabeth Swayne, "Soviet Advertising: Communism Imitates Capitalism to Survive," in *The Role of Advertising: A Book of Readings*, ed. C. H. Sandage and Vernon Fryburger (Homewood, IL: Richard D. Irwin, 1960), 97.

92. M. R. Morolev, *Sovetskaia pechatnaia vneshnetorgovaia reklama* (Moscow: Zaochnii institut sovetskoi torgovli, 1964), 3–9; Markham, "Is Advertising Important," 35.

93. Juliane Fürst, "The Importance of Being Stylish: Youth, Culture, and Identity in Late Stalinism," in *Late Stalinist Russia*, 209–30, and *Stalin's Last Generation: Soviet Post-War Youth and the Emergence of Mature Socialism* (Oxford: Oxford University Press, 2010), 217–35.

94. Karpova, *Comradely Objects*, 49.

95. Timothy Ryback, *Rock around the Bloc: A History of Rock Music in Eastern Europe and the Soviet Union* (New York: Oxford University Press, 1990), 10, as referenced in Crowley and Reid, "Style and Socialism," 15.

96. Hixson, *Parting the Curtain*, 116.

97. This was true of many western goods (Chernyshova, *Soviet Consumer Culture*, 113–20).

98. Sinel'nikov, *Delo—Tabak*, 104; L. Khudiakov, "Obez'iany" cover for *Boevoi karandal*, no. 38 (1957), as featured in G. Demosfenova, A. Nurok, and N. Shantyko, *Sovetskii politicheskii plakat* (Moscow: Iskusstvo, 1962), 410.

99. Brian LaPierre, *Hooligans in Khrushchev's Russia: Defining, Policing, and Producing Deviance during the Thaw* (Madison: University of Wisconsin Press, 2012), 36–37.

100. Sinel'nikov, *Delo—Tabak*, 54, 97, 123–24, 222, 231.

101. McCallum, *Fate of the New Man*, 1–20; Robert Dale, "Rats and Resentment: The Demobilization of the Red Army in Postwar Leningrad, 1945–1950," *Journal of Contemporary History* 45, no. 1 (2010): 119.

102. Starks, *Smoking under the Tsars*, 147–48.

103. McCallum, *Fate of the New Man*, 42.

104. Zubkova, *Russia after the War*, 28.

105. McCallum, *Fate of the New Man*, 26, 33–34; Ethan Pollock, *Without the Banya We Would Perish: A History of the Russian Bathhouse* (New York: Oxford University Press, 2019), 198–99.

106. McCallum, *Fate of the New Man*, 149.

107. Editors, "50 geroicheskikh let," *Tabak*, no. 1 (1967): 4–5.

8. PARTNERED

1. Sinel'nikov, *Delo—Tabak*, 61–74, 96, 126.

2. Sinel'nikov, *Delo—Tabak*, 210.

3. Sinel'nikov, email correspondence to author, November 1, 2019.

4. Gorchakova, "Iava Tobacco Factory," 213. Susan E. Reid, "This Is Tomorrow! Becoming a Consumer in the Soviet Sixties," in *The Socialist Sixties: Crossing Borders in the Second World War*, ed. Anne E. Gorsuch and Diane P. Koenker (Bloomington: Indiana University Press, 2013), 28.

5. Helena Goscilo, "Luxuriating in Lack: Plentitude and Consuming Happiness in Soviet Paintings and Posters, 1930s–1953," in *Petrified Utopia: Happiness Soviet Style*, ed. Marina Balina and Evgeny Dobrenko (London: Anthem, 2009), 53–78; Natalya Chernyshova, "Consumers as Citizens: Revisiting the Question of Public Disengagement in the Brezhnev Era," in *Reconsidering Stagnation in the Brezhnev Era: Ideology and Exchange*, ed. Dina Fainberg and Artemy Kalinovsky (Lanham, MD: Lexington Books, 2016), 3–5.

6. Reid, "Cold War in the Kitchen," 222–23.

7. GARF f. R-5587, op. 19, d. 1095, l. 8.

8. Sinel'nikov, *Delo—Tabak*, 198.

9. Sinel'nikov, *Delo—Tabak*, 199.

10. Sinel'nikov, *Delo—Tabak*, 199. Similar import of machinery happened for wine (Bittner, *Whites and Reds*, 208).

11. Sinel'nikov, *Delo—Tabak*, 207–8.

12. Sinel'nikov, *Delo—Tabak*, 196.

13. Milov, *Cigarette*, 47–116.

14. H. J. Maidenberg, "Tobacco Men are Seeking Ways to Spur Export Volume," March 14, 1964, https://www.industrydocuments.ucsf.edu/docs/sndv0024.

15. P. Shepherd, "Transnational Corporations and the International Cigarette Industry," *Market Structure and Industrial Performance* 15 (1994): 164–65; National Center for Chronic Disease Prevention and Health Promotion, (US) Office on Smoking and Health, "The Health Consequences of Smoking—50 Years of Progress: A Report of the Surgeon General," https://www.ncbi.nlm.nih.gov/pubmed/24455788.

16. *Tobacco Reporter*, "Soviet Union 'Demanding' Better Made Foreign Cigarettes," March 1975, https://www.industrydocuments.ucsf.edu/docs/psfb0020, esp. 40. On the "Iron Curtain of taste," see Neuburger, *Balkan Smoke*, 199–200.

17. Neuburger, *Balkan Smoke*, 214, 274n71.

18. Milov, *Cigarette*, 89–94.

19. World Tobacco, "Soviet Union: Machinery on Display," June 1972, https://www.industrydocuments.ucsf.edu/docs/znvg0117; Shepherd, "Transnational Corporations," 162.

20. J. Heymans, "Report Visit to Moscow," June 26 1964, 3–5, https://www.industrydocuments.ucsf.edu/docs/ntml0127.

21. Neuburger, *Balkan Smoke*, 211. See also with wine (Bittner, *Whites and Reds*, 179).

22. *Tobacco Reporter*, "Russia's Demand for Imports," August 1972, https://www.industrydocuments.ucsf.edu/docs/npgj0127.

23. The Tobacco Institute (f. 1958), an offshoot of the Tobacco Industry Research Committee (f. 1954), was heavily involved in the creation of a haze of distrust for the science around tobacco danger through publications that declared the science inconclusive. The group sponsored tobacco research but focused largely on nontobacco-related disease, preferring instead to find work that blamed heredity, infection, nutrition, hormones, nervous strain, and environment (Proctor, *Golden Holocaust*, 257–63).

24. Neuburger, *Balkan Smoke*, 211–14; Mateusz Zygmunt Zatoński, "State, Society, and the Politics of Smoking in Poland, during and after Communism (1960–2000)" (PhD diss., University of London, 2018), 32–33.

25. Richard Halloran, "Six U.S. Firms Defy Boycott Threat for Importing Yugoslav Tobacco," October 12, 1965, https://www.industrydocuments.ucsf.edu/docs/tmyk0016; R. J. Reynolds Tobacco Company, December 27, 1966, https://www.industrydocuments.ucsf.edu/docs/#id=qjnw0043. See also https://www.industrydocuments.ucsf.edu/docs/tpyk0016; https://www.industrydocuments.ucsf.edu/docs/fhjd0130; and https://www.industrydocuments.ucsf.edu/docs/tsbc0102.

26. US Department of Commerce, "Overseas Business Reports," January 1974, https://www.industrydocuments.ucsf.edu/docs/rxcy0124, quotations 1, 3, 11, 15. Increased initiatives for trade were seen across the bloc (Neuburger, *Balkan Smoke*, 221).

27. A. G. Buzzi, A. Gembler, D. A. Morse, and W. S. Surrey, "Philip Morris Mission to Moscow—Confidential Report," June 17, 1973, https://www.industrydocuments.ucsf.edu/tobacco/docs/lrhb0048.

28. H. Wakeham, "Project Red Carpet," October 16, 1973, https://www.industrydocuments.ucsf.edu/docs/gfhj0127. The preliminary plan for the "Mission to Moscow" expanded on work by representatives of PM-Europe and the Washington, DC, law firm of Surrey, Karasik, and Morse (Buzzi et al., "Philip Morris Mission to Moscow").

29. Buzzi et al., "Philip Morris Mission to Moscow," 7–10.

30. Buzzi et al., "Philip Morris Mission to Moscow," 14–15.

31. Buzzi et al., "Philip Morris Mission to Moscow," 15–16.

32. PM and BAT would be the primary combatants, with RJR a lesser challenger. Ligget and Lorillard were not as successful (Shepherd, "Transnational Corporations," 165–66). The Soviets mention RJR to the PM executives in "Major Issues: Philip Morris Mission to Moscow," March 18–22, 1974, https://www.industrydocuments.ucsf.edu/docs/qlhj0127, quotations 6, 7.

33. John Thompson, "Memo: Russia," June 25, 1973, https://www.industrydocuments. ucsf.edu/docs/zzgj0127.

34. The IRI was started in 1938 under the National Research Council and was organized to help private company research and development teams (H. Fusfeld, "I.R.I. Representatives," July 2, 1973, https://www.industrydocuments.ucsf.edu/docs/hsgj0127; R. A. Ioanes, letter to H. Kornegay, "Tobacco Institute, Inc.," July 25, 1973, https://www.industry documents.ucsf.edu/docs/nljw0130; H. Kornegay, "Letter to J. F. Cullman," August 1, 1973, https://www.industrydocuments.ucsf.edu/docs/fxld0131).

35. H. Wakeham, "USSR Project," August 8, 1973, https://www.industrydocuments. ucsf.edu/docs/jfhj0127.

36. "U.S.S.R.—Tobacco," July 25, 1973, https://www.industrydocuments.ucsf.edu/ docs/ftbb0114.

37. For more on the American attempts to trade Pepsi for Soviet goods, see Bittner, "Problem of Taste," 317–23, and *Whites and Reds*, 178–207; A. Gembler and S. W. Surrey, "Philip Morris: Second Mission to Moscow," September 9, 1973, http://industry documents.library/ucsf.edu/tobacco/docs/krhb0048; and "Annual Report for PepsiCo, Inc.," March 1, 1975, https://www.industrydocuments.ucsf.edu/docs/npfw0229.

38. Gembler, "Second Mission," 10.

39. Gembler, "Second Mission," 20–21.

40. Gembler, "Second Mission," 25–26.

41. Philip Morris Incorporated (hereafter PMI), "Mission to Moscow," December 7, 1973, https://www.industrydocuments.ucsf.edu/docs/hfhj0127.

42. Castillo, *Cold War on the Home Front*, 133.

43. "Report of Meetings with Soviet Tobacco Representatives," December 18, 1973, https://www.industrydocuments.ucsf.edu/docs/nldb0106; "Summary of December Trip to Moscow," December 11, 1973, https://www.industrydocuments.ucsf.edu/docs/ nnhj0127.

44. "Report of Meetings with Soviet Tobacco Representatives," quotations 31, 34.

45. State Committee of the Council of Ministers of the USSR for Science and Technology and PMI, "Agreement," December 27, 1973, https://www.industrydocuments.ucsf. edu/docs/yyby0124.

46. Ward, "Moscow Symposium," February 7, 1974, https://www.industrydocuments. ucsf.edu/docs/fyvy0124.

47. "Philip Morris Symposium Tobacco Presentation Introduction," February 15, 1974, https://www.industrydocuments.ucsf.edu/docs/klhj0127; English with Russian (and some visuals) at Philip Morris Symposium, "Tobacco Presentation Introduction," February 15, 1974, https://www.industrydocuments.ucsf.edu/docs/hnhj0127.

48. See, briefly, Malinin, *Tabachnaia istoriia Rossii*, 165; Korno and Kitainer, *Balkanskaia zvezda*, 161. On visa problems, see H. Wakeham and H. B. Merritt, "Report of Meetings with USSR Tobacco Representatives," April 17, 1974, https://www.industry documents.ucsf.edu/docs/xxcy0124, quotations 1, 3.

49. Wakeham and Merritt, "Report," 1, 3.

50. Wakeham and Merritt, "Report."

51. Wakeham and Merritt, "Report."

52. H. Cullman, "USSR Strategy," April 19, 1974, https://www.industrydocuments. ucsf.edu/docs/zmby0124.

53. A. G. Buzzi, "Urgent," May 21, 1974, https://www.industrydocuments.ucsf.edu/ docs/jmby0124.

54. Buzzi, "Urgent."

55. Buzzi, "Urgent."

56. S. Ward. "Moscow Mission," September 9,1974, https://www.industrydocuments. ucsf.edu/docs/rghj0127.

57. Kifuriak, *Tabachnaia fabrika "Iava,"* 29.

58. Sinel'nikov, *Delo—Tabak*, 189–90.

59. Wakeham and Merritt, "Report"; "Visit to Yritskago Factory," March 22, 1974, https://www.industrydocuments.ucsf.edu/docs/gyhj0127.

60. Sinel'nikov, *Delo—Tabak*, 189–90.

61. Sinel'nikov, *Delo—Tabak*, 192.

62. "Pervyi chelovek v otkrytom kosmose byl khudozhnikom," *Novaia gazeta*, October 11, 2019, https://www.novayagazeta.ru/articles/2019/10/11/82319-dvazhdy-geroy-rossii-pervyy-chelovek-v-otkrytom-kosmose-i-hudozhnik-fantast.

63. J. L. Ems. Brown and Williamson Tobacco Company, "Apollo/Soyuz," October 1, 1975 https://www.industrydocuments.ucsf.edu/docs/hmjj0197.

64. V. B. Lougee, III, "Apollo-Soyuz Cigarettes Developed by Philip Morris, Inc., and Glavtabak, U.S.S.R.," September 19, 1975, http://industrydocuments.library.ucsf.edu/ tobacco/docs/hnfm0134.

65. The Finns, because of postwar reparation payments, had early entry into the Soviet market and industrial cooperation (Kochetkova, "'Shop Window,'" 4–14; Sinel'nikov, *Delo—Tabak*, 53).

66. "Notes re U.S.S.R. Ministry of Food Apollo Soyuz Cigarette Project," June 9, 1975, https://www.industrydocuments.ucsf.edu/docs/mskd0068.

67. Sinel'nikov, *Delo—Tabak*, 192.

68. Sinel'nikov, *Delo—Tabak*, 192.

69. "Commemorative Cigarette Brands," July 18, 1975, https://www.industry documents.ucsf.edu/docs/jgxx0127.

70. Jack Mills, "Dear Jim," August 5, 1975, https://www.industrydocuments.ucsf.edu/ docs/zmmd0047.

71. "Synopsis of Press, Radio and Television Coverage," July 15, 1975, https://www. industrydocuments.ucsf.edu/docs/gfdm0087.

72. Philip Morris Inc., "Circular no. 444 Amended," July 14, 1975, https://www.industry documents.ucsf.edu/docs/jhbj0099.

73. The Americans had sent special carton-packing machines to the Soviets, but these were not sufficient (Sinel'nikov, *Delo—Tabak*, 193; A. Gembler, A. Beuchat, and P. Greenfield, "Trip to Moscow," October 1975, https://www.industrydocuments.ucsf.edu/docs/ qzpn0124).

74. N. E. Lincoln, "Corporate Products Committee Meeting," December 14, 1976, https://www.industrydocuments.ucsf.edu/docs/rldy0108.

75. *Philip Morris News*, "Marlboro to Be Marketed under License in the USSR," March 1977, https://www.industrydocuments.ucsf.edu/docs/tpdb0102.

76. *Wall Street Journal*, "Philip Morris Says Soviet to Make Own Marlboros," January 18, 1977, https://www.industrydocuments.ucsf.edu/docs/tjyk0040.

77. Malinin, *Tabachnaia istoriia Rossii*, 165n72; Moiseev, *Tabak i tabachnaia industriia*, 122.

78. GARF f. R-8009, op. 50, d. 9245, ll. 94–95.

79. Sinel'nikov details many of the issues with consistency in Gorchakova, "Iava Tobacco Factory," 211–12.

80. Brandt, *Cigarette Century*, 69–100.

81. Sinel'nikov, email correspondence to author, July 1, 2019.

82. Neuburger, *Balkan Smoke*, 209–12; Starks, "Taste, Smell, and Semiotics," 97–116; Sinel'nikov, email correspondence to author, July 1, 2019.

83. Sinel'nikov, *Delo—Tabak*, 35.

84. Proctor, *Golden Holocaust*, on marketing 56–77; on filter "flim-flam," 340–56; on nicotine "freebasing," 39–405. See also Cross and Proctor, *Packaged Pleasures*, 84–87; and Terrell Stevenson, "The Secret and Soul of Marlboro: Phillip [sic.] Morris and the Origins, Spread, and Denial of Nicotine Freebasing," *American Journal of Public Health* 98, no. 7 (2008): 1184–94. On possible changes in style brought on by nicotine intensity, see Neuburger, *Balkan Smoke*, 217.

85. Milov, *Cigarette*, 89.

86. Sinel'nikov, *Delo—Tabak*, 104.

87. Neuburger, *Balkan Smoke*, 225.

88. James T. Andrews, "Getting Ready for Khrushchev's *Sputnik*: Russian Popular Culture and National Markers at the Dawn of the Space Age," in *Into the Cosmos: Space Exploration and Soviet Culture*, ed. James T. Andrews and Asif A. Siddiqi (Pittsburgh: University of Pittsburgh Press, 2011), 44.

89. Bogdanov, *Dym otechestva*, 233; Cathleen S. Lewis, "From the Kitchen into Orbit: The Convergence of Human Spaceflight and Khrushchev's Nascent Consumerism," in *Into the Cosmos*, 213–39; Gabrielle Cornish, "Music and the Making of the Cosmonaut Everyman," *Journal of Musicology* 36, no. 4 (2019): 477; Sinel'nikov, *Delo—Tabak*, 125.

90. Amy Nelson, "Cold War Celebrity and the Courageous Canine Scout: The Life and Times of Soviet Space Dogs," in *Into the Cosmos*, 133–58.

91. On the connection of the generation of the 1960s to space achievement, see Alexei Kojevnikov, "The Cultural Spaces of the Soviet Cosmos," in *Into the Cosmos*, 25–27.

92. Erica L. Fraser, *Military Masculinity and Postwar Recovery in the Soviet Union* (Toronto: University of Toronto Press, 2019), 146, 143–61; Slava Gerovitch, *Soviet Space Mythologies: Public Images, Private Memories, and the Making of a Cultural Identity* (Pittsburgh: University of Pittsburgh Press, 2015), 128–54; Slava Gerovitch, "The Human inside a Propaganda Machine: The Public Image and Professional Identity of Soviet Cosmonauts," in *Into the Cosmos*, 77–106.

93. The lyric was changed after pressure. Marching songs and other musical tributes featured prominently in the press campaigns surrounding the cosmonauts (Cornish, "Music and the Making of the Cosmonaut," 464–97).

94. Gately, *Tobacco*, 337.

95. Po-Chitatel', "Listaia stranitsy: Dali prikurit'!" *Krokodil*, no. 20 (1958): 14.

96. Unnamed Bulgarian tobacco official from 1960s quoted in Neuburger, *Balkan Smoke*, 214.

97. Alexei Yurchak, *Everything Was Forever, until It Was No More: The Last Soviet Generation* (Princeton, NJ: Princeton University Press, 2006), 185–86, 198; Juliane Fürst, *Flowers through Concrete: Explorations in Soviet Hippieland* (Oxford: Oxford University Press, 2021), 13, 40–41, 55.

98. Neuburger, *Balkan Smoke*, 216–17.

99. Sergey Kolobenov, "Moscow Sociological Agency: Gender Consumer Survey Uzbekistan," April 30, 1979, https://www.industrydocuments.ucsf.edu/docs/hnnj0212.

100. Sinel'nikov, *Delo—Tabak*, 247.

101. Zatoński, "State Society and Politics of Smoking," 142–48.

102. Anna Gilmore, "Tobacco and Transition: The Advent of the Transnational Tobacco Companies," and Judyth L. Twigg, "Up in Smoke? The Politics and Health Impact of Tobacco in Today's Russia," in *Tobacco in Russian History*, 244–66 and 267–82, respectively.

103. Chernyshova, *Soviet Consumer Culture*, 21, 28.

104. Sinel'nikov, *Delo—Tabak*, 172–73, 191.

105. James Heinzen, *The Art of the Bribe: Corruption under Stalin, 1943–1953* (New Haven: Yale University Press, 2016), 84.

106. Bittner, *Whites and Reds*, 146.

107. Sinel'nikov, *Delo—Tabak*, 210.

108. Sinel'nikov denied that Moldavian tobacco made it into Iava cigarettes, saying it all came from Switzerland (*Delo—Tabak*, 208).

109. Sinel'nikov, email correspondence to author, November 1, 2019.

9. PRESSURED

1. Boris Urlanis, "Beregite muzhchin!," *Literaturnaia gazeta*, July 24, 1968, 12.

2. Urlanis, "Beregite muzhchin!"

3. Urlanis, "Beregite muzhchin!"

4. Box Folder 1/2 A–D and Box Folder 2/3 A–D, Anatolii Zakharovich Rubinov Papers.

5. "Diskussionnyi klub," *Literaturnaia gazeta*, October 9, 1968, 12.

6. Brandt makes this argument regarding antismoking propaganda in the west (*Cigarette Century*, 57).

7. E. Zdravomyslova and A. Temkina, "Krizis maskulinnosti v pozdnesovetskom diskurse," in *O muzhe(i)stvennosti*, ed. S. Ushakin (Moscow: Novoe literaturnoe obozrenie, 2002), 432–41; quotations 434, 435.

8. Goscilo and Lanoux, "Introduction," 17; Dan Healey, *Russian Homophobia from Stalin to Sochi* (London: Bloomsbury, 2018), 138–39.

9. Utrata, *Women without Men*, 27–29.

10. Urlanis, "Beregite muzhchin!"

11. L. V. Orlovskii, comp. *O raz"iasnenii naseleniiu vreda kureniia i upotrebleniia nasa* (Moscow: Kommunar, 1972).

12. Deber, "The Limits of Persuasion," 120.

13. Brandt, *Cigarette Century*, 216. For the Royal College of Physicians report, see https://www.rcplondon.ac.uk/projects/outputs/smoking-and-health-1962. For the Surgeon General's Report, see https://profiles.nlm.nih.gov/ps/access/nnbbmq.pdf.

14. D. I. Reitynbarg, "Kurenie i zdorov'e," *Sovetskoe zdravookhranenie*, no. 6 (1965): 78.

15. Naomi Oreskes and Erik M. Conway, *Merchants of Doubt: How a Handful of Scientists Obscured the Truth on Issues from Tobacco Smoke to Global Warming* (London: Bloomsbury, 2010), 136–68.

16. G. M. Pivovarov, S. P. Arzumanov, and N. K. Azbekian, "Peresmotret' instruktsiiu po uchetu tabaka i tary," *Tabak*, no. 3 (1953): 57–60; L. N. Shakhnovskii, "K voprosu o soderzhanii nikotina i vkusovykh kachestvakh kuritel'nykh izdelii," *Tabak*, no. 1 (1959): 32–33; K. A. Zonov, "Snizit' soderzhanie nikotina v makhorochnykh izdeliiakh," *Tabak*, no. 2 (1959): 17–18; Ia. I. Semenov, "Pop povodu stat'i N. I. Rainysha 'O vypuske kuritel'nykh izdelii vysokogo kachestva s nizkim soderzhaniem nikotina," *Tabak*, no. 2 (1959): 18–19; Editors, "Po povodu predlozheniia t. Rainysha o snizhenii soderzhaniia nikotina v kuritel'nykh izdeliiakh," *Tabak*, no. 2 (1959): 20–23.

17. Wood, *Baba and the Comrade*, 106–11.

18. Nakachi, *Replacing the Dead*, 153–215; Christopher Burton, "Minzdrav, Soviet Doctors, and the Policing of Reproduction during Late Stalinism, 1943–53," *Russian History* 27, no. 2 (2000): 197–221; Edward D. Cohn, "Sex and the Married Communist: Family Troubles, Marital Infidelity, and Party Discipline in the Postwar USSR, 1945–65," *Russian Review* 68, no. 3 (2009): 429–50; Amy E. Randall, "'Abortion Will Deprive You of Happiness!' Soviet Reproductive Politics in the Post-Stalin Era," *Journal of Women's History* 23, no. 3 (2011): 13–38.

19. Schrad, *Vodka Politics*, 245; Brandon Gray Miller, "The New Soviet *Narkoman*: Drugs and Youth in Post-Stalinist Russia," *REGION: Regional Studies of Russia, Eastern Europe, and Central Asia* 4:1 (2014): 45–69.

20. Schrad, *Vodka Politics*, 251.

21. Aleksandr Latsis, "Lotereia neobriavlennykh proigryshei," *Literaturnaia gazeta*, July 29, 1965, 2.

22. Transchel, *Under the Influence*, 154–55.

23. Schrad, *Vodka Politics*, 245.

24. "Tabachnaia promyshlennost' za 40 let."

25. Malinin, *Tabachnaia istoriia Rossii*, 158–60.

26. "Tabachnaia promyshlennost' za 40 let"; Malinin, *Tabachnaia istoriia Rossii*, 159–60.

27. K. S. Kosiakov, *Pochemu vredno kurit'* (Moscow: Medgiz, 1957), 28; Beliaev, "Bor'ba s kureniem," 88.

28. National Center for Chronic Disease Prevention and Health Promotion (US) Office on Smoking and Health, *The Health Consequences of Smoking—50 Years of Progress: A Report of the Surgeon General* (Atlanta, GA: Centers for Disease Control and Prevention, 2014).

29. "Smoking Statistics: Who Smokes and How Much," *Ash Fact Sheet* (February 2016), 1, http://ash.org.uk/wp-content/uploads/2016/06/Smoking-Statistics-Who-Smokes-and-How-Much.pdf.

30. Zorii Shokin, "Kuril'shik: V sotsiologicheskom i meditsinskom aspektakh," *Literaturnaia gazeta*, August 18, 1971, 13.

31. G. I. Ivakhno, "Nekotorye voprosy organizatsii bor'by s kureniem," *Vrachebnoe delo*, no. 11 (1966): 128–29.

32. Loranskii and Popova, "Kurenie i ego vliianie na zdorov'e cheloveka," 49.

33. Lillard and Dorofeeva, "Smoking in Russia and Ukraine," 117–40.

34. A. N. Novikov, "Mezhdunarodnoe znachenie sovetskoi onkologii," *Sovetskoe zdravookhranenie*, no. 6 (1962): 9–10.

35. D.N. Mats, L. E. Miziak, V. M. Uglova, and A. V. Chaklin, "Nekotorye dannye po statistike raka legkikh," *Voprosy onkologii*, no. 5 (1957): 611–12; L. M. Shabad, "Aktual'nye voprosy etnologii i patogeneza raka legkikh," *Voprosy onkologii*, no. 4 (1957): 387–93.

36. A. I. Rakov, "Nekotorye voprosy problem raka legkogo," *Voprosy onkologii*, no. 4 (1957): 404–10; Ia. M. Grushko, "Rak legkikh i ego profilaktika," *Voprosy onkologii*, no. 5 (1957): 624–33.

37. I. J. Beffinger, "Investigaciones del humo del tabaco," Philip Morris Records, 1967, https://www.industrydocuments.ucsf.edu/docs/hjgc0106.

38. P. P. Grabovskii, G. Iu. Voronaia, and S. A. Davydov, "K voprosu o rasprostranennosti raka organov dykhaniia v Ukrainskoi SSR," *Sovetskoe zdravookhranenie*, no. 7 (1967): 32–36.

39. V. N. Demin, "Kurenie i rak legkogo," *Zdorov'e*, no. 8 (1967): 32.

40. M. V. Dzvonik and P. I. Zaborovskaia, "Kuriashchie o kurenii," *Sovetskaia meditsina*, no. 7 (1980): 93–95.

41. Murray Feshbach, "The Soviet Union: Population Trends and Dilemmas," *Population Bulletin* 37, no. 3 (1982): 36.

42. L. P. Zaits, *Brosaite kurit'!* (Sverdlovsk: Sverdlovskoe knizhnoe izdatel'stvo, 1960), 16.

43. Nikolai Krementsov, *The Cure: A Story of Cancer and Politics from the Annals of the Cold War* (Chicago: University of Chicago Press, 2004), 8; Anna Geltzer, "Stagnant Science? The Planning and Coordination of Biomedical Research in the Brezhnev Era," in *Reconsidering Stagnation in the Brezhnev Era*, 105–21; Proctor, *Nazi War on Cancer*, 174–90; Alfredo Morabia, "Quality, Originality, and Significance of the 1939 'Tobacco Consumption and Lung Carcinoma' Article by Mueller, Including Translation of a Section of the Paper," *Preventive Medicine* 53, no. 3 (2012): 171–77. Similarly, the 1943 study by German doctors did not find a strong representation in a Soviet press distanced politically from the German medical community and plagued further by publishing difficulties from

the war (Alfredo Morabia, "'Lung Cancer and Tobacco Consumption': Technical Evaluation of the 1943 Paper by Schairer and Schoeniger Published in Nazi Germany," *Journal of Epidemiology and Community Health* 67 [2013]: 208–12).

44. B. D. Petrov, "Sanitarnoe prosveshchenie na novom etape," *Sovetskoe zdravookhranenie*, no. 7 (1963): 3–6; I. N. Alekperov, E. K. Andreeva, and A. I. Seidbekov, "Sanitarno-prosvetitel'naia rabota po zavodskomu radioveshchaniiu," *Sovetskoe zdravookhranenie*, no. 7 (1963): 25–28; V. S. Ershov, L. A. Zlotnikov, and I. B. Rostotskii, "Kino kaka effektivnaia forma gigienicheskogo vospitaniia naseleniia," *Sovetskoe zdravookhranenie*, no. 8 (1964): 51–53; Anna Toropova, "Science, Medicine, and the Creation of a 'Healthy' Soviet Cinema," *Journal of Contemporary History* 55, no. 1 (2019): 3–28.

45. A. D. Ostrovskii, *Pravda o tabake (Konspekt lektsii)* (Moscow: Institut sanitarnogo prosveshcheniia, 1959), 1–18, alcohol and tobacco 26, quotation 17, conclusion 31–33.

46. Alex Inkeles, *Public Opinion in Soviet Russia: A Study in Mass Persuasion* (Cambridge, MA: Harvard University Press, 1967), 40, as quoted in Fox, "'Tobacco Is Poison!,'" 199.

47. Fox, "'Tobacco Is Poison!,'" 193.

48. Budanova, "Problema tabakokureniia v otechestvennom plakate," 37.

49. GARF f. R-8009, op. 50, d. 9265, l. 68; for reviews of some of these, see V. Lagutina, "Novye filmy," *Zdorov'e*, no. 3 (1971): 32.

50. Fox, "'Tobacco Is Poison!,'" 194–96.

51. Francis K. Decker, Letter, August 9, 1968, https://www.industrydocuments.ucsf.edu/docs/yspj0045.

52. Fox made this point regarding the name in "'Tobacco Is Poison!,'" 194.

53. Iurii Aleksandrov, *Zelenaia pogibel'* (Moscow: Znanie, 1964), 58–59; A. Perolaeva-Makovskaia, L. A. Persov, and D. K. Popov, "K voprosu o soderzhanii poloniia-210 v tabake," *Gigiena i sanitariia*, no. 12 (1965): 40–43; Shokin, "Kuril'shik," 13; V. A. Bogoslovskii, *O vrede kureniia (Konspekt lektsii)* (Moscow: Institut sanitarnogo prosveshcheniia, 1965), 11; V. A. Frolov, *Kurit' zdorov'iu vredit'* (Moscow: Meditsina, 1969), 5–18; I. P. Bazhenov, *Tabak gubit zdorov'e* (Moscow: Meditsina, 1964); L. V. Orlovskii, "Kurit'—ne tol'ko sebia gubit'," *Gigiena i sanitariia*, no. 9 (1969): 39; "Zdorov'e sovetuet: Ne kurite natoshchak," *Zdorov'e*, no. 1 (1973): 30.

54. A. V. Chaklin, *Vrednye privychki i rak* (Moscow: Znanie, 1969), quotations 4, 9–10, and 11.

55. Kosiakov, *Pochemu vredno kurit'*, 30.

56. I. I. Beliaev, "Bor'ba s kureniem tabaka—aktual'naia sotsial'no-gigienicheskaia problema sovremennosti," *Gigiena i sanitariia*, no. 2 (1965): 88.

57. Anon., "Dotianulsia," *Zdorov'e*, no. 8 (1960): 32.

58. Zaits, *Brosaite kurit'!*, 16.

59. Boris Filippov, "Ot tsigarki dym udavom," *Zdorov'e*, no. 5 (1961): 33.

60. Kosiakov, *Pochemu vredno kurit'*, 29.

61. V. Lagutina, "Novye filmy," *Zdorov'e*, no. 3 (1971): 32.

62. Tamtam, "O vrede tabaka," *Krokodil*, no. 24 (1967): 12.

63. M. M. Bubnova, "Mozhno li kormiashchei materi kurit'?," *Zdorov'e*, no. 7 (1960): 13.

64. Bogoslovskii, *O vrede kureniia*, 16–17, 21, 31.

65. Galina Serikova and Darikha Khodzhikova, "Chitatel' stavit vopros: Ne pora li ogranichit' kuril'shchikov?," *Zdorov'e*, no. 9 (1972): 8.

66. "Vozvrashchaias' k napechatannomu: Ne pora li ogranichit' kuril'shchikov?," *Zdorov'e*, no. 2 (1973): 20.

67. "Vozvrashchaias' k napechatannomu," 21.

68. "Po sledam nashikh vystuplenii: Ne pora li ogranichit' kuril'shchikov?," *Zdorov'e*, no. 3 (1973): 6.

69. "Po sledam nashikh vystuplenii," 6.

70. "Po sledam nashikh vystuplenii," 10.

71. E. Shcheglov, "Prima," *Krokodil*, no. 29 (1974): cover.

72. Mikh. Khodanov, "Trubka protiv kureniia," *Krokodil*, no. 30 (1976): 11.

73. V. Mikhailov, "Tabachnaia smert'," *Literaturnaia gazeta*, April 2, 1975, 13.

74. Mikhailov, "Tabachnaia smert'," 13; Aleksandra M. Brokman, "Creating a Medical Speciality: Psychotherapy in the Post-war Soviet Healthcare System," *Journal of Health Inequalities* 5, no. 2 (2019): 203–9.

75. Urlanis, "Beregite muzhchin!," concentrated on underage smoking. See Aleksandr Lapis, "Lotereia neob"iavlennykh proigryshei," *Literaturnaia gazeta*, July 29, 1965, 2; Sergei Mikhailov, "Blagorodnoe serdtse," *Literaturnaia gazeta*, December 10, 1969, 10.

76. N. Gerasimenko, "Bros'te sigaretu: Sluzhba zdorov'ia," *Pravda*, September 7, 1974, 3.

77. V. Petrovskii, "Kurenie i rak," *Pravda*, April 15, 1978, 3.

78. Mikhailov, "Tabachnaia smert'," 13.

79. Mikhailov, "Tabachnaia smert'," 13.

80. Jean-Francois Etter, "Cytisine for Smoking Cessation: A Literature Review and a Meta-analysis," *Archives of Internal Medicine* 166, no. 15 (2006): 1553–54.

81. Mikhailov, "Tabachnaia smert'," 13.

82. The full section was titled "Dym unosiashchii zdorov'e" and included I. Prokopov, "Serditoe pis'mo"; L. Orlovskii, "Kategoricheski protivopokazano: Chitateliu otvechaet doktor meditsinskikh nauk L. Orlovskii"; "K slovu skazat': Kak pokonchit' s vrednoi privychkoi"; and Otdel nauki "LG," "Anketa 'LG': 13 voprosov dlia kuriashchikh i nekuri-ashchikh," *Literaturnaia gazeta*, June 18, 1975, 13.

83. Prokopov, "Serditoe pis'mo."

84. Orlovskii, "Kategoricheski protivopokazano."

85. Otdel nauki "LG," "Anketa 'LG': Protsent nadezhdy," *Literaturnaia gazeta*, March 24, 1976, 13.

86. Kluger, *Ashes to Ashes*, 224, 259.

87. "K slovu skazat'."

88. Otdel nauki "LG," "Anketa 'LG': Protsent nadezhdy."

89. Otdel nauki "LG," "Anketa 'LG': Protsent nadezhdy."

90. Oleg Moroz, "Khotim li my ne kurit'?," *Literaturnaia gazeta*, March 24, 1976, 13.

91. "USSR: Little War against 'Tabagism,'" *La Suisse*, July 19, 1977; Philip Morris Records, http://www.industrydocuments.ucsf.edu/docs/trfx0117; Deber, "The Limits of Persuasion," 120.

92. B. Urlanis, "I snova beregite muzhchin: K iubileiu gazetnoi stat'i," *Literaturnaia gazeta*, June 7, 1978, 7.

93. K. Fagerstrom, "Determinants of Tobacco Use and Renaming the FTND to the Fagerstrom Test for Cigarette Dependence," *Nicotine Tobacco Research* 14 (2012): 75–78.

94. G. B. Tkachenko, "Kurenie tabaka i zdorov'e naseleniia v Rossii," in *Kurenie ili zdorov'e v Rossii*, 38.

95. Mark G. Field quickly outlines the problem of health decline in the Soviet Union in "The Health and Demographic Crisis in Post-Soviet Russia: A Two-Phase Development," in *Russia's Torn Safety Nets: Health and Social Welfare during the Transition*, ed. Mark G. Field and Judyth L. Twigg (New York: Palgrave, 2000), 21–23; William C. Cockerham, "The Social Determinants of the Decline of Life Expectancy in Russia and Eastern Europe: A Lifestyle Explanation," *Journal of Health and Social Behavior* 38, no. 2 (1997): 117–30.

96. V. Ia. Kiselev, "Izuchenie sotsial'no-gigienicheskikh aspektov kureniia u studentov-medikov," *Sovetskoe zdravookhranenie,* no. 5 (1983): 33; V. P. Vtiurin, K. L. Poliakov, and V. E. Starodubtsev, "O kurenii vrachei i merakh bor'by s nim," *Sovetskoe zdravookhranenie,* no. 7 (1989): 24–26.

97. Murray Feshbach and Alfred Friendly, Jr., *Ecocide in the USSR: Health and Nature under Siege* (New York: Basic Books, 1991), 183–85; for alcohol 187–89; for cancer and circulatory disease, 189–90. For discussions of the demographic crisis of the 1970s, see Christopher Davis and Murray Feshbach, *Rising Infant Mortality in the USSR in the 1970s,* Series P-25, no. 74 (Washington, DC: US Bureau of the Census, September 1980); and Murray Feshbach, *The Soviet Union: Population Trends and Dilemmas. Population Bulletin* 37, no. 3 (Washington, DC: Population Reference Bureau, August 1982).

98. GARF f. R-8009, op. 50, d. 2349, ll. 1–4, 18–61, quotation l. 3, survey l. 4.

99. GARF f. R-8009, op. 50, d. 2349, ll. 1–4, survey ll. 16–21, quotations ll. 23, 26.

100. Witold Zatoński and Mateusz Zatoński, "Cytisine versus Nicotine for Smoking Cessation," *New England Journal of Medicine* 372, no. 11 (2015): 1072.

101. The document referenced a 1971 Minzdrav methodological recommendation, "O raz"iasneniiakh naselenii vreda kureniia i upotrebleniia nasa."

102. GARF f. R-8009, op. 50, d. 4908, l. 62.

103. GARF f. R-5462, op. 32, d. 1793, ll. 69, 69 ob., 70.

104. GARF f. R-5462, op. 32, d. 1793, l. 70.

105. GARF f. R-5462, op. 32, d. 1793, l. 74; Zakarpatskii obkom, ll. 89–90; Zaporozhskii oblast, ll. 91–92; Ivanovskii oblast, ll. 93–95.

106. GARF f. R-5462, op. 32, d. 1793, l. 76.

107. "O merakh po dal'neishemu uluchsheniiu narodnogo zdravookhraneniia," in *Spravochnik partiinogo rabotnika,* ed. K. M. Bogoliubov, P. G. Mishunin, E. Z. Razumov, and Ia. V. Storozhev (Moscow: Politicheskaia literatura, 1978), 18: 316–19; excerpts from Tkachenko, "Kurenie tabaka i zdorov'e," 38–39.

108. GARF f. R-5446, op. 136, d.1129, ll. 1–6.

109. GARF f. R-5446, op. 136, d. 1129, ll. 31, 39–40, 45, 53.

110. GARF f. R-5446, op. 136, d. 1129, ll. 55–56.

111. GARF f. R5446, op. 136, d. 1129, ll. 150–55; Deber, "Limits of Persuasion," 123.

112. V. I. Kozlova, "Poluchenie sortov tabaka s nizkim soderzheniem nikotina," *Tabak,* no. 1 (1965): 30–31.

113. Filtered cigarettes are not safer but engineered to compensate for the lighter taste with more nicotine (Kluger, *Ashes to Ashes,* 188).

114. GARF f. R-5446, op 136, d. 1129, l. 57.

115. Sinel'nikov, *Delo—Tabak,* 211–12.

116. Kifuriak, *Tabachnaia fabrika "Iava,"* 25–28.

117. "Preduprezhdenie kuril'shchikam," *Zdorov'e,* no. 5 (1978): 28.

118. Sinel'nikov, *Delo-Tabak,* 231–32.

119. Gorchakova, "Iava Tobacco Factory," 213; Sinel'nikov, *Delo—Tabak,* 230–31.

120. Deber, "Limits of Persuasion," 121; World Health Organization, "Survey on Smoking and Health in the European Region, 1974–75," British American Tobacco Records, https://www.industrydocuments.ucsf.edu/docs/ljvn0212.

121. Golubev, *Things of Life,* 90–112.

122. Schlögel, *Scent of Empires,* 21–30.

123. GARF f. R-8009, op. 50, d. 6998, ll. 1–2.

124. GARF f. R-8009, op. 50, d. 6998, ll. 3–4.

125. GARF f. R-5446, op 136, d. 1129, ll. 159–63; "O merakh po usileniiu bor'by s kureniem," in *Spravochnik partiinogo rabotnika,* 21, 316–19.

126. GARF f. R-5465, op. 26, d. 5669a (1981) l. 2; Bogoliubov et. al., *Spravochnik partiinogo rabotnika*, 433–39.

127. Aleksandra M. Brokman, "Creating a Medical Specialty: Psychotherapy in the Post-War Soviet Healthcare System," *Journal of Health Inequalities* 5, no. 2 (2019): 203–9.

128. GARF f. R-5465, op. 26, d. 5669a, l. 7.

129. GARF f. R-5465, op. 26, d. 5669a, ll. 12–16; GARF f. 7901, op. 3, d. 4656, ll. 70–72.

130. GARF f. A-259, op. 48, d. 5890, l. 3.

131. The warning read, "Kurenie opasno dlia vashego zdorov'ia i zdorov'ia okruzhaiushchikh vas liudei i ne ukrashaet vas kak cheloveka."

132. GARF f. R-5446, op. 150, d. 1375, ll. 1–3, 5–7.

133. GARF f. R-5446, op. 150, d. 1375, l. 8.

134. GARF f. R-5446, op. 150, d. 1375, l. 35–40 agriculture, l. 66 finance.

135. V. Sudakov, "Pervyi den' bez tabaka," *Pravda*, April 4, 1988, 3.

136. Demin et al., *Rossiia*, 60.

137. Demin et al., *Rossiia*, 60.

138. GARF f. R-8009, op. 51, d. 5054, l. 4.

139. Demin et al., *Rossiia*, 52–55.

140. Milov, *Cigarette*, 1–11.

141. Richard Cooper, "Around Europe: Smoking in the Soviet Union," *British Medical Journal* 285 (August 21, 1982): 549.

142. Loranskii and Popova, "Kurenie i ego vliianie na zdorov'e cheloveka," 49; Lillard and Dorofeeva, "Smoking in Russia and Ukraine," 124, 117–40.

EPILOGUE

1. A. Pivovarov, "Delo-Tabak," *Krokodil*, no. 5 (1983): 12; "Poleznye sovety," *Krokodil*, no. 5 (1986): 12; Sinel'nikov, *Delo—Tabak*, 196, 229, 244–45.

2. Bittner, *Whites and Reds*, 230. Schrad, *Vodka Politics*, 263–64.

3. Tkachenko, "Kurenie tabaka i zdorov'e," 49.

4. Neuburger, *Balkan Smoke*, 227.

5. William Moskoff, *Hard Times: Impoverishment and Protest in the Perestroika Years. The Soviet Union, 1981–1991* (Armonk, NY: M. E. Sharpe, 1993), 40, 61–62.

6. "Vstrechi s kommunistami Frunzenskogo raiona stolitsy," *Pravda*, May 12, 1990, 5; V. Parfenov, "Delo tabak?" *Pravda*, July 10, 1990, 8; A. Aksenov, A. Androshin, B. Pipiia, A. Sarkisian, "Bol'shoi perekur, "*Pravda*, July 26, 1990, 4; A. Urvantsev, "Ataka . . . na tabachnyi kiosk," *Pravda*, August 25, 1990, 2; Z. Kadymbekov, "Tabachnyi nokaut," *Pravda*, September 3, 1990, 6; V. Larin, "Serpantin: Davai zakurim," *Pravda*, September 7, 1990, 6; "V sovete ministrov SSSR," *Pravda*, September 16, 1990, 1.

7. Unknown, "Moscow Smokers Revolt and Get Results," August 22, 1990, https://www.industrydocuments.ucsf.edu/docs/yylm0026.

8. Sinel'nikov, email correspondence to author, July 4, 2019; Gorchakova, "Iava Tobacco Factory," 220–21; Sinel'nikov, *Delo—Tabak*, 353.

9. Gorchakova, "Iava Tobacco Factory," 220–21; Sinel'nikov, *Delo—Tabak*, 351–56; Anthony Ramirez, "Two U.S. Companies Plan to Sell Soviets 34 Billion Cigarettes," *New York Times,* September 14, 1990, https://www.nytimes.com/1990/09/14/business/two-us-companies-plan-to-sell-soviets-34-billion-cigarettes.html.

10. James Rupert and Glenn Frankel, "In Ex-Soviet Markets, U.S. Brands Took on Role of Capitalist Liberator," *Washington Post*, November 19, 1996, A01; Kluger, *Ashes to Ashes*, 717–18; Gilmore, "Tobacco and Transition," 245; Anthony Ramirez, "Tobacco Industry Sees Boon in Sales to Soviets," *New York Times*, September 17, 1990, http://www.nytimes.com/1990/09/17/business/tobacco-industry-sees-boon-in-sales-to-soviets.html.

11. Lillard and Dorofeeva, "Smoking in Russia and Ukraine," 120.

12. Gilmore, "Tobacco and Transition," 244–47; Lillard and Dorofeeva, "Smoking in Russia and Ukraine," 124–25.

13. Lillard and Dorofeeva, "Smoking in Russia and Ukraine," 132.

14. Vedomosti, ""Sigaretu na kolenke ne sdelaesh," and "Leonid Sinel'nikov, predsedatel' soveta direktor 'BAT-Iavy,'" *Rambler—Finansy*, March 12, 2009, http://finance.rambler.ru/news/economics/57543529.html.

15. N. G. Brookes, "Yava Tobacco Factory-Moscow," 1992, https://www.industrydocuments.ucsf.edu/docs/xpxc0205.

16. Sinel'nikov, *Delo—Tabak*, 322–26, 390, 411–12, 439–40.

17. Gilmore, "Tobacco and Transition," 250.

18. Sinel'nikov, *Delo—Tabak*, 390.

19. Gilmore, "Tobacco and Transition," 249, 255; Lillard and Dorofeeva, "Smoking in Russia and Ukraine," 120–21.

20. Twigg, "Up in Smoke?," 276–77.

21. Michael Janofsky, "The Media Business: Advertising; Moscow Draws Line on Cigarette and Liquor Ads," *New York Times*, July 20, 1993, D1; Rupert and Frankel, "In Ex-Soviet Markets." For enforcement, see Tkachenko, "Kurenie tabaka i zdorov'e," 63.

22. Kluger, *Ashes to Ashes*, 219.

23. Gilmore, "Tobacco and Transition," 254.

24. Twigg, "Up in Smoke?," 271.

25. Figures taken from the WHO, http://www.who.int/tobacco/media/en/Russian_Federation.pdf.

26. Sinel'nikov, *Delo—Tabak*, 399; Lillard and Dorofeeva, "Smoking in Russia and Ukraine," 136.

27. Jeremy Morris, "The Empire Strikes Back: Projections of National Identity in Contemporary Russian Advertising," *Russian Review* 64, no. 4 (2005): 2–20.

28. Gilmore, "Tobacco and Transition," 253–54, 256–60.

29. Twigg, "Up in Smoke?," 269.

30. Tkachenko, "Kurenie tabaka i zdorov'e," 63.

31. Jean-Noël Kapferer, *(Re)inventing the Brand: Can Top Brands Survive the New Market Realities?* (London: Kogan Page, 2001), 49.

32. Field, "Health and Demographic Crisis," 23; Judyth L. Twigg, "Unfulfilled Hopes: The Struggle to Reform Russian Health Care and Its Financing," in *Russia's Torn Safety Nets*, 43–64.

33. Maria Neufeld et. al., "Alcohol Control Policies in Former Soviet Union Countries: A Narrative Review of Three Decades of Policy Changes and Their Apparent Effects," *Drug and Alcohol Review* 40, no. 3 (2020): 1–18.

34. Field, "Health and Demographic Crisis," 16–20.

35. Per Carlson, *An Unhealthy Decade: A Sociological Study of the State of Public Health in Russia, 1990–1999* (Stockholm: Alqvist & Wiksell, 2000), 29. See also R. A. Galkin, V. N. Mal'tsev, N. P. Lopukhov, and O. L. Nikitin, eds., *Tabak ili zhizn': Aktual'nye problemy profilaktiki kureniia* (Samara: Perspektiva, 2000).

36. Elizabeth A. Swanson and Ann M. Valentine, "Health Education on Wellness Centered Living: Maximizing Women's Potential in the United States and Russia," in *Medical Issues and Health Care Reform in Russia*, ed. Vicki L. Hesli and Margaret H. Mills (Lewiston, ME: Edwin Mellen Press, 1999), 302.

37. Gilmore, "Tobacco in Transition," 258; Brian P. Hinote, William C. Cockerham, and Pamela Abbott, "Post-Communism and Female Tobacco Consumption in the Former Soviet States," *Europe-Asia Studies* 61, no. 9 (2009): 1543–55.

38. Tkachenko, "Kurenie tabaka i zdorov'e," 102–8.

39. Judy Twigg, "A Habit That's Hard to Kick: The Evolution of Tobacco Control Policy in Russia," *Russian Analytical Digest*, no. 35 (2008): 2–3.

40. Iurii Krupnov, "Prekratite nas berech'!," *Literaturnaia gazeta*, January 17, 2007, 12.

41. Twigg, "Up in Smoke?," 269.

42. Amy E. Randall, "Soviet and Russian Masculinities: Rethinking Soviet Fatherhood after Stalin and Renewing Virility in the Russian Nation under Putin," *Journal of Modern History* 92, no. 4 (2020): 859–98; Valerie Sperling, *Sex, Politics, and Putin: Political Legitimacy in Russia* (Oxford: Oxford University Press, 2015).

43. Twigg, "Up in Smoke?," 273.

44. Henry St. George Brooke and Jordan Gans-Morse, "Putin's Crackdown on Mortality: Rethinking Legal Nihilism and State Capacity in Light of Russia's Surprising Public Health Campaigns," *Problems of Post-Communism* 63, no. 1 (2015): 2–3.

45. Brooke and Gans-Morse, "Putin's Crackdown on Mortality," 5.

46. Kathryn Stoner, "Social Foundations of Tobacco Smoking in Russia," *American Journal of Public Health* 109, no. 4 (2019): 524.

Bibliography

ARCHIVES
Russia

Gosudarstvennyi arkhiv Rossiisskoi Federatsii (GARF)
Rossiiskii gosudarstvennyi arkhiv sotsial'no-politicheskoi istorii (RGASPI)
Tsentral'nyi arkhiv obshchestvennykh dvizhenii Moskvy (TsAODM)
Tsentral'nyi munitsipal'nyi arkhiv Moskvy (TsMAM)

United States

Anatolii Zakharovich Rubinov Papers at the Library of Congress
Harvard Project on the Soviet Social System
Industry Documents Archive, University of California—Santa Barbara
Zosa Szajkowski Collection, Bakhmeteff Archive of Russian and East
    European Culture, Rare Book and Manuscript Library, Columbia
    University Libraries

JOURNALS AND NEWSPAPERS
Russian

Agitator i propagandist Krasnoi Armii
Biulleten' NKZ
Den' respubliki
Gigiena i epidemiologiia
Gigiena i sanitariia
Gigiena i zdorov'e rabochei i krest'ianskoi sem'i (GiZRiKS)
Gigiena i zdorov'e rabochei sem'i (GiZRS)
Izvestiia
Izvestiia Narodnogo komissariata zdravookhraneniia
Komsomol'skaia pravda
Kooperativnoe delo
Krokodil
Literaturnaia gazeta
Meditsina: Ezhemesiachnyi zhurnal dlia usovershenstvovaniia
Molodaia gvardiia

Pamiatka tabakovoda
Pravda
Rabotnitsa
Rambler-Finansy
Sotsiologicheskie issledovaniia
Sovetskoe zdravookhranenie
Tabachnaia promyshlennost'
Tabak (formerly Tabachnaia promyshlennost')
Trezvost' i kul'tura
Vestnik tabachnoi promyshlennosti
Voprosy istorii
Voprosy kul'turologii
Voprosy narkologii
Voprosy onkologii
Vrachebnoe delo
Za novyi byt (ZNB)
Zdorov'e

English and French

American Historical Review
American Journal of Public Health
Annals of Surgery
Archives of Internal Medicine
Biochemical Pharmacology
British Journal of Psychiatry
British Medical Journal
Cahiers du monde russe et soviétique
Canadian Journal of Public Health
Drug and Alcohol Review
European Journal of Psychotherapy and Counselling
European Review
International Labor and Working-Class History
Journal of Cancer Research and Clinical Oncology
Journal of Cold War Studies
Journal of Contemporary History
Journal of Design History
Journal of Epidemiology and Community Health
Journal of Health and Social Behavior
Journal of Health Inequalities
Journal of the History of Medicine and Allied Sciences
Journal of Marketing

Journal of Musicology
Journal of Policy History
Journal of Public Health
Journal of Social History
Journal of Women's History
Journalism Quarterly
Kritika: Explorations in Russian and Eurasian History
Market Structure and Industrial Performance
Medical History
New England Journal of Medicine
New York Times
Nicotine Tobacco Research
Osiris
Pharmacological Reports
Philip Morris News
Preventive Medicine
Population Bulletin
Problems of Post-Communism
REGION: Regional Studies of Russia, Eastern Europe, and Central Asia
Russian Analytical Digest
Russian History
Russian Review
Scandinavian Journal of History
Slavic and East European Review
Slavic Review
Soviet Studies
Suisse, La
Times of London
Tobacco Reporter
Wall Street Journal
Washington Post
World's Paper Trade Review

BOOKS AND DISSERTATIONS

Primary Sources

Aleksandrov, Iurii. *Zelenaia pogibel'*. Moscow: Znanie, 1964.
Babel, Isaac. *The Complete Works of Isaac Babel*. Edited by Nathalie Babel. New York: W. W. Norton, 2002.
Basserman, L. M., ed. *Trud, zdorov'e, byt Leningradskoi rabochei molodezhi*. Vol. 1: *Rabochie podrostki i shkoly fabzavucha (po dannym obsledovanii 1923–24 gg.)*. Leningrad: Izdatel'stvo Sanprosveta Leningradskogo gubzdravotdela, 1925.
Bazhenov, I. P. *Tabak gubit zdorov'e*. Moscow: Meditsina, 1964.

Bekhterev, V. M. *Gipnoz, vnushenie, telepatiia.* Reprinted Moscow: Mysl', 1994.

Belousov, V. V. *Izuchenie truda v tabachnom proizvodstve.* Petersburg: Gosizdat, 1921.

Beraud, Henri. *The Truth about Moscow: As Seen by A French Visitor.* Translated by John Peile. London: Faber and Gwyer, 1925.

Berman, E. I. *O stol' tsenimom tabake i trudovom molodniake: S pit'iu diagrammami v tekste.* Moscow: Zhizn' i znanie, 1926.

Bliumenau, E. B. *Okhmeliaiushchie durmany: Tabak, opii i morfii, kokain, efir i gashish, ikh vred i posledstviia.* Leningrad: Seiatel', 1925.

Boginskii, S. N. *Tabak i ego kurenie.* Nizhnii Novgorod: Nizhpoligraf, 1925.

Bogolepov, N. K. *Voprosy nevro-psikhiatricheskoi dispansernoi praktiki.* Moscow: Moskovskii gorodskoi otdel zdravookhrnaneniia, 1936.

Bogoliubov, K. M., P. G. Mishunin, E. Z. Razumov, and Ia. V. Storozhev, eds. *Spravochnik partiinogo rabotnika.* Moscow: Politicheskaia literatura, 1978.

Bogoslovskii, V. A. *O vrede kureniia (Konspekt lektsii).* Moscow: Institut sanitarnogo prosveshcheniia, 1965.

Bohlen, Charles E. *Witness to History, 1929–1969.* New York: W. W. Norton, 1973.

Bordonos, V. *Opyt raboty fabrichnogo komiteta Khar'kovskoi tabachnoi fabriki pro organizatsiiu sotsialisticheskogo sorevnovaniia.* Kiev: URSPS, 1954.

Brennan, William Augustine. *Tobacco Leaves: Being a Book of Facts for Smokers.* Menasha, WI: Index Office, 1915.

Brokgauz, F. A., and I. A. Efron, eds. *Entsiklopedicheskii slovar'.* St. Petersburg: I. A. Efron, 1901.

Bulgakov, Mikhail. *Notes on the Cuff and Other Stories.* Translated by Alison Rice. Ann Arbor, MI: Ardis, 1991.

Chaklin, A.V. *Vrednye privychki i rak.* Moscow: Znanie, 1969.

Chekhov, A. P. *Zagadochnaia natura: Rasskazy.* Moscow: Izdatel'stvo Narodnogo komissariata oborony, 1944.

Dreiser, Theodore. *Dreiser Looks at Russia.* New York: Horace Liveright, 1928.

Dzhervis, M. V. *Russkaia tabachnaia fabrika v XVIII i XIX vekakh.* Leningrad: Akademiia nauk SSSR, 1933.

Egiz, S. A., ed. *Sbornik statei i materialov po tabachnomu delu.* Peterburg: V. F. Kirshbaum, 1913.

Epshtein, M., ed. *Za novyi byt: Posobie dlia gorodskikh klubov.* Moscow: Doloi negramotnost', 1925.

Formakov, Arsenii. *Gulag Letters.* Edited and translated by Emily D. Johnson. New Haven: Yale University Press, 2017.

Frolov, V. A. *Kurit' zdorov'iu vredit'.* Moscow: Meditsina, 1969.

Galkin, R. A., V. N. Mal'tsev, N. P. Lopukhov, and O. L. Nikitin, eds. *Tabak ili zhizn': Aktual'nye problemy profilaktiki kureniia.* Samara: Perspektiva, 2000.

Gastev, A. *Iunost' idi!* Moscow: VTsSPS, 1923.

Give the Boy a Square Deal! Annual Report. Chicago: Anti-Cigarette International League, 1921.

Gol'bert, Ia. M., ed. *Tabachnaia promyshlennost' i tabakovodstvo.* Moscow: Mospoligraf, 1926.

Goldman, Emma. *My Disillusionment in Russia.* Mineola, NY: Dover Publications, 1923.

Gol'dshtein, S. A., ed. *Tabachnaia promyshlennost'.* Moscow: RIO TsK VSRPVP, 1929.

Gorokhov, K. *Zlaia travka (tabachnoe zasil'e).* Odessa: Avtora, 1929.

Greene, F. V. *Sketches of Army Life in Russia.* New York: Charles Scribner's Sons, 1880.

Grigor'ian, V. *Tabak: Pavil'ion gruzinskoi SSR.* Tbilisi: Zaria vostoka, 1935.

Grossman, Vasily. *A Writer at War: A Soviet Journalist with the Red Army, 1941–1945.* New York: Vintage Books, 2005.

Il'inskii, A. I. *Tri iada: Tabak, alkogol' (vodka) i sifilis.* 2nd ed. Moscow: Kh. Barkhudarian, 1898.

Kagan, A. G. *Rabochaia molodezh' na otdykhe.* Leningrad: Priboi, n.d.

Kal'manson, S., and D. Bekariukov. *Beregi svoe zdorov'e! Sanitarnaia pamiatka dlia rabochikh podrostkov.* Leningrad: Molodaia gvardiia, 1925.

Kaplan, K. *Ne kuri.* Khar'kov: Nauchnaia mysl', 1930.

Kogan, B. B., and M. S. Lebedinskii. *Byt rabochei molodezhi.* Moscow: Moszdravotdel, 1929.

Kosiakov, K. S. *Pochemu vredno kurit'.* Moscow: Medgiz, 1957.

Kovgankin, B. S. *Komsomol na bor'bu s narkotizmom: Kak molodezhi pobedit' bolezni byta. P'ianstvo i kurenie tabaka.* Moscow: Molodaia gvardiia, 1929.

Krasnaia Moskva. Moscow: Izdatel'stvo Moskovskogo soveta RKiKrD, n.d.

Kratkii ocherk tabakokureniia v Rossii, v minuvshev 19-m stoletii: Za period vremeni s 1810 po 1906 god. Kiev: Petr Varskii, 1906.

Krymskii, E. S. *Vred dlia zdorov'ia ot kureniia i niukhaniia tabaku i sredstva perestat' kurit'.* Evenigorodka: E. S. Krymskii, 1889.

Lenin, V. I. *Collected Works.* Moscow: Progress Publishers, 1960–1970.

Lenin, V. I. *Polnoe sobranie sochinenii.* Moscow: Gosizdat, 1958.

Lifshits, Ia. I. *Doloi kurenie i p'ianstvo!* Kharkov: Nauchnaia mysl', 1928.

Listov, K. (music) and M. Ruderman (lyrics). *Makhorochka.* Translated by Paula Stone. New York: Russian-American Music Publishers, 1943.

Lukashevich, D. N. *"Nevinnaia privychka" (tabakokurenie).* Leningrad: Priboi, 1925.

Lukovnikov, A. *Druz'ia-odnopolchane: Rasskazy pesniakh, rozhdennykh voinoi, melodii i teksty.* Moscow: Muzak, 1985.

Maiakovskii, V. V. *Polnoe sobranie sochinenii.* Moscow: Khudozhestvennaia literatura, 1958.

Markovich, K. *Otchet: Po sboru papiros, tabaku i kuritel'nykh prinadlezhnostei, proizvedennomu v g. Rostove n/D. i po nekotorym stantsiiam Vladinavnazskoi zheleznoi dorogi.* Rostov-on-Don: S. P. Iakovlev, 1904.

Mendel'son, A. L. *Vospitanie voli.* Leningrad: Leningradskaia pravda, 1928.

Morolev, M. R. *Sovetskaia pechatnaia vneshnetorgovaia reklama.* Moscow: Zaochnii institute sovetskoi torgovli, 1964.

Narkir'er, S. *Proizvodstvo tabachnykh fabrik RSFSR v 1919 godu (v tsifrakh): Po materialam Statisticheskogo otdela Glavnogo upravleniia gosudarstvennoi tabachnoi promyshlennosti.* Moscow: Vysshii sovet narodnogo khoziastva, 1921.

Nechaev, A. P. *Tabak i ego vliianie na umstvennuiu deiatel'nost' vzroslykh i detei.* Moscow: Zhizn' i znanie, 1925.

Nezlin, S. *O vrede kureniia tabaka.* Moscow: Doloi negramotnost', 1926.

Novikova, V. G., and N. N. Shchemelev, *Nasha marka: Ocherki istorii Donskoi gosudarstvennoi tabachnoi fabriki.* Rostov-on-Don: Rostovskoe knizhnoe izdatel'stvo, 1968.

Orlovskii, L. V., ed. *O raz"iasnenii naseleniiu vreda kureniia i upotrebleniia nasa.* Moscow: Kommunar, 1972.

Ostrovskii, A. D. *Pravda o tabake (Konspekt lektsii).* Moscow: Institut sanitarnogo prosveshcheniia, 1959.

Panomareva, N. A. *O lechenii lits, kuriashchikh tabak (instruktivno-metodicheskoe pis'mo).* Moscow: Rosglavpoligrafprom, 1965.

Petrov, N. N. *Chto nado znat' o rake.* Leningrad: Leningradskaia pravda, n.d.

Polianskii, A., ed. *Deistvie tabachnago dyma na zhivotnykh i cheloveka (Stoit'-li kurit'? Kak rekomenduetsia kurit'?)*. Novo-Nikolaevsk: Soiuz-Bank, 1919.

Pomerantsev, N. P. *O tabake i vrede ego kureniia*. Moscow: M. M. Tarchigin, 1908.

Popov, S. P. *Vred tabakokureniia: Sotsial'no-gigienicheskii ocherk*. Perm: Sanprosveta Permskogo okradrava, 1926.

Pridonov, I. A., ed. *Bros'te kurit'! Populiarnoe izlozhenie o vrede tabaka*. Kostroma: Gosudarstvennaia tipo-litografiia, 1922.

Priklonskii, Ivan Ivanovich. *Upotrebelenie tabaka i ego vrednoe na organizm cheloveka vliianie*. Moscow: K. Tikhomivor, 1909.

Putevoditel' po Muzeiu zdravookhraneniia Leningradskogo obzdravotdela. Leningrad: Leningradskii meditsinskii zhurnal, 1928.

Radek, Karl. *Through Germany in the Sealed Coach*. Translated by Ian Birchall (2005). https://www.marxists.org/archive/radek/1924/xx/train.htm.

Rapoport, A. M. *Tabak i ego vliianie na organizm*. Moscow: Gosmedizdat, 1929.

Reed, John. *Ten Days That Shook the World*. New York: Vintage, 1960.

Rokau, Dr. *Interesnaia i liubopytnaia istoriia kurivshikh, niuchavshikh i zhevashikh tabak: S legendarnym pravdivym skazaniem o ego pagubnom vliianiia na zdorovy cheloveka*. Moscow: Tipografiia byvshei A. V. Kudriavtsevoi, 1885/1886.

Rossiiskii, D. M. *O tabake i vrede ego kureniia*. Moscow: G. F. Mirimanov, 1925.

Rozenbaum, N. D. *Tabachnoe proizvodstvo: Sanitarno-gigienicheskie ocherki*. Moscow: Voprosy truda, 1924.

Rozhnov, A. A. *Sbornik materialov po tabachnoi promyshlennosti*. Moscow: Gosudarstvennoe tekhnicheskoe izdatel'stvo, 1930.

Sandage, C. H., and Vernon Fryburger, eds. *The Role of Advertising: A Book of Readings*. Homewood, IL: Richard D. Irwin, 1960.

Sazhin, I. V. *Pravda o kurenii*. Leningrad: Leningradskaia pravda, (1926) 1930.

Sbornik dekretov, postanovlenii, instruktsii, Sovnarkoma, VTsIKa i dr. organov pravitel'stvennoi vlasti, noiabr'–dekabr', 1921. Novo-Nikolaevsk: Sibirskoe otdelenie tsentrosoiuza, 1921.

Schmuk, A. A. *The Chemistry and Technology of Tobacco*. Moscow: Pishchepromizdat, 1953.

Semashko, N. A., ed. *Desiat' let oktiabria i sovetskaia meditsina*. Moscow: NKZ RSFSR, 1927.

Semashko, N. A. *Health Protection in the USSR*. London: Victor Gollancz, 1934.

Semashko, N. A. *Nezabyvaemyi obraz*. Moscow: Gosizdat, 1959.

Semashko, N. A. *Sotsial'nye bolezni i bor'ba s nimi*. Moscow: Voprosy truda, 1925.

Semenova, Nina Ivanovna. "Issledovanie aromaticheskikh veshchestv tabaka i ikh izmenenie v protsessakh tekhnologicheskoi pererabotki." PhD diss., Krasnodarskii politekhnicheskii institut, 1975.

Serebriakov, S. V. *Organizatsiia i tekhnika sovetskoi torgovli*. Moscow: Gostorgizdat, 1956.

Sholomovich, A. S. *Detskii pokhod na vzroslykh*. Moscow: Moszdravotdel, 1926.

Shostak, Ia. E. *Kurevo*. Ul'ianovsk: Izdatel'stvo Ul'ianovskogo gubzdravotdela, 1925.

Sigal, B. *I. Sud nad pionerom kuril'shchikom i II. Sud nad neriashlivym pionerom: Dve intsenorovki*. Moscow: Zhizn' i znanie, 1927.

Sigal, B. *Trud i zdorov'e rabochei molodezhi*. Leningrad: Molodaia gvardiia, 1925.

Sigal, B. *Vrednaia privychka (Kuren'e tabaka)*. Moscow: Gosmedizdat, 1929.

Sigerist, Henry. *Medicine and Health in the Soviet Union*. New York: Citadel Press, 1947.

Sinel'nikov, Leonid. *Delo—Tabak: Polveka fabriki "Iava" glazami ee rukovoditelia*. Moscow: Delo, 2017.

Sinelnikov, Leonid. *Smoke and Mirrors: From the Soviet Union to Russia, the Pipedream Meets Reality*. London: Unicorn Publishing, 2020.

Smith, Jessica. *Women in Soviet Russia*. New York: Vanguard Press, 1928.

Sokolnikov, Gregory Y. *Soviet Policy in Public Finance, 1917–1928*. Stanford, CA: Stanford University Press, 1931.

Stalin, I. V. *Collected Works*. Moscow: Foreign Languages Publishing House, 1954.

Stal'skii, I., ed. *Donskaia gosudarstvennaia tabachnaia fabrika: Ocherk po materialam starykh kadrovikov DGTF A. K. Vasil'eva, E. I. Riabininoi, O. P. Ogarenko i V. I. Shcherbakova* (Rostov-on-Don: Gosizdat, 1938).

Sukhanov, N. N. *The Russian Revolution, 1917*. Edited and translated by Joel Carmichael. Princeton, NJ: Princeton University Press, 1984.

Telegina, M. Ia., ed. *Pervyi opyt Stakhanovtsev DGTF*. Rostov-on-Don: Stachin, 1935.

Tiapugin, N. P. *Pochemu i kak dolzhna molodezh' borot'sia s tabakom*. Moscow: Gosmedizdat, 1930.

Tolstoy, L. N. *Polnoe sobranie sochinenii*. Moscow: Gosizdat, 1937.

Trakhman, M. G. *Materialy po zdravookhraneniiu na transporte za 1924 god*. Moscow: Mediko-sanitarnyi otdel putei soobshcheniia Narodnogo komissariata zdravookhraneniia RSFSR, 1926.

Tregubov, I. *Normal'nyi sposob brosit' kurit'*. Batum: D. L. Kapelia, 1912.

Trofimov, V. A. *Tabak—vrag zdorov'ia*. Leningrad: Meditsinskaia literatura, 1959.

Trotsky, Leon. *The Military Writings of Leon Trotsky*. New York: New Park Publications, 1979.

Trotsky, Leon. *My Life*. New York: Pathfinder Press, 1930.

Trotsky, Leon. *Problems of Everyday Life: And Other Writings on Culture and Science*. New York: Monad, 1973.

United States President. *Eighteenth Report to Congress on Lend-Lease Operations*. Washington, DC: Government Printing Office, 1944.

Uporov, I. G. *Tabak, ego kurenie i vliianie na organizm*. Sverdlovsk: Izdatel'stvo Sanepida Sverdlovskogo okzdravotdela, 1925.

Utekhin, A. S. *Doloi kurevo, s 8 risunkami*. Leningrad: Fizkul'tura i sport, 1930.

Varushkin, I. M. *Pochemu vreden tabak*. Moscow: Gosizdat, 1926.

Vasilevskii, L. M. *Gigiena molodoi devushki*. Moscow: Novaia Moskva, 1926.

Vasilevskii, L. M. *Gigiena pionera*. Moscow: Novaia Moskva, 1925.

Vasilevskii, L. M. *Gigiena propagandista (Agitatora, lektora, prepodavatelia)*. Moscow: Molodaia gvardiia, 1924.

Violin, Ia. A. *Tabak i ego vred dlia zdorov'ia*. Kazan: Shtaba zapasnoi armii, 1920.

Volkova, Nina. *Dostignutoe ne predel!* Moscow: Pishchepromizdat, 1935.

Vsia Moskva. Moscow: Moskovskii rabochii, 1928.

Wicksteed, Alexander. *Life under the Soviets*. London: John Lane the Bodley Head, 1928.

Zaits, L. P. *Brosaite kurit'!* Sverdlovsk: Sverdlovskoe knizhnoe izdatel'stvo, 1960.

Zolotnitskii, V. N. *O vrede kureniia tabaka*. Moscow: G. F. Mirimanov, 1925.

Zoshchenko, Mikhail Mikhailovich. *Shestaia povest' Belkina*. Moscow: Vremia, 2008.

Secondary Sources

Acton, Edward, Vladimir Iu. Cherniaev, and William G. Rosenberg, eds. *Critical Companion to the Russian Revolution, 1914–1921*. Bloomington: Indiana University Press, 1997.

Alexopoulos, Golfo. *Stalin's Outcasts: Aliens, Citizens, and the Soviet State, 1926–1936*. Ithaca, NY: Cornell University Press, 2003.

Andrews, James T., and Asif A. Siddiqi, eds. *Into the Cosmos: Space Exploration and Soviet Culture.* Pittsburgh: University of Pittsburgh Press, 2011.

Appadurai, Arjun, ed. *The Social Life of Things.* Cambridge: Cambridge University Press, 1986.

Armstrong, John, ed. *The Soviet Partisans in World War II.* Madison: University of Wisconsin Press, 1964.

Ashurkov, E. D., et al., eds. *N. A. Semashko: Izbrannye zdravookhraneniia.* Moscow: Meditsinskaia literatura, 1954.

Avdeichik, I. P., and G. K. Iukhnovich, eds. *Plakaty pervykh let sovetskoi vlasti i sotsialisticheskogo stroitel'stva (1918–1941).* Minsk: Plymia, 1985.

Balina, Marina, and Evgeny Dobrenko, eds. *Petrified Utopia: Happiness Soviet Style.* London: Anthem, 2009.

Barber, John, and Mark Harrison. *The Soviet Home Front, 1941–1945: A Social and Economic History of the USSR in World War II.* London: Longman, 1991.

Barkhatova, E. V. *Iz istorii russkogo plakata: "Okna" ROSTA i Glavpolitprosveta 1919–1922.* St. Petersburg: Rossiskaia natsional'naia biblioteka, 2000.

Beer, Daniel. *Renovating Russia: The Human Sciences and the Fate of Liberal Modernity, 1880–1930.* Ithaca, NY: Cornell University Press, 2008.

Beevor, Anthony. *The Second World War.* Boston: Little, Brown, 2012.

Benedict, Carol. *Golden-Silk Smoke: A History of Tobacco in China, 1550–2010.* Berkeley: University of California Press, 2011.

Bennett, Jane. *Vibrant Matter: A Political Ecology of Things.* Durham, NC: Duke University Press, 2010.

Bernstein, Frances Lee. *The Dictatorship of Sex: Lifestyle Advice for the Soviet Masses.* DeKalb: Northern Illinois University Press, 2007.

Bernstein, Frances Lee, Christopher Burton, and Dan Healey, eds. *Soviet Medicine: Culture, Practice, and Science.* DeKalb: Northern Illinois University Press, 2010.

Bernstein, Seth. *Raised under Stalin: Young Communists and the Defense of Socialism.* Ithaca, NY: Cornell University Press, 2017.

Bialer, Seweryn, ed. *Stalin and His Generals: Soviet Military Memoirs of World War II.* New York: Pegasus, 1969.

Bittner, Stephen V. *Whites and Reds: A History of Wine in the Lands of Tsar and Commissar.* Oxford: Oxford University Press, 2021.

Bius, Joel R. *Smoke 'em if You Got 'em: The Rise and Fall of the Military Cigarette Ration.* Annapolis, MD: Naval Institute Press, 2018.

Bogdanov, Igor'. *Dym otechestva, ili kratkaia istoriia tabakokureniia.* Moscow: Novoe literaturnoe obozrenie, 2007.

Bonnell, Victoria. *Iconography of Power: Soviet Political Posters under Lenin and Stalin.* Berkeley: University of California Press, 1997.

Bonnell, Victoria, ed. *The Russian Worker: Life and Labor under the Tsarist Regime.* Berkeley: University of California Press, 1983.

Borenstein, Eliot. *Men without Women: Masculinity and Revolution in Russian Fiction, 1917–1929.* Durham, NC: Duke University Press, 2000.

Borrero, Mauricio. *Hungry Moscow: Scarcity and Urban Society in the Russian Civil War, 1917–1921.* New York: Peter Lang, 2003.

Boym, Svetlana. *Common Places: Mythologies of Everyday Life in Russia.* Cambridge, MA: Harvard University Press, 1994.

Brake, Michael. *The Sociology of Youth Culture and Youth Subcultures.* New York: Routledge, 2013.

Brandt, Allan M. *The Cigarette Century: The Rise, Fall, and Deadly Persistence of the Product That Defined America.* New York: Basic Books, 2007.

Bren, Paulina, and Mary Neuburger, eds. *Communism Unwrapped: Consumption in Cold War Eastern Europe*. Oxford: Oxford University Press, 2012.

Brovkin, Vladimir. *Behind the Front Lines of the Civil War: Political Parties and Social Movements in Russia, 1918–1922*. Princeton, NJ: Princeton Legacy Library, 1994.

Brovkin, Vladimir. *The Mensheviks after October: Socialist Opposition and the Rise of the Bolshevik Dictatorship*. Ithaca, NY: Cornell University Press, 1991.

Bruisch, Katja, ed. *Biulleten' Germanskogo istoricheskogo instituta v Moskve*. Moscow: Germanskii istoricheskii institut v. Moskve, 2012.

Bucher, Greta. *Women, the Bureaucracy, and Daily Life in Postwar Moscow, 1945–1953*. Boulder, CO: East European Monographs, 2006.

Buralenko, A. Kh. *Razvitie sovetskoi torgovoi reklamy*. L'vov: n.p. 1959.

Burnham, John C. *Bad Habits: Drinking, Smoking, Taking Drugs, Gambling, Sexual Misbehavior, and Swearing in American History*. New York: New York University Press, 1993.

Cameron, Sarah. *The Hungry Steppe: Famine, Violence, and the Making of Soviet Kazakhstan*. Ithaca, NY: Cornell University Press, 2020.

Carlson, Per. *An Unhealthy Decade: A Sociological Study of the State of Public Health in Russia, 1990–1999*. Stockholm: Alqvist & Wiksell, 2000.

Carroll, Jennifer J. *Narkomania: Drugs, HIV, and Citizenship in Ukraine*. Ithaca, NY: Cornell University Press, 2019.

Cassiday, Julia A. *The Enemy on Trial: Early Soviet Courts on Stage and Screen*. DeKalb: Northern Illinois University Press, 2000.

Castillo, Greg. *Cold War on the Home Front: The Soft Power of Midcentury Design*. Minneapolis: University of Minnesota Press, 2010.

Cavanaugh, Cassandra. "Backwardness and Biology: Medicine and Power in Russian and Soviet Central Asia, 1868–1934." PhD diss., Columbia University, 2001.

Chase, William J. *Workers, Society, and the Soviet State: Labor and Life in Moscow, 1918–1929*. Urbana: University of Illinois Press, 1987.

Chernyshova, Natalya. *Soviet Consumer Culture in the Brezhnev Era*. London: Routledge, 2013.

Clements, Barbara Evans, Rebecca Friedman, and Dan Healey, eds. *Russian Masculinities in History and Culture*. New York: Palgrave Macmillan, 2002.

Colton, Timothy J. *Moscow: Governing the Socialist Metropolis*. Cambridge, MA: Harvard University Press, 1996.

Conquest, Robert. *Harvest of Sorrow: Soviet Collectivization and the Terror-Famine*. New York: Oxford University Press, 1986.

Courtwright, David T. *The Age of Addiction: How Bad Habits Became Big Business*. Cambridge, MA: Belknap, 2019.

Courtwright, David T. *Forces of Habit: Drugs and the Making of the Modern World*. Cambridge, MA: Harvard University Press, 2002.

Cox, Randi Barnes. "The Creation of the Socialist Consumer: Advertising, Citizenship, and NEP." PhD diss., Indiana University, 1999.

Cross, Gary S., and Robert N. Proctor. *Packaged Pleasures: How Technology and Marketing Revolutionized Desire*. Chicago: University of Chicago Press, 2014.

David, Michael Zdenek. "The White Plague in the Red Capital: The Control of Tuberculosis in Russia, 1900–1941." PhD diss., University of Chicago, 2007.

David-Fox, Michael. *Showcasing the Great Experiment: Cultural Diplomacy and Western Visitors to the Soviet Union, 1921–1941*. Oxford: Oxford University Press, 2012.

Davies, R. W. *The Soviet Economy in Turmoil, 1929–1930*. Cambridge, MA: Harvard University Press, 1989.

Davis, Christopher, and Murray Feshbach. *Rising Infant Mortality in the USSR in the 1970s*. Series P-25, no. 74. Washington, DC: US Bureau of the Census, September 1980.

Demin, A. K. *Kurenie ili zdorov'e v Rossii*. Moscow: Fond "Zdorov'e i okruzhaiushchaia sreda," 1996.

Demin, A.K., et al. *Rossiia: Delo tabak. Rassledovanie massovogo ubiistva*. Moscow: Rossiiskaia assotsiatsiia obshchestvennogo zdorov'ia, 2012.

Demosfenova, A. Nurok, and N. Shantyko, *Sovetskii politicheskii plakat*. Moscow: Iskusstvo, 1962.

Dodge, Norton T. *Women in the Soviet Economy: Their Role in Economic, Scientific, and Technical Development*. Baltimore: Johns Hopkins University Press, 1966.

Dunham, Vera. *In Stalin's Time: Middleclass Values in Soviet Fiction*. New York: Cambridge University Press, 1976.

Fainberg, Dina, and Artemy Kalinovsky, eds. *Reconsidering Stagnation in the Brezhnev Era: Ideology and Exchange*. Lanham, MD: Lexington Books, 2016.

Federenko, L. N. *Kurenie v Rossii*. Armavir: Slavianskii filial Armavirskogo gosudarstvennogo pedagogicheskogo instituta, 2002.

Feshbach, Murray. *The Soviet Union: Population Trends and Dilemmas. Population Bulletin* 37, no. 3. Washington, DC: Population Reference Bureau, August 1982.

Feshbach, Murray, and Alfred Friendly, Jr. *Ecocide in the USSR: Health and Nature under Siege*. New York: Basic Books, 1991.

Field, Deborah A. *Private Life and Communist Morality in Khrushchev's Russia*. New York: Peter Lang, 2007.

Field, Mark G., and Judyth L. Twigg, eds. *Russia's Torn Safety Nets: Health and Social Welfare during the Transition*. New York: Palgrave, 2000.

Filtzer, Donald A., and Wendy Z. Goldman, eds. *Hunger and War: Food Provisioning in the Soviet Union during World War II*. Bloomington: Indiana University Press, 2015.

Fisher, Ralph Talcott, Jr. *Pattern for Soviet Youth: A Study of the Congresses of the Komsomol, 1918–1954*. New York: Columbia University Press, 1959.

Fitzpatrick, Sheila. *Education and Social Mobility in the Soviet Union, 1921–1934*. Cambridge: Cambridge University Press, 1979.

Fitzpatrick, Sheila. *Everyday Stalinism: Ordinary Life in Extraordinary Times. Soviet Russia in the 1930s*. New York: Oxford University Press, 1999.

Fitzpatrick, Sheila. *The Russian Revolution*. Oxford: Oxford University Press, 2001.

Fitzpatrick, Sheila, Alexander Rabinowitch, and Richard Stites, eds. *Russia in the Era of NEP: Explorations in Soviet Society and Culture*. Bloomington: Indiana University Press, 1991.

Fitzpatrick, Sheila, and Yuri Slezkine, eds. *In the Shadow of Revolution: Life Stories of Russian Women from 1917 to the Second World War*. Princeton, NJ: Princeton University Press, 2000.

Fizeler [Fieseler], Beate, and Rodzher D. Markvik [Roger D. Markwick], eds. *Sovetskii tyl 1941–1945: Povsednevnaia zhizn' v gody voiny*. Moscow: Rosspen, 2019.

Fraser, Erica L. *Military Masculinity and Postwar Recovery in the Soviet Union*. Toronto: University of Toronto Press, 2019.

Fürst, Juliane. *Flowers through Concrete: Explorations in Soviet Hippieland*. Oxford: Oxford University Press, 2021.

Fürst, Juliane, ed. *Late Stalinist Russia: Society between Reconstruction and Reinvention*. London: Routledge, 2006.

Fürst, Juliane, *Stalin's Last Generation: Soviet Post-War Youth and the Emergence of Mature Socialism*. Oxford: Oxford University Press, 2010.

Gately, Iain. *Tobacco: The Story of How Tobacco Seduced the World*. New York: Grove, 2001.

Gerovitch, Slava. *Soviet Space Mythologies: Public Images, Private Memories, and the Making of a Cultural Identity*. Pittsburgh: University of Pittsburgh Press, 2015.

Getty, J. Arch, and Roberta T. Manning, eds. *Stalinist Terror: New Perspectives*. Cambridge: Cambridge University Press, 1993.

Gilman, Sander L., and Zhou Xun, eds. *Smoke: A Global History of Smoking*. London: Reaktion Books, 2004.

Gleason, Abbott, Peter Kenez, and Richard Stites, eds. *Bolshevik Culture: Experiment and Order in the Russian Revolution*. Bloomington: Indiana University Press, 1985.

Goldman, Wendy Z. *Women at the Gates: Gender and Industry in Stalin's Russia*. Cambridge: Cambridge University Press, 2002.

Goldman, Wendy Z., and Donald Filtzer. *Fortress Dark and Stern: The Soviet Home Front during World War II*. New York: Oxford University Press, 2021.

Golubev, Alexey. *The Things of Life: Materiality in Late Soviet Russia*. Ithaca, NY: Cornell University Press, 2020.

Goodman, Jordan. *Tobacco in History: The Cultures of Dependence*. London: Routledge, 1993.

Gorsuch, Anne E., and Diane P. Koenker, eds. *The Socialist Sixties: Crossing Borders in the Second World War*. Bloomington: Indiana University Press, 2013.

Goscilo, Helen, and Andrea Lanoux, eds. *Gender and National Identity in Twentieth-Century Russian Culture*. DeKalb: Northern Illinois University Press, 2006.

Grant, Susan, ed. *Russian and Soviet Health Care from an International Perspective: Comparing Professions, Practice, and Gender, 1880–1960*. Basingstoke: Palgrave Macmillan, 2017.

Gronow, Jukka. *Caviar with Champagne: Common Luxury and the Ideals of the Good Life in Stalin's Russia*. Oxford: Berg, 2003.

Hahn, Barbara. *Making Tobacco Bright: Creating an American Commodity, 1617–1937*. Baltimore: Johns Hopkins University Press, 2011.

Halfin, Igal. *Intimate Enemies: Demonizing the Bolshevik Opposition, 1918–1928*. Pittsburgh: University of Pittsburgh Press, 2007.

Halfin, Igal. *Terror in My Soul: Communist Autobiographies on Trial*. Cambridge, MA: Harvard University Press, 2003.

Hanson, Philip. *Advertising and Socialism: The Nature and Extent of Consumer Advertising in the Soviet Union, Poland, Hungary, and Yugoslavia*. White Plains, NY: International Arts and Sciences Press, 1974.

Hanson, Philip. *The Rise and Fall of the Soviet Economy*. London: Longman, 2003.

Harris, Steven. *Communism on Tomorrow Street: Mass Housing and Everyday Life after Stalin*. Baltimore: Johns Hopkins University Press, 2013.

Harrison, Mark. *Accounting for War: Soviet Production, Employment, and the Defense Burden, 1940–1945*. Cambridge: Cambridge University Press, 1996.

Healey, Dan. *Homosexual Desire in Revolutionary Russia: The Regulation of Sexual and Gender Dissent*. Chicago: University of Chicago Press, 2002.

Healey, Dan. *Russian Homophobia from Stalin to Sochi*. London: Bloomsbury, 2018.

Heinzen, James. *The Art of the Bribe: Corruption under Stalin, 1943–1953*. New Haven: Yale University Press, 2016.

Hellbeck, Jochen. *Revolution on My Mind: Writing a Diary under Stalin*. Cambridge, MA: Harvard University Press, 2009.

Henningfield, Jack E., Emma Calvento, and Sakire Pogun. *Nicotine Psychopharmacology*. Bethesda, MD: Springer, 2009.

Herlihy, Patricia. *The Alcoholic Empire: Vodka and Politics in Late Imperial Russia.* Oxford: Oxford University Press, 2002.

Herring, Jr., George C. *Aid to Russia, 1941–1946: Strategy, Diplomacy, the Origins of the Cold War.* New York: Columbia University Press, 1973.

Hesli, Vicki L., and Margaret H. Mills, eds. *Medical Issues and Health Care Reform in Russia.* Lewiston, ME: Edwin Mellen, 1999.

Hessler, Julie. *A Social History of Soviet Trade: Trade Policy, Retail Practices, and Consumption, 1917–1953.* Princeton, NJ: Princeton University Press, 2004.

Hillis, Faith. *Utopia's Discontents: Russian Émigrés and the Quest for Freedom, 1830s–1930s.* New York: Oxford University Press, 2021.

Hilton, Matthew. *Smoking in British Popular Culture, 1800–2000.* Manchester: Manchester University Press, 2000.

Hixson, Walter L. *Parting the Curtain: Propaganda, Culture, and the Cold War, 1945–1961.* New York: St. Martin's Griffin, 1997.

Hoffmann, David L. *Cultivating the Masses: Modern State Practices and Soviet Socialism, 1914–1939.* Ithaca, NY: Cornell University Press, 2011.

Hoffmann, David L. *Peasant Metropolis: Social Identities in Moscow, 1929–1941.* Ithaca, NY: Cornell University Press, 1994.

Hoffmann, David L. *Stalinist Values: The Cultural Norms of Soviet Modernity, 1917–1941.* Ithaca, NY: Cornell University Press, 2003.

Holmes, Larry E. *Stalin's World War II Evacuations: Triumph and Troubles in Kirov.* Lawrence: University Press of Kansas, 2017.

Horn, David G. *The Criminal Body: Lombroso and the Anatomy of Deviance.* New York: Routledge, 2003.

Howes, David. *Empire of the Senses: The Sensual Culture Reader.* London: Bloomsbury Academic, 2005.

Inkeles, Alex. *Public Opinion in Soviet Russia: A Study in Mass Persuasion.* Cambridge, MA: Harvard University Press, 1967.

Ironside, Kristy. *A Full-Value Ruble: The Promise of Prosperity in the Postwar Soviet Union.* Cambridge, MA: Harvard University Press, 2021.

Ivanova, E. A., ed. *Rumiantsevskie chteniia—2015.* Moscow: Pashkov dom, 2015.

Jones, D. G. Brian, and Mark Tadajewski, eds. *The Routledge Companion to Marketing History.* New York: Routledge, 2016.

Joravsky, David. *Russian Psychology: A Critical History.* Oxford: Basil Blackwell, 1989.

Kafengauz, Lev Borisovich. *Evoliutsiia promyshlennogo proizvodstva Rossii (posledniaia tret' XIX v.–30-e gody XX v.).* Moscow: Epifaniia, 1994.

Kalantarova, N. A., N. V. Ponomarev, et al. *Moskva v fotografiiakh, 1920–1930-e gody.* St. Petersburg: Liki Rossii, 2010.

Kapferer, Jean-Noël. *(Re)inventing the Brand: Can Top Brands Survive the New Market Realities?* London: Kogan Page, 2001.

Karpova, Yulia. *Comradely Objects: Design and Material Culture in Soviet Russia, 1960s–1980s.* Manchester: Manchester University Press, 2020.

Kelly, Catriona. *Children's World: Growing up in Russia, 1890–1991.* New Haven: Yale University Press, 2007.

Kelly, Catriona. *Refining Russia: Advice Literature, Polite Culture, and Gender from Catherine to Yeltsin.* Oxford: Oxford University Press, 2001.

Kiaer, Christina. *Imagine No Possessions: The Socialist Objects of Russian Constructivism.* Cambridge, MA: MIT Press, 2005.

Kiaer, Christina, and Eric Naiman, eds. *Everyday Life in Early Soviet Russia.* Bloomington: Indiana University Press, 2006.

Kiernan, Victor Gordon. *Tobacco: A History.* London: Hutchinson Radius, 1991.

Kifuriak, S. V. *Tabachnaia fabrika "Iava."* Moscow: Pishchevaia promyshlennost', 1978.

Kindler, Robert. *Stalin's Nomads: Power and Famine in Kazakhstan.* Pittsburgh: University of Pittsburgh Press, 2018.

Kluger, Richard. *Ashes to Ashes: America's Hundred-Year Cigarette War, the Public Health, and the Unabashed Triumph of Philip Morris.* New York: Knopf, 1996.

Koenker, Diane. *Moscow Workers and the 1917 Revolution.* Princeton, NJ: Princeton University Press, 1981.

Koenker, Diane, William G. Rosenberg, and Ronald Grigor Suny, eds. *Party, State and Society in the Russian Civil War: Explorations in Social History.* Bloomington: Indiana University Press, 1989.

Kohrman, Matthew, Gan Quan, Liu Wennan, and Robert N. Proctor, eds. *Poisonous Pandas: Chinese Cigarette Manufacturing in Critical Historical Perspectives.* Stanford, CA: Stanford University Press, 2018.

Koloskova, E. E. *Moskva v fotografiiakh, 1941–1945.* St. Petersburg: Liki Rossii, 2015.

Kopovalova, N. *Konstantin Stepanovich Mel'nikova (1890–1974).* Moscow: Komsomol'skaia pravda, 2016.

Korno, V. I., and M. I. Kitainer, *Balkanskaia zvezda: Stranitsy istorii.* Iaroslavl: Niuans, 2000.

Kotkin, Stephen. *Magnetic Mountain: Stalinism as a Civilization.* Berkeley: University of California Press, 1995.

Kovrigin, M. D., ed. *Okhrana narodnogo zdorov'ia v SSSR.* Moscow: Meditsinskaia literatura, 1957.

Kowalski, Ronald I. *The Russian Revolution, 1917–1921.* London: Routledge, 1997.

Krementsov, Nikolai. *The Cure: A Story of Cancer and Politics from the Annals of the Cold War.* Chicago: University of Chicago Press, 2004.

Krementsov, Nikolai. *A Martian Stranded on Earth: Alexander Bogdanov, Blood Transfusions, and Proletarian Science.* Chicago: University of Chicago Press, 2011.

Krementsov, Nikolai. *Revolutionary Experiments: The Quest for Immortality in Bolshevik Science and Fiction.* Oxford: Oxford University Press, 2014.

Krementsov, Nikolai, and Yvonne Howell, eds. *The Art and Science of Making the New Man in Early-Twentieth-Century Russia.* London: Bloomsbury, 2021.

Kuptsov, Vasilii Petrovich. "Problemy perestroiki narodnogo khoziastva i evakuatsii mirnogo naseleniia v gody velikoi otechestvennoi voiny." Doctor of Historical Sciences diss., Rossiiskaia ekonomicheskaia akademiia im. G. V. Plekhanova, Moscow, 2002.

LaPierre, Brian. *Hooligans in Khrushchev's Russia: Defining, Policing, and Producing Deviance during the Thaw.* Madison: University of Wisconsin Press, 2012.

Lebina, N. B. *Rabochaia molodezh' Leningrada: Trud i sotsial'nyi oblik, 1921–1925 gody.* Leningrad: Nauka, 1982.

Liakov, V. N. *Sovetskii reklamnyi plakat i reklamnaia grafika, 1933–1973.* Moscow: Sovetskii khudozhnik, 1977.

Lillard, Dean, and Rebekka Christopoulou, eds. *Life Course Smoking Behavior: Patterns and National Context in Ten Countries.* Oxford: Oxford University Press, 2015.

Lindenmeyr, Adele, Christopher Read, and Peter Waldron, eds. *Russia's Home Front in War and Revolution, 1914–22.* Book 2: *The Experience of War and Revolution.* Bloomington, IN: Slavica Publishers, 2016.

Linz, Susan J., ed. *The Impact of World War II on the Soviet Union.* Totowa, NJ: Rowman and Allanheld, 1985.

Lock, Stephen, Lois Reynolds, and E. M. Tanesey, eds. *Ashes to Ashes: The History of Smoking and Health.* Amsterdam: Rodopi, 1988.

Malinin, A. V. *Tabachnaia istoriia Rossii*. Moscow: Russkii tabak, 2006.

Malinin, A. V. *Tabak: O chem umolchal MINZDRAV*. Moscow: Russkii tabak, 2003.

Mally, Lynn. *Revolutionary Acts: Amateur Theater and the Soviet State, 1917–1938*. Ithaca, NY: Cornell University Press, 2000.

Manley, Rebecca. *To the Tashkent Station: Evacuation and Survival in the Soviet Union at War*. Ithaca, NY: Cornell University Press, 2009.

Matich, Olga. *Erotic Utopia: The Decadent Imagination in Russia's Fin de Siècle*. Madison: University of Wisconsin Press, 2005.

McCallum, Claire E. *The Fate of the New Man: Representing and Reconstructing Masculinity in Soviet Visual Culture, 1945–1965*. DeKalb: Northern Illinois University Press, 2018.

McGeever, Brendan. *Antisemitism and the Russian Revolution*. Cambridge: Cambridge University Press, 2019.

Merridale, Catherine. *Ivan's War: Life and Death in the Red Army, 1939–1945*. New York: Metropolitan Books, 2006.

Michaels, Paula. *Curative Powers: Medicine and Empire in Stalin's Central Asia*. Pittsburgh: University of Pittsburgh Press, 2003.

Michaels, Paula. *Lamaze: An International History*. Oxford: Oxford University Press, 2014.

Miller, Daniel. *Stuff*. Cambridge: Polity, 2010.

Miller, Martin Allan. *Freud and the Bolsheviks: Psychoanalysis in Imperial Russia and the Soviet Union*. New Haven: Yale University Press, 1998.

Milov, Sarah. *The Cigarette: A Political History*. Cambridge, MA: Harvard University Press, 2019.

Mitrofanova, A. V., ed. *Rabochii klass SSSR, 1966–1970*. Moscow: Nauka, 1979.

Moiseev, I. V. *Tabak i tabachnaia industriia: Vchera, segodnia, zavtra*. Moscow: Russkii tabak, 2002.

Moskoff, William. *The Bread of Affliction: The Food Supply in the USSR during World War II*. Cambridge: Cambridge University Press, 1990.

Moskoff, William. *Hard Times: Impoverishment and Protest in the Perestroika Years. The Soviet Union, 1981–1991*. Armonk, NY: M. E. Sharpe, 1993.

Naiman, Eric. *Sex in Public: The Incarnation of Early Soviet Ideology*. Princeton, NJ: Princeton University Press, 1997.

Nakachi, Mie. *Replacing the Dead: The Politics of Reproduction in the Postwar Soviet Union*. New York: Oxford University Press, 2021.

National Center for Chronic Disease Prevention and Health Promotion (US) Office on Smoking and Health. *The Health Consequences of Smoking—50 Years of Progress: A Report of the Surgeon General*. Atlanta, GA: Centers for Disease Control and Prevention, 2014.

Naumov, V. P., and A. A. Kosakovskii, eds. *Kronshtadt 1921*. Moscow: Fond "Demokratiia," 1997.

Neuburger, Mary C. *Balkan Smoke: Tobacco and the Making of Modern Bulgaria*. Ithaca, NY: Cornell University Press, 2013.

Oreskes, Naomi, and Erik M. Conway. *Merchants of Doubt: How a Handful of Scientists Obscured the Truth on Issues from Tobacco Smoke to Global Warming*. London: Bloomsbury, 2010.

Overy, Richard. *Russia's War: A History of the Soviet War Effort, 1941–1945*. New York: Penguin, 1997.

Patenaude, Bertrand M. *The Big Show in Bololand: The American Relief Expedition to Soviet Russia in the Famine of 1921*. Stanford, CA: Stanford University Press, 2002.

Pearson, Michael. *The Sealed Train*. New York: G. P. Putnam's Sons, 1975.

Pennock, Pamela E. *Advertising Sin and Sickness: The Politics of Alcohol and Tobacco Marketing, 1950–1990*. DeKalb: Northern Illinois University Press, 2007.

Peri, Alexis. *The War Within: Diaries from the Siege of Leningrad*. Cambridge, MA: Harvard University Press, 2017.

Petrone, Karen. *The Great War in Russian Memory*. Bloomington: Indiana University Press, 2011.

Petrova, Anna, ed. *Arkhitektor Konstantin Mel'nikov: Pavil'ony, garazhi, kluby i zhil'e sovetskoi epokhi*. Moscow: Gosudarstvennyi muzei arkhitektury im. A. V. Shchuseva, 2015.

Phillips, Laura L. *Bolsheviks and the Bottle: Drink and Worker Culture in St. Petersburg, 1900–1929*. DeKalb: Northern Illinois University Press, 2000.

Pollock, Ethan. *Without the Banya We Would Perish: A History of the Russian Bathhouse*. New York: Oxford University Press, 2019.

Proctor, Robert N. *Golden Holocaust: Origins of the Cigarette Catastrophe and the Case for Abolition*. Berkeley: University of California Press, 2011.

Proctor, Robert N. *The Nazi War on Cancer*. Princeton, NJ: Princeton University Press, 1999.

Rabinowitch, Alexander. *The Bolsheviks Come to Power: The Revolution of 1917 in Petrograd*. New York: W. W. Norton, 1978.

Rabinowitch, Alexander. *Prelude to Revolution: The Petrograd Bolsheviks and the July 1917 Uprising*. Bloomington: Indiana University Press, 1991.

Randall, Amy E. *The Soviet Dream World of Retail Trade and Consumption in the 1930s*. New York: Palgrave, 2008.

Reid, Susan E., and David Crowley, eds. *Style and Socialism: Modernity and Material Culture in Post-War Eastern Europe*. Oxford: Berg, 2000.

Retish, Aaron. *Russia's Peasants in Revolution and Civil War: Citizenship, Identity, and the Creation of the Soviet State, 1914–1922*. Cambridge: Cambridge University Press, 2008.

Rigby, T. H. *Lenin's Government: Sovnarkom, 1917–1922*. Cambridge: Cambridge University Press, 1979.

Roberts, Graham H. *Material Culture in Russia and the USSR: Things, Values, Identities*. London: Bloomsbury, 2017.

Romaniello, Matthew P., Alison K. Smith, and Tricia Starks, eds. *The Life Cycle of Russian Things: From Fish Guts to Fabergé, 1600–Present*. London: Bloomsbury, 2021.

Romaniello, Matthew P., and Tricia Starks, eds. *Russian History through the Senses: From 1700 to the Present*. London: Bloomsbury, 2016.

Romaniello, Matthew P., and Tricia Starks, eds. *Tobacco in Russian History and Culture: From the Seventeenth Century to the Present*. New York: Routledge, 2009.

Rudy, Jarret. *The Freedom to Smoke: Tobacco Consumption and Identity*. Montreal: McGill-Queen's University Press, 2005.

Ryback, Timothy. *Rock around the Bloc: A History of Rock Music in Eastern Europe and the Soviet Union*. New York: Oxford University Press, 1990.

Salisbury, Harrison E. *The 900 Days: The Siege of Leningrad*. New York: Harper and Row, 1969.

Saushin, F. S. *Khleb i sol'*. Iaroslavl: Verkhne-Volzhskoe, 1983.

Schechter, Brandon Michael. "Governmental Issue: The Material Culture of the Red Army, 1941–1945." PhD diss., University of California, Berkeley, 2015.

Schechter, Brandon Michael. *The Stuff of Soldiers: A History of the Red Army in World War II through Objects*. Ithaca, NY: Cornell University Press, 2019.

Schlögel, Karl. *The Scent of Empires: Chanel No. 5 and Red Moscow*. Translated by Jessica Spengler. Cambridge: Polity, 2020.

Schrad, Mark Lawrence. *Vodka Politics: Alcohol, Autocracy, and the Secret History of the Russian State*. New York: Oxford University Press, 2014.

Sebelius, Kathleen. *How Tobacco Smoke Causes Disease: The Biology and Behavioral Basis for Smoking-Attributable Disease. A Report of the Surgeon General*. Rockville, MD: US Department of Health and Human Services, 2010.

Siegelbaum, Lewis H., ed. *Borders of Socialism: Private Spheres of Soviet Russia*. New York: Palgrave, 2006.

Siegelbaum, Lewis H. *Cars for Comrades: The Life of the Soviet Automobile*. Ithaca, NY: Cornell University Press, 2008.

Siegelbaum, Lewis H. *Soviet State and Society between Revolutions, 1918–1929*. New York: Cambridge University Press, 1992.

Siegelbaum, Lewis H. *Stakhanovism and the Politics of Productivity in the USSR, 1935–41*. New York: Cambridge University Press, 1988.

Sirotkina, Irina. *Diagnosing Literary Genius: A Cultural History of Psychiatry in Russia, 1880–1930*. Baltimore: Johns Hopkins University Press, 2002.

Slepyan, Kenneth. *Stalin's Guerrillas: Soviet Partisans in World War II*. Lawrence: University Press of Kansas, 2006.

Slezkine, Yuri. *The House of Government: A Saga of the Russian Revolution*. Princeton, NJ: Princeton University Press, 2017.

Snopkov, Aleksandr, Pavel Snopkov, and Aleksandr Shkliaruk, eds. *Reklama v plakate: Russkii torgovo-promyshlennyi plakat za 100 let (Advertising Art in Russia)*. Moscow: Kontakt-kul'tura, 2007.

Snopkov, Aleksandr, Pavel Snopkov, and Aleksandr Shkliaruk, eds. *Sovetskii reklamnyi plakat, 1923–1941/Soviet Advertising Posters*. Moscow: Kontakt, 2013.

Solomon, Susan Gross, and John F. Hutchinson, eds. *Health and Society in Revolutionary Russia*. Bloomington: Indiana University Press, 1990.

Sperling, Valerie. *Sex, Politics, and Putin: Political Legitimacy in Russia*. Oxford: Oxford University Press, 2015.

Starks, Tricia. *The Body Soviet: Propaganda, Hygiene, and the Revolutionary State*. Madison: University of Wisconsin Press, 2008.

Starks, Tricia. *Smoking under the Tsars: A History of Tobacco in Imperial Russia*. Ithaca, NY: Cornell University Press, 2018.

Stites, Richard. *Revolutionary Dreams: Utopian Visions and Experimental Life in the Russian Revolution*. New York: Oxford University Press, 1988.

Strigaleva, A. A., and I. V. Kokkinaki, eds. *Konstantin Stepanovich Mel'nikov*. Moscow: Iskusstvo, 1985.

Todes, Daniel P. *Ivan Pavlov: A Russian Life in Science*. Oxford: Oxford University Press, 2014.

Transchel, Kathy S. *Under the Influence: Working-Class Drinking, Temperance, and Cultural Revolution in Russia, 1895–1932*. Pittsburgh: University of Pittsburgh Press, 2006.

Ushakin, S., ed. *O muzhe(i)stvennosti*. Moscow: Novoe literaturnoe obozrenie, 2002

Utrata, Jennifer. *Women without Men: Single Mothers and Family Change in the New Russia*. Ithaca, NY: Cornell University Press, 2015.

Varga-Harris, Christine. *Stories of House and Home: Soviet Apartment Life during the Khrushchev Years*. Ithaca, NY: Cornell University Press, 2016.

Vashik, Klaus, and Nina Baburina. *Real'nost' utopii: Iskusstvo russkogo plakata XX veka*. Moscow: Progress-Traditsiia, 2003.

Vihavainen, Timo, and Elena Bogdanova, eds. *Communism and Consumerism: The Soviet Alternative to the Affluent Society.* Leiden: Brill, 2015.

Viola, Lynne. *The Best Sons of the Fatherland: Workers in the Vanguard of Soviet Collectivization.* Oxford: Oxford University Press, 1987.

Viola, Lynne. *Peasant Rebels under Stalin: Collectivization and the Culture of Peasant Resistance.* New York: Oxford University Press, 1996.

Weeks, Albert L. *Russia's Life-Saver: Lend-Lease Aid to the U.S.S.R in World War II.* Lanham, MD: Lexington Books, 2004.

White, Stephen. *Russia Goes Dry: Alcohol, State and Society.* Cambridge: Cambridge University Press, 1996.

Widdis, Emma. *Socialist Senses: Film, Feeling, and the Soviet Subject, 1917–1940.* Bloomington: Indiana University Press, 2017.

Willimott, Andy. *Living the Revolution: Urban Communes and Soviet Socialism, 1917–1932.* Oxford: Oxford University Press, 2017.

Wood, Elizabeth. *The Baba and the Comrade: Gender and Politics in Revolutionary Russia.* Bloomington: Indiana University Press, 1997.

Wood, Elizabeth. *Performing Justice: Agitation Trials in Early Soviet Russia.* Ithaca, NY: Cornell University Press, 2005.

Yurchak, Alexei. *Everything Was Forever, until It Was No More: The Last Soviet Generation.* Princeton, NJ: Princeton University Press, 2006.

Zatoński, Mateusz Zygmunt. "State, Society, and the Politics of Smoking in Poland, during and after Communism (1960–2000)." PhD diss., University of London, 2018.

Zubkova, Elena. *Russia after the War: Hopes, Illusions, and Disappointments, 1945–1957.* Armonk, NY: M. E. Sharpe, 1998.

Index

Abkhaziia, 35, 113

addiction, 5, 8–9, 94, 103, 147, 167, 176, 187, 210, 215, 232, 234, 247, 262, 289. *See also* dependency

additives. *See* saucing

advertising, 6, 9–10, 53, 56–62, 68, 73, 77, 119, 121, 182, 186–88, 200, 209; restrictions on, 165–70, 201, 212, 227–30

Agit-Reklam, 59

agriculture, 7–9, 12–15, 33–36, 56, 60, 89, 109, 113–18, 134, 140, 145, 147, 158, 176, 180–82, 197, 213, 219–26. *See also* collectivization

air quality, 5, 19, 24, 27–28, 47, 95–96, 100–101, 108, 127, 212

alcohol, 6, 8, 13–18, 21, 28–29, 33, 37, 41–42, 44, 52, 81, 92–97, 101–3, 107, 113, 121, 125, 128, 147–48, 191, 195–206, 215, 223–30

alcoholism, 18, 27, 92, 96, 100, 103, 110, 215

Aleksei Mikhailovich, 16

All-Russia Congress of Soviet Workers, 16

All-Union Institute of Tobacco and Makhorka Production, 116

America. *See* United States

anarchists, 48

Andijan, 218

Andropov, Iurii, 225

Anti-Cigarette League (United States), 105, 109

anxiety, 8, 28–29, 197–97

Apollo-Soyuz: cigarettes, 175–76, 181–86, 192; joint mission, 175, 181–82

Asmolov, V. I., 32–33, 158. *See also* Don State Tobacco Factory

Babel, Isaac, 34

Balkan Star Factory, 36, 40, 115, 158

Bekhterev, Vladimir, 15, 103, 200

Belomorkanal, 7, 123, 141, 145, 160, 169, 209–10

black market, 42, 145, 151, 192

Bolshevik Revolution, 2, 5, 170

Bonch-Bruevich, Vladimir, 2

bourgeoisie, 48, 108

Brezhnev, Leonid, 156, 162, 164, 169–70, 179, 186, 197, 200

budget. *See* taxes

Bukharin, Nikolai, 1, 17, 75

Bulgaria, 148, 151, 167, 174–78, 188, 192, 215, 226

Bulgakov, Mikhail, 81, 107

cancer: general, 9–12, 27, 130, 177, 199, 205; lung, 5, 27, 130, 156, 163, 173, 195, 209, 214; mouth, 27, 129–30

capitalism, 3, 6, 9, 18, 32–33, 57–60, 68–69, 73, 81, 91, 96–97, 111–13, 132, 140, 163, 167, 174, 192–93, 220, 227

cardiovascular disease, 156, 199, 205

Caucasus, 14, 34, 35

Central Committee of the Communist Party, 44, 177, 218, 220, 222

cessation, 2–3, 5–6, 10, 13, 16–19, 21–26, 29, 31, 34, 59, 69, 92–95, 99–113, 127, 130, 132–35, 160, 196–97, 200–205, 210, 213–19, 221–24, 228, 258n117, 262n90, 265n58

Chekhov, A. P., 151, 200

Chernenko, Konstantin, 225

Chernigov, 136, 151

children: generally, 17, 69–71, 96, 98, 118, 145, 161, 197; as laborers, 46–49, 141–42; as smokers, 30–31, 96–101, 107, 110, 113, 121, 173, 196, 200, 212–15, 219, 228; as victims, 19, 75, 26, 128–32. *See also* pioneers; komsomol

cigarettes, 2–4, 7–8, 10, 36, 44, 75, 138–40, 156, 161–97, 205, 213–16, 220–30, 232n19, 265n58, 276n113

cigars, 20, 57, 168

cytisine, 151, 215, 218, 262n90

civil war: Russian, 9, 16, 31, 31,-39, 98, 139; Spanish, 139

Cold War, 8, 174–77, 200

collectivization, 113–15, 156

Commission to Fight Smoking, 15

Communist Party of the Soviet Union, 177, 218, 220

conditioned reflex. *See* reflexology

consumption, 3–4, 11, 15, 34, 41, 47, 53–91, 104, 108, 124, 139, 145–48, 156–64, 178–82, 198, 224–30. *See also* tuberculosis

Cossacks, 55

CPSIA information can be obtained
at www.ICGtesting.com
Printed in the USA
LVHW071811030123
736352LV00011B/542